CLEARLY
KETO

Also by Mary T. Newport

*The Complete Book of Ketones: A Practical Guide
to Ketogenic Diets and Ketone Supplements*

*The Coconut Oil and Low Carb Solution for Alzheimer's,
Parkinson's, and Other Diseases: A Guide to Using Diet and
a High-Energy Food to Protect and Nourish the Brain*

*Alzheimer's Disease: What If There Was
a Cure? The Story of Ketones*

CLEARLY
KETO

For Healthy
Brain Aging
and Alzheimer's
Prevention

Mary T. Newport, M.D.
Author of *The Complete Book of Ketones*

Foreword by Dominic D'Agostino, Ph.D.,
and Milene Brownlow, Ph.D.

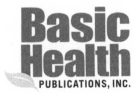

Basic Health
PUBLICATIONS, INC.

BASIC HEALTH
AN IMPRINT OF TURNER PUBLISHING COMPANY
Nashville, Tennessee
www.turnerpublishing.com

Clearly Keto: For Healthy Brain Aging and Alzheimer's Prevention

Text and cover design by William Ruoto
Charts and images drawn by Joanna Newport

Library of Congress Cataloging-in-Publication Data
Names: Newport, Mary T., 1952- author.
Title: Clearly keto : for healthy brain aging and Alzheimer's prevention / Mary T. Newport, M.D.
Description: Nashville, Tennessee : Basic Health, an imprint of Turner Publishing Company [2022] | Includes bibliographical references and index.
Identifiers: LCCN 2022008317 (print) | LCCN 2022008318 (ebook) | ISBN 9781684428342 (paperback) | ISBN 9781684428359 (hardcover) | ISBN 9781684428366 (epub)
Subjects: LCSH: Alzheimer's disease—Diet therapy. | Ketones. | Ketogenic diet. | Fatty acids—Therapeutic use.
Classification: LCC RC523 .N5357 2022 (print) | LCC RC523 (ebook) | DDC 616.8/310654—dc23/eng/20220401
LC record available at https://lccn.loc.gov/2022008317
LC ebook record available at https://lccn.loc.gov/2022008318

Printed in the United States of America

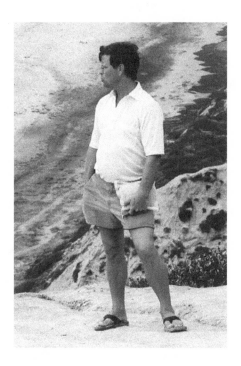

Steven Jerry Newport, my husband, my best friend, and a wonderful father to our children, 1950 to 2016.

This book is dedicated to my husband and best friend, Steven Jerry Newport, who fought with all his might against early-onset Alzheimer's disease but lost the battle on January 2, 2016.

This book is also dedicated to the memories of Richard L. Veech, MD, D.Phil., Theodore B. VanItallie, MD, and George Cahill, Jr., MD: three extraordinary ketone researchers whose studies and writings were instrumental in Steve's recovery and better life.

CONTENTS

FOREWORD

By Dominic D'Agostino, PhD, and Milene Brownlow, PhD

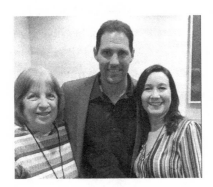

Left to right, Mary Newport, MD, Dominic D'Agostino, PhD, Milene Brownlow, PhD, enjoying the Metabolic Health Summit, January 2020.

Alzheimer's disease is considered the sixth-leading cause of death in the United States (second in the United Kingdom), currently affecting 6.2 million Americans. This number is projected to reach 12.7 million by 2050 as the population of Americans aged 65 and older is projected to continue growing (Alzheimer's Association 2021). These numbers, coupled with decades of pharmaceutical research that has resulted in few treatments, which merely address symptoms, highlight an urgent need for better approaches to optimize brain health and preserve cognitive function with age.

For well over a decade, Dr. Newport has played an instrumental role in advancing the field of Nutritional Neuroscience by expanding the use of ketogenic diets and supplementation beyond their traditional use as metabolic therapies for epilepsy. Her personal story and educational outreach have inspired researchers and brought hope for many families and caregivers, empowering them to be their own health advocates and taking steps to improve their own prognosis. She was, after all, that caregiver, faced with an impossible situation when her husband Steve, at age fifty-one, started developing early-onset Alzheimer's and Lewy body dementia. As Steve's cognition deteriorated with alarming speed, Dr. Newport began a desperate search for anything that could bring her husband back. Through her tireless efforts, she stumbled upon research indicating that a hallmark of Alzheimer's disease is impaired brain energy (glucose) metabolism. Further investigation led her to early research conducted by Dr. George Cahill (Harvard), Dr. Richard L. Veech (NIH) (Veech 2001), and Dr. Samuel Henderson. Collectively, their research suggested that ketone bodies (β-hydroxybutyrate and acetoacetate) could function as an alternative fuel to preserve and enhance brain-energy metabolism. Dr. Newport tested this hypothesis on her husband by administering coconut oil, a source of medium-chain triglycerides which convert to ketones when ingested and induce hyperketonemia, more commonly known as ketosis. Remarkably, this relatively modest elevation in ketone levels resulted in positive changes in Steve's mood and objective measures, including the Mini-Mental Status Exam and clock-drawing test. Dr. Newport's observations garnered local media attention, including a 2008 St. Petersburg Times article about their experience using this nutritional therapy (Hosley-Moore 2008).

As a faculty member at the University of South Florida Morsani College of Medicine, Dr. Newport's story about ketones piqued my interest from a personal and research perspective. I (D'Agostino) had personally witnessed Steve's positive response to acute ketogenic supplementation, and it greatly inspired my interest in this topic. We had gone out to lunch after Dr. Newport guest-lectured at USF, and Steve joined us. Just prior to eating, Steve consumed a small vial of coconut/medium-chain triglyceride oil mixture. Shortly after, he became more engaged and talkative, and his fine tremors stopped. From a research perspective, I had previously proposed using a ketogenic diet as a strategy to prevent central nervous system oxygen toxicity seizures, a limitation for Navy SEAL divers breathing high concentrations of oxygen; however, the Office of Naval Research was concerned about the safety, efficacy, and logistics of feeding divers this type of diet under operational constraints. Therefore, the possibility of using supplemental ketosis (without dietary restriction) as a neuroprotective strategy was appealing to me and later became a major focus of several research projects. Shortly after I became aware of this story, another article highlighting Dr. Newport's success with ketone supplementation surfaced in 2009, and Dr. Dave Morgan, PhD, the CEO of the University of South Florida Byrd Alzheimer's Institute, organized a meeting. This collaborative meeting was organized to discuss investigating the efficacy and mechanism of ketogenesis for Alzheimer's disease.

Dr. Newport is the reason I (Brownlow) became passionate about the topic of ketogenic diets and metabolic therapies for brain health. Back in 2009, I was a first-year doctoral student at the Byrd Alzheimer's Institute in search for a thesis topic. My background in behavioral neuroscience had previously focused on specific brain areas that control food intake and metabolism. After joining an Alzheimer's Research Laboratory with a strong focus on immunology, I was intent on finding a connection between brain health and metabolism, and I soon learned that type 2 diabetes is a strong risk factor for cognitive decline. As I was digging through the literature and trying to piece together a reasonable research question, Dr. Dave Morgan invited me to join in the aforementioned meeting to hear about Dr. Newport's personal experience.

From that conversation, a collaborative research project was formed to test the hypothesis that a low-carbohydrate ketogenic diet rich in medium-chain triglycerides could slow or reverse the neuropathological and behavioral features of Alzheimer's mouse models. Our experiments used two different transgenic mouse models that each focused on well-established hallmarks of Alzheimer's pathology: amyloid-beta and tau proteins. As rodents do not develop dementia, these transgenic models are genetically engineered to overexpress these proteins that aggregate in the brain and are associated with disease onset and progression. We tested adult mice that already had established pathology to address the question of whether our intervention could attenuate or reverse disease once it was already underway. This way, we could mimic Steve's experience with testing an intervention once symptoms were established.

The mice loved their new diet, promptly eating the ketogenic food provided multiple times a week. We did not restrict calories, and despite the transgenic mice eating more than their controls on a standard rodent diet, we did not see overall differences in body weight. It has since been reported that these transgenic lines tend to present hyperactivity and increased metabolic rate that, at the time, prevented us from seeing the weight loss and satiety effects that are now consistently reported in human clinical studies testing ketogenic diets for metabolic health. The most striking result reported was a greatly improved motor performance by the mice consuming the ketogenic diet (Brownlow 2013). Because we did not see improvements in memory tests or neuropathology, this finding could have easily become sidelined or gone unnoticed. However, two key points came up as we worked on data analysis and interpretation. First, as mentioned above, these transgenic mice carry mutations that replicate early-onset or autosomal dominant Alzheimer's disease, and these represent approximately 1 percent of diagnosed cases (Alzheimer's Association 2020), suggesting that a genetic model is likely not representative of a majority of patients or even optimal to address our central question of whether the cerebral hypometabolism can be mitigated by ketones as alternative brain fuel. Second, improvements in motor performance may immensely improve quality of life for many patients and caregivers. It could be the difference between being bedridden and getting dressed by yourself, preventing a fall, or even filling your own glass of water. As any caregiver or family member with a loved one undergoing a dementia diagnosis could probably attest, these small steps can slowly add up and amount to more good days than not.

Dr. Newport has propelled biomedical research in ketogenic diets; but, more importantly, her work has inspired many to take control of their seemingly impossible situations. While Alzheimer's remains a neurodegenerative disease with more pharmaceutical failures than successes, Dr. Newport's story and continued efforts encourage others to become their own health advocates by using nutrition and targeted supplementation to care for Alzheimer's and other dementias. In times when healthy eating is viewed as costly and labor-intensive, Dr. Newport proposes that wellness and cognitive health can start at home, in your very own kitchen, and that starting earlier will pay big dividends later in life. When I was growing up, I often heard my mother say she would rather spend on food than on medicine. I am often reminded of her motto when I am contemplating healthcare costs (for my small family of three or even for the nation amid a global pandemic) and whenever I am at the grocery store.

PAST, PRESENT, AND FUTURE

After its use in treating epilepsy for over one hundred years and its resurgence in the 1990s due to the heroic efforts of Jim Abrahams and the Charlie Foundation, the ketogenic diet has rapidly expanded as a more accepted metabolic-based therapy for seizures and for managing other neurological diseases, type 2 diabetes, and even brain cancer (Clini calTrials.gov 2021). It takes many years for a new treatment to gain acceptance or to be repurposed for other medical applications. Sadly, many doctors who are accustomed to prescribing pharmaceuticals still view diet therapy as snake oil. However, diet therapy was the prevailing practice long before the ketogenic diet was shown to effectively manage (and cure, in some cases) ⅔ of epilepsy patients after they failed multiple anti-seizure drugs. The consensus today is that the ketogenic diet's effects are multifaceted and synergistic, and work independently of any known drug mechanism. It shifts metabolic physiology and brain-energy metabolism, and it targets signaling pathways (e.g., ion channels, neurotransmitters, epigenetics) that help restore brain homeostasis. Although epilepsy patients are acutely and overtly responsive, it is becoming clear that these beneficial changes also occur in those with Alzheimer's and other neurodegenerative and neuropsychiatric diseases. Evidence of this is demonstrated in figures 1 and 2. No doubt the science

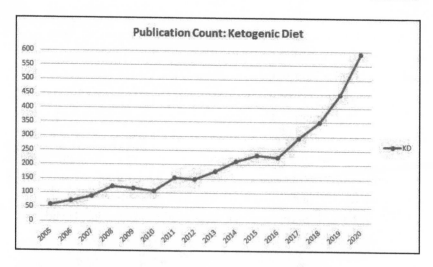

FIGURE 1. Publication by year (from PubMed as of 8.6.21). Overall increasing publication count for the term: "ketogenic diet," 2005 to 2020.

of ketogenic therapies will continue to increase for many years to come, not only as a therapy but as a preventative lifestyle approach.

For decades, Alzheimer's-disease therapies and research focused on transgenic rodent models that assume the aggregation and deposition of amyloid beta and tau protein is the root cause of the disease. Although the targeting of amyloid beta and tau protein is the primary research focus, it does not address all neuropathological features and has consistently shown translational shortcomings in drug trials. The presence of amyloid plaques and tau tangles are important features of this chronic condition, but the true cause of Alzheimer's remains largely unknown and debated. Emerging data suggest that factors such as metabolic dysregulation, insulin resistance, chronic inflammation, or a chronic infectious agent (viral or bacterial) could trigger and precede the development of amyloid beta and tau pathologies (Abbott 2020; Irwin 2019; Butterfield 2019). When viewed from this perspective, the amyloid beta, tau, and even Lewy-body pathologies may simply be a downstream reactive response to inflammation or infection (Pastore 2020). Although the cause of Alzheimer's disease remains elusive,

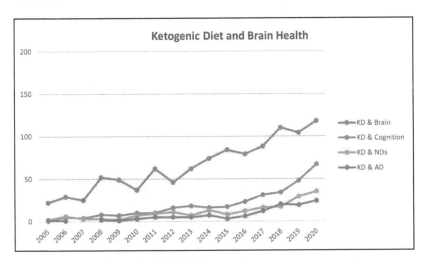

FIGURE 2. Publication by year (from PubMed as of 8.6.21). Increasing publication count for the terms "ketogenic diet" and "brain," "cognition," "neurodegenerative disease," and "Alzheimer's disease," 2005 to 2020. KD: Ketogenic diet; NDs: neurodegenerative diseases; AD: Alzheimer's disease.

investigators like Dr. Stephen Cunnane, PhD and others have further validated the observations Dr. Newport saw in Steve (Fortier 2021; Broom 2019).

By sharing her story and science-based, family-friendly research, Dr. Newport continues to be a beacon of hope offering a path forward to many of us. In Clearly Keto for Healthy Brain Aging and Alzheimer's Prevention, she has compiled all the latest information on this topic and synthesized it into a user-friendly plan to treat and prevent Alzheimer's disease and age-related cognitive decline. It is an exciting time for those of us working on the front lines of ketogenic diet research, and we are very grateful for Dr. Newport's tireless effort to advance the science and practical application of ketogenic therapies.

PREFACE

Over the past century, the average lifespan has more than doubled worldwide, from just thirty to more than seventy years, thanks to advances in surgical techniques, medical practice, pharmaceuticals, and especially in the prevention and treatment of infection. Industrialization, urbanization, and advances in transportation have improved many aspects of our lives, but they have also polluted our air and soil, resulting in significant health threats. Humans on average are taller and stronger, thanks to an abundance of food. However, the global population explosion has required escalation of food production, and food quality has deteriorated. Over the past half century, Alzheimer's and other dementias have become epidemic, along with diabetes and obesity. Much of this can be blamed on the very changes that have made our lives easier.

Keynote speakers at recent Alzheimer's Association International Conferences have reported that modifiable lifestyle risk factors account for at least 30 percent of dementia cases, of which Alzheimer's is the most common. Poor diet is the greatest risk factor for development of chronic diseases, dementia, and premature death, and may seriously impact the second half of our extended lives. In this book, we will discuss dietary and other lifestyle risk factors and changes that we can make to try to prevent age-related cognitive decline and improve symptoms in people who already have mild cognitive impairment, dementia, or other brain-related problems. People who are diabetic or prediabetic may also benefit from this approach, since diabetes accelerates brain aging and is a major risk factor for dementia.

In part 1, we will discuss the problems of insulin resistance and the "brain-energy gap," how a low-carb ketogenic diet could help, and how to adopt a reasonable, healthy Mediterranean-style diet to sustain mild-to-moderate nutritional ketosis. We will also discuss other ketogenic strategies and a few supplements that make sense. Part 2 delves deeply into other lifestyle-risk factors, positive changes you can make, and some things to avoid that may cause, trigger, or accelerate Alzheimer's and other dementias and impact healthy brain aging. Part Three provides a comprehensive review of the pathologies in the Alzheimer's brain and how each brain cell type is affected. You will learn that insulin resistance leads to many different pathological changes in the brain, which then further worsen insulin resistance—vicious cycles that could explain the progressive downward spiral that is Alzheimer's.

Alzheimer's is the most studied of brain diseases, but insulin resistance with poor glucose uptake occurs in many other types of dementia and neurodegenerative diseases, diabetes, Down syndrome, migraines, and certain psychiatric disorders. The heart could also benefit from ketones as fuel for congestive heart failure and for recovery from a heart attack.

The Clearly Keto approach will not require you to spend a fortune on frequent doctor visits, prescribed supplements, and monthly newsletters. However, if you have a medical condition, I encourage you to find a doctor who recognizes the importance of good nutrition to support and monitor you. People with epilepsy or cancer could also benefit from a strict very-high-fat version of the ketogenic diet, in which case I strongly recommend working with a dietitian trained in the ketogenic diet. Of course, anyone could benefit from the help of a knowledgeable dietitian. It is never too late to make beneficial lifestyle changes, but the sooner, the better.

My previous books go into much greater detail about my husband Steve's story and the large body of science behind this concept. A companion booklet is also available on my website (coconutketones.com) with recipes and color photos to help you plan healthy and delicious Mediterranean-style ketogenic meals.

INTRODUCTION

STEVE'S REPRIEVE FROM ALZHEIMER'S DISEASE

"Physicians have long been taught to fear ketosis . . . This fear of ketosis may be exaggerated. Mild ketosis can have therapeutic potential in a variety of disparate disease states."
—Richard L. Veech, MD, D.Phil. (Veech 2001)

Steven Jerry Newport's battle with early-onset Alzheimer's does not have a happy ending, but there is a happy middle in this story.

My husband Steve and I grew up in Cincinnati, Ohio, and started dating when I was a high school senior. We were married after he graduated with a BS in business administration from Xavier University, while I was still in pre-medicine there. He stuck with me patiently through medical school and years of training in pediatrics and neonatology (the care of sick and premature newborns). When we decided to have children, he volunteered to work from home as the manager and accountant for my medical practice, which made it possible for me to be a mother and a doctor. I owe all of that to Steve, and he often said taking care of our two girls was the best job he ever had.

Steve was a physically active, creative man who loved gardening, kayaking, and reading Stephen King and Clive Cussler novels. He always had the latest, fastest computer for his accounting work, and when he was not working on his computer, he was playing on it. As an accountant he was a perfectionist and kept the business end of my practice flowing smoothly. Steve was not someone you would ever expect to get Alzheimer's disease.

At age fifty-one, Steve began to show signs of a serious memory problem. He missed deadlines for simple quarterly tax returns and appointments for our children; soon he began forgetting whether he had been to the bank and post office, which was part of his daily work routine for many years. At first, his doctor thought depression explained his memory problems, which was likely exacerbated by his awareness that his brain was struggling. The memory problems steadily worsened, and he was diagnosed with early-onset Alzheimer's disease in 2004 at age fifty-four. This was devastating news, since we fully expected to retire, travel, and live to a ripe old age together. Instead, our world was forever turned upside-down. Steve took the usual Alzheimer's medications for years, but we did not see any difference.

By 2006, Steve could no longer read a map and stopped driving after turning up three hours away on the opposite coast of Florida; fortunately, he still remembered how to use his cell phone. By the end of that year, he could no longer do any accounting, use a calculator, do very simple math, or even remember how to turn on his computer. By mid-2007, Steve was losing weight and unable to prepare meals for himself. He was very distractible, often dismantling things like the vacuum cleaner and his lawn tractor and misplacing the parts. He had trouble finishing his sentences, could barely write a short word or two, and forgot how to tie his shoes. He had tremors in his hands and jaw when he tried to eat and speak. Steve had a slow, stiff gait and could no longer pick up his feet to run. The physical symptoms were most likely due to the further complication of Lewy Body dementia, which brain donation later confirmed.

Two clinical trials became available at the same time in our area in the spring of 2008. Steve was spiraling downhill, and we were very hopeful that one of these drugs would be the long-promised "cure" for Alzheimer's. He was scheduled for screenings two days in a row on May 20 and 21, 2008. On the evening of May 19, while searching online for risks and benefits of the two drugs, semagacestat and bapineuzumab, I happened upon a press release for a medical food called AC-1202 (now Axona), which was about one year away from FDA recognition. In their studies, nearly half of the people with Alzheimer's taking AC-1202 experienced improved memory and cognition after a single dose pilot study and during a 90-day study.

Digging deeper, in the AC-1202 patent application I learned that a key feature of Alzheimer's is diabetes of the brain, which results in poor glucose uptake into cells in the affected brain areas. With no fuel, these brain cells malfunction and eventually die. Furthermore, ketones could bypass the problem of getting glucose into the brain and potentially help somebody with Alzheimer's disease (see figure 1). The only active ingredient in AC-1202 was simply medium-chain triglyceride (MCT) oil, which is converted partly to ketones in the liver after it is consumed. The brain eagerly takes up ketones from the bloodstream, which enter the same chemical pathway as glucose to make the energy molecule ATP (adenosine triphosphate), which cells require to function. I also learned that MCT oil is usually extracted from coconut oil or palm-kernel oil.

This information hit me like a bolt of lightning. As a newborn specialist, I was quite familiar with MCT oil, which was added to the feedings of our tiniest premature newborns in the late 1970s to the mid-1980s to help them grow faster. Then formula manufacturers began to add MCT, coconut oil, and/or palm-kernel oil directly to infant formulas for premature and larger infants to mimic those found in human breast milk, which contains about 10 to 17 percent medium-chain triglycerides.

People consuming a typical American diet do not usually have ketones in their blood, and glucose is the main fuel to the brain and other organs. Ketosis begins naturally

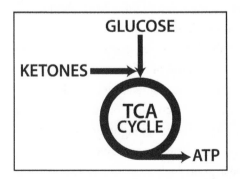

FIGURE 1. Ketones and glucose enter the TCA cycle to make ATP.

after about ten hours of fasting, as the glucose stored in our liver is depleted and the ketone level steadily increases thereafter. At that point, stored fat is converted to fatty acids, which provide fuel to the heart, muscles, and most other organs but do not cross easily into the brain, which then needs another source of fuel. Fortunately, fatty acids can be converted to ketones in the liver and used by the brain as fuel. If fasting or starvation is prolonged, ketone levels increase substantially and can provide up to two-thirds of the fuel required by the brain. Without fat and ketones, even with water available, we would likely die in a matter of seven to ten days. Use of our stored fat substantially increases how long we can live during starvation.

Finding the press release and patent for AC-1202 gave me an idea to help Steve, but at this point it was about 1:00 a.m., and he was scheduled at 9:00 a.m. for his first clinical trial screening. We were very disappointed after the screening in St. Petersburg, Florida, since Steve came up two points short of the sixteen needed to qualify on the simple thirty-point Mini-Mental State Exam (MMSE). On a clock drawing, a specific test for Alzheimer's disease, Steve drew just a few random circles and four numbers, and the doctor advised me that he was on the verge of severe Alzheimer's (see figure 2).

Thinking "What do we have to lose?" we stopped at a health-food store to pick up coconut oil. In medical school, I was taught that coconut oil was an "artery-clogging" fat, but then wondered why it was sold in health food stores. When we arrived home, I reviewed online which fatty acids were classified as medium chains. From the USDA website, I learned that coconut oil is about 60 percent medium-chain triglycerides and calculated that about seven teaspoons (just over two tablespoons) would equal the 20-gram dose of AC-1202.

The following day, with the second screening scheduled for 1:00 p.m., Steve ate seven teaspoons of coconut oil in oatmeal for breakfast. Four hours later in Tampa, he scored eighteen out of thirty points and qualified for the study! Obviously, we were extremely happy. I wondered if this result was just good luck, prayers, or the coconut oil, but decided to continue this new dietary intervention and I set out to learn everything I could about coconut oil and cooking with it. I

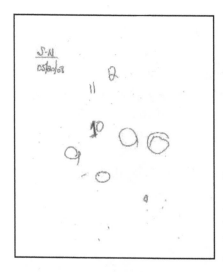

FIGURE 2. Steve's clock drawing on May 20, 2008, the day before starting coconut oil. The doctor advised us that the disorganized pattern indicated that Steve was on the verge of severe Alzheimer's.

questioned whether one dose daily was adequate if his brain needed ketones 24/7. Thereafter, I gave Steve just over two tablespoons each morning at breakfast and added coconut oil to most other meals and snacks.

Over the next few days, things changed very rapidly. Steve was no longer sluggish and could carry on a good conversation, and was back to whistling and joking. His tremors nearly stopped except in the morning before he had his coconut oil. Steve said that on the day he started coconut oil, it was like a light switch came back on in his brain. His mood improved dramatically, and he expressed hope for his future.

I began calling and emailing Richard Veech, MD, D.Phil., a world expert on ketones working at the National Institutes of Health (NIH) near Washington, D.C. Veech had spent years developing a ketone ester and needed funding for mass production to conduct clinical trials for Alzheimer's. Two weeks after starting coconut oil, Steve drew a second clock that was remarkably improved from the day before he started consuming coconut oil (see figure 3). The clock was a single full circle with all the numbers in the correct order, though there were numerous hands on the clock. I faxed the clock to Dr. Veech, who immediately called and said this was "unexpected." He thought it would take much higher levels of ketones to produce any improvement in someone with Alzheimer's disease.

Dr. Veech encouraged us to add MCT oil to try to achieve higher ketone levels. I found MCT oil available online, began mixing coconut oil and MCT oil together, and slowly increased the amount Steve was taking to maximize his ketone levels. I soon learned that a 4:3 ratio (4 parts MCT oil to 3 parts coconut oil) stays liquid at room temperature and can be used in almost any type of food, hot or cold.

About two months after starting the coconut oil, Steve rescreened and qualified for the other clinical trial with twenty out of thirty points

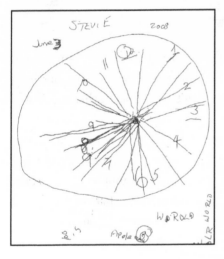

FIGURE 3. Steve's clock drawing on June 3, 2008, 14 days after starting coconut oil. This drawing is a big improvement from fourteen days earlier.

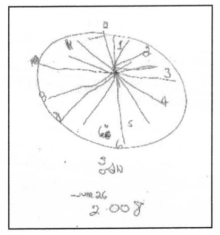

FIGURE 4. Steve's clock drawing on July 26, 2008, just over two months after starting coconut oil. The clock continued to improve, with better organization, and was less messy.

on the MMSE. He drew a third clock that was even better (see figure 4, clock dated July 26, 2008). The dietary intervention with coconut and MCT oil did not disqualify him, and Steve started the trial shortly after. During that first year, he improved by six of seventy-five points on more detailed cognitive testing and by fourteen of seventy-eight points on Activities of Daily Living, which, for Steve, meant he could "do things better." Two months after starting coconut oil and then adding MCT oil, he was able to walk normally and run again. By four months, he could read again after a visual tremor stopped. and by ten months, he could remember details of what he'd read several hours earlier. Steve improved so much that he began to volunteer in the supply warehouse of the hospital where I worked, which made him very happy (see photo 1).

Unlike many people with dementia, Steve was always very aware that he had Alzheimer's, what he once had been able to do, and what he could no longer do. Eventually, we learned that he had been receiving the placebo for at least the first twelve months of the clinical trial. So we could attribute his improvement to ketones and possibly other effects of coconut oil and MCT oil, the only other factors that had changed that year. Over several months, Steve worked up to nine to ten tablespoons of coconut and MCT oil per day, while eliminating most carbs and starchy foods, except vegetables and very small servings of

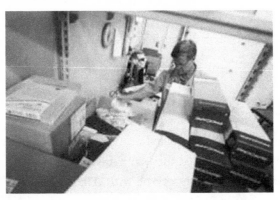

PHOTO 1. Steve Newport working as a volunteer in a hospital supply warehouse in fall 2009.

berries and whole-grain rice. He was effectively on a ketogenic diet by virtue of the low-carbohydrate and high-healthy-fat content, though at-home blood ketone level testing was not yet available to prove it.

Steve was quite stable for another year, but then had a setback in early 2010. At that point, we believed he had crossed over to the clinical trial drug, because his hair was growing out lighter, a known side effect. He also had other alarming side effects, such as wounds that would not heal and a fainting episode, and some dementia symptoms returned, like requiring supervision with bathing, shaving, and picking out clothes. Imagine how difficult this setback was after two very hopeful years. We decided to withdraw from the study and were advised a few months later that the entire clinical trial had been stopped because the drug (semagacestat) was found to accelerate Alzheimer's disease. The irony was that Steve's improvement from consuming coconut oil led to his qualifying for a study drug that likely harmed him.

In April 2010, due to this serious setback, Dr. Veech proposed that Steve become the sole participant in a pilot study of his ketone ester. Since I am a physician, he felt comfortable allowing me to conduct this study with Steve. Dr. Veech sent the raw material, which, I can attest, tasted very much like jet fuel, and left it to me to make it drinkable. Steve took the ester willingly and with great excitement, but he shuddered every time, despite trying various flavors and sweeteners to hide the taste. During the first two hours after the first dose of ester, Steve recited and wrote out the entire alphabet for the first time in months, after trying repeatedly for twenty minutes. Within twenty-four hours, he took a shower, shaved, brushed his teeth, and picked out clothes, which he put on correctly without step-by-step instructions. Nearly all the new symptoms he'd experienced with this setback reversed over about six weeks. The ketone ester kept Steve stable for another twenty months before the next serious setback. Between the coconut oil, MCT oil, and ketone ester, Steve gained nearly four years of better quality of life than he had experienced the year before he started the coconut oil.

Eventually, Steve lost his battle with Alzheimer's and Lewy Body dementia on January 2, 2016. This began with a head injury that occurred when he fell back during his first-ever seizure, a common occurrence in the later stages of Alzheimer's and Lewy body dementia. During that first twenty-minute seizure, he stopped breathing and turned blue. This was too much for his already-fragile brain. He did not recover well, was totally dependent, and most of his speech was gone. We continued the ketone ester, coconut oil, MCT oil, and the healthy Mediterranean diet. Steve ate well and maintained a healthy weight. He always knew my voice, and he would hold my hand whenever we sat together. Steve was in home hospice care for about one and a half years and passed away peacefully at home while listening to a playlist of his favorite music that our daughter Joanna prepared for that moment.

In May 2008, when Steve improved so dramatically from simply adding coconut oil to his diet, I knew others would improve as well, and there were 35 million other people in the world and their families dealing with dementia. I became a messenger for ketones at that point and now dedicate my life to carrying on Steve's legacy. It is gratifying that so many others are now spreading the message of ketones. Since 2008, ketone research has grown exponentially for Alzheimer's and many other conditions that share the problem of insulin resistance with poor glucose uptake into the brain and other organs.

PART **ONE**

How a Mediterranean-Style Diet and Ketogenic Strategies Could Change Your Life and Health Span

CHAPTER ONE

GET READY TO CHANGE YOUR LIFE AND YOUR BRAIN

"Let food be thy medicine, and let medicine be thy food."
—Attributed to Hippocrates, c. 400 B.C.

LET FOOD BE THY MEDICINE

Soon after starting medical school in 1974, I realized that science had barely uncovered what causes disease and how to treat it. Given how rapidly medical science was (and still is) advancing, I cringed upon reading about treatments for newborns in a decades-old medical textbook with "modern" in the title, then laughed at the "far superior" information in a slightly newer "contemporary" textbook. In the 1970s, words like "neuroinflammation" and "microbiome" were not yet part of the medical vernacular. Like other medical students, I took the Hippocratic Oath to "first do no harm." Despite his teachings, the typical medical curriculum, then and now, focuses on pharmaceuticals, which do save many lives, but the curriculum seriously neglects nutrition, which could prevent disease altogether, reduce disability, and save many more lives. During four years of medical school, my total education on how diet affects health and disease consisted of just three hours on a single afternoon.

While rotating through the basic medical fields, I learned that many diseases could not be treated effectively and seemed hopeless—invasive cancers, many psychiatric disorders, and all neurodegenerative diseases. I chose a satisfying field of great hope, neonatology, the care of sick and premature newborns. As a neonatal doctor or nurse, you save lives and usher many families from utter fear to hope and promise. My pediatrics and neonatology nutrition training centered much more on what infant formula to prescribe than why, without much critical consideration of the evidence that led to the formulations. As a neonatologist, I encouraged breastfeeding, worked to maximize oral feedings, and wrote out formulas for intravenous nutrition daily. Breast milk is incredibly complex, with thousands of different nutrients, and infant formulas contain only a fraction of these nutrients. I came to recognize that, if a natural substance is consistently present in breast milk, it is likely an important building block for cells or has another important biological function in the developing human. This is relevant here, because breast milk contains significant amounts of medium-chain triglycerides, an important part of the Clearly Keto diet.

For decades, I followed the AHA and USDA low-fat dogma—no eggs, butter, or cream. I was shocked and overjoyed when the first USDA Food Pyramid was published in 1992 (see figure 1.1), which encouraged six to eleven servings per day of grains at its base, with a tiny point of fat and sweets at the top with advice to "use sparingly." I was "on a diet," counting calories every day and always hungry. I drank skim milk and ate low-fat everything, like "heart-healthy" cereals, margarine, and overly processed packaged foods that typically contained trans fat, high-fructose corn syrup, and synthetic chemicals. I repeatedly lost, then slowly regained, very large amounts of weight. At age fifty-four in 2006, my BMI was just above the cutoff for "morbid obesity," my fasting blood sugar was elevated, and my heart was enlarged. I was on the pathway to diabetes.

With Steve's symptoms progressing rapidly, I came across a study of improved survival for people with Alzheimer's who consumed a Mediterranean-style diet (Scarmeas 2007). I read every book and scientific study I could to devise a plan using this new information. Up until

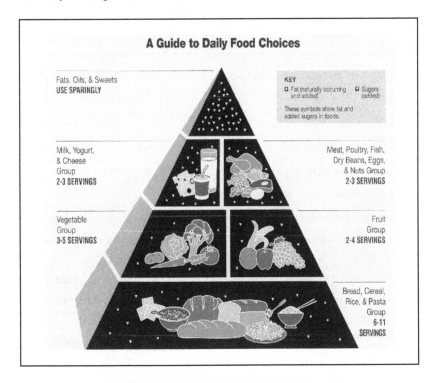

FIGURE 1.1. USDA Food Pyramid, 1992.

then, we had eaten a "convenience-food diet." We dined out often, including fast-food restaurants, and were fond of easy frozen family meals. As a physician, I am embarrassed at how poorly we fed our growing daughters and ourselves and that we were so far off-track from a healthy diet. We quickly transitioned to a whole-food Mediterranean-style diet with much fewer carbohydrates and more healthy fat intake, mainly as olive oil, and began to take fish oil. We removed the sweets and refined grains from our house. We ate a variety of colors of fresh vegetables and fruit, much more fish, and whole-grain rice, pasta, and breads in small servings.

Over the next two years, coupling the diet with more intense exercise, I lost ninety-four pounds and easily got my fasting blood sugar back to normal. However, Steve's Alzheimer's symptoms steadily worsened, and it is impossible to know whether the diet slowed the disease progression. Then, in 2008, armed with new information about Alzheimer's as diabetes of the brain and ketones as an alternative fuel to glucose, we incorporated ketogenic oils (coconut oil and MCT oil), followed by a dramatic steady improvement in Steve's symptoms. Within the year, we transitioned further to a lower-carb ketogenic diet. We maintained a ketogenic whole-food Mediterranean-style diet throughout Steve's life, and I have continued thereafter.

THE MEDITERRANEAN-STYLE DIET

The specific foods in the Mediterranean diet differ greatly among populations of Europe and are far from exclusive to Europe. Therefore, I refer to it as a "Mediterranean-style" diet, which includes daily consumption of vegetables, fruits, whole grains, and adequate protein as poultry, legumes, eggs, moderate portions of whole-fat dairy or goat-milk products, intake of fatty fish at least weekly, and limited intake of red meat. Healthy fat is a "mainstay" of the diet, emphasizing olive oil, and I also include coconut oil and MCT oil on the healthy fats list. Eating this way can substantially lower the amount of carbohydrates in the diet. We will discuss the specifics of the Mediterranean-style ketogenic diet in much more detail in chapter 4 and coconut and MCT oil in chapter 5.

The whole-food Mediterranean-style diet is easily adaptable to a reasonable low-carb, ketogenic diet, as are the Paleo, vegetarian, vegan, and traditional diets of many cultures. It is even possible to eat a "junk-food" ketogenic diet if there is too much reliance on overly processed packaged foods, and I strongly discourage that for obvious reasons.

First Steps to Go Keto and Clean Up Your Diet

To help kick-start nutritional ketosis and clean up your diet, I suggest the following:

- Consult with your physician before making any radical change in your diet, especially if you have medical conditions, if you are taking medications, or if you are elderly, pregnant, breastfeeding, or helping a child with the diet.

- Consider this as dietary advice to discuss with your physician, and not as medical advice.
- Do not stop or change any medications without consulting your physician. If you are diabetic, you need to know that a low-carb diet can drop your blood sugar quickly. Monitor your blood sugar more often, and discuss medication changes with your doctor to avoid hypoglycemia.
- If you are taking warfarin (an anti-blood-clotting medication), you should be aware of foods and supplements that could throw off your INR test. Consult with your doctor before instituting dietary changes or adding supplements suggested in the book.
- A very high-fat diet is not for you if you have severe liver disease or liver failure, or certain rare enzyme defects involving fat metabolism.
- If you are allergic to coconut oil, do not eat it . . . or any other food you are allergic to, for that matter.

First Steps to Kick-Start Nutritional Ketosis

- Add virgin organic coconut oil and MCT oil (which is extracted from coconut oil) to your diet.
- Since MCT oil is more ketogenic, I suggest starting with coconut oil and then consider combining MCT oil with virgin coconut oil to smooth out the ups and downs of ketone levels that may occur when taking just MCT oil. You can make your own mixture or look at my website (see Resources) for commercial options.
- To avoid diarrhea, which can happen if you are not used to larger amounts of oils, start with one teaspoon of coconut oil two or three times a day with food, and increase by this amount every few days as tolerated.
- Mixture: 4 ounces MCT oil to each 3 ounces of virgin organic coconut oil. Warm the coconut oil until it is liquid, and use a funnel

to add the oils to the same bottle. Invert the bottle a few times to mix. Store at room temperature. The mixture is stable for up to two years and can be added to many types of food, warm or cold, and used to cook at low to low-medium heat.

- Increase MCT oil, or the mixture, as for coconut oil above. For prevention, work up slowly to at least 3 tablespoons daily, or more as tolerated. If you have a brain disease or brain fog, you might (with doctor's permission) increase to 5 to 9 tablespoons daily, as tolerated, divided between meals and snacks.
- If you are thin, simply add these oils to your diet, and you may gain weight.
- If you are overweight, substitute these oils for other fats, or, even better, reduce carbs as you add the oils, which we will talk about next.
- Consider adding an exogenous ketone supplement, such as ketone salts or ketone esters. Exogenous means originating from outside the body, as opposed to the ketones you make in your body from breaking down fat or on a ketogenic diet or from adding coconut and MCT oil to your diet. Chapter 5 will cover this at length.

Next Steps

- Avoid eating during the night and start narrowing down the window during which you eat in the daytime. You could begin with a 12-hour overnight fast (drinking sugar-free liquids is fine and important), then slowly work toward a "window of eating" of six to ten hours. This strategy can help you wake up in mild ketosis, and then you can build on that with what you eat and by adopting other keto strategies like exercise.
- Eliminate sugary drinks and obvious sweets. Avoid adding extra sugar to anything.
- Remove tempting sweets, high-carb foods, and junk food from your pantry and refrigerator, and donate unopened packages to a food pantry.

- Begin to cut down your portions of starchy foods like bread, pasta, rice, and cereals, and replace refined flours and grains with whole grains. Cut your portions of these foods in half, and then, when you are used to that, cut the portions in half again.
- If you eat out, turn down the breadbasket, and consider adding a second vegetable in place of the potato or pasta. Learn to say "no, thank you" to the dessert menu.
- Begin to increase your intake of healthy fats and oils like olive oil, coconut oil, butter, cream, and high-fat foods like nuts, seeds, avocados, eggs, and olives. Substitute these fats for other less healthy vegetable oils and, especially, carbohydrates.
- If you eat dairy, choose whole-fat versions, like milk, cheese, and yogurt, preferably from pasture-raised, grass-fed animals.
- Do not be afraid to eat the fat of grass-fed and pasture-raised meats and poultry, and consider eating more fatty fish and poultry and less beef and pork.
- Consider choosing organically grown vegetables and fruits and non-GMO as available.
- Consider eating gluten-free foods, as excessive gluten may cause a leaky gut, which could affect your brain.
- Choose oils and fats that are organic and cold-pressed or expeller-pressed whenever available, since they have not been subjected to high heat during processing. Also, look for virgin coconut oil and for extra-virgin olive oil that are less processed and retain maximum nutritional value. Organic versions are available for MCT oil, chicken fat, lard, beef tallow, and most refined oils.
- Consider taking your whole family on this journey with you. They will benefit, and there will be less tempting food in the house for all of you. A younger couple in my family embraced a whole-food, low-carb lifestyle more than three years ago, and they are leaner and feel healthier, and their teenage son has grown perfectly into his height by eating what his parents eat. Figure 1.2 summarizes how to clean up your diet as you begin on your journey to a healthier brain.

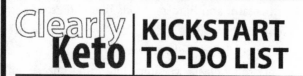

KICKSTART TO-DO LIST

Add more healthy fats to your diet, along with a variety of types and colors of **vegetables and fruits**.

Begin coconut and/or MCT oil separately or mixed.
- Start with 1 tsp (5 gm) 2-3 time/day with food.
- Increase **slowly** as tolerated.

Avoid eating overnight and narrow your daytime "window of eating" to between 6-12 hours.

Avoid sugary drinks, obvious sweets, starchy snacks, and refined grains.

Remove tempting foods from your house.

Reduce portions of starchy vegetables, breads, cereals, pasta, and rice.

Consider adding an exogenous ketone supplement.

FIGURE 1.2. Clearly Keto Kickstart To-Do List.

CHAPTER TWO

WHY GO KETO? FUEL, ENERGY, AND THE AGING BRAIN

"Energy is the difference between being alive and being dead."
—Douglas C. Wallace, PhD

WHAT IS ENERGY, AND WHERE DOES IT COME FROM?

When we contemplate what energy is, most of us think about our energy level. Do we carry out mental and physical activities with strength and focus, or are we sluggish and slow to react? At any age, our energy level fluctuates throughout the day, but many elderly people are quite slow, both physically and mentally.

At a deeper level, nearly every cell in our body needs energy to carry out its functions—specifically, the energy molecule adenosine triphosphate (ATP)—and each cell requires fuel to make ATP. Like a whole person, a given cell can have low or high energy, depending on how much fuel is available and if the apparatus to make ATP is functioning properly. You might think of your overall energy level as the sum of the energy levels of the trillions of cells in your body at that moment. When it comes to your energy level, your mind and body work together. It is unlikely that your body will move with high energy if your brain feels sluggish.

The fuel to make ATP ultimately comes from food. As we digest food, it is broken down into much smaller components—sugars, proteins, fats, and other nutrients, such as vitamins and minerals. We eliminate what we do not need and store what might be useful. Sugars, proteins, and fats are further broken down to be used as fuel (mainly glucose, fatty acids, and ketones) or to be rearranged into new materials to build and operate cells and communicate between cells. We might also hang on to potentially harmful substances from our food and store them in our fat, liver, brain, and other tissues. This whole very complex process is called metabolism. How well we age depends greatly on what we feed into our metabolism.

On a typical American high-carb diet, glucose is the main fuel the brain and other organs use to produce ATP. During prolonged fasting or starvation, glucose stores in the liver and muscles are used up within a couple of days. To provide an alternative source of fuel, our metabolism turns to stored fat, which is converted to long-chain fatty acids that can provide fuel to the heart, kidneys, muscles, and other organs. However, long-chain fatty acids do not readily cross the blood–brain barrier, and some fatty acids are converted in the liver to ketones, which are small molecules that easily cross the blood–brain barrier. Brain cells can instantaneously switch from using glucose to ketones as fuel. This metabolic fact is the foundation for lifestyle changes we will discuss throughout the book. Consuming a ketogenic diet, medium-chain triglyceride oil, coconut oil, exercise, and overnight fasting can increase ketone production within the body (called endogenous ketones). Exogenous ketone supplements contain the same natural ketones and increase blood ketone levels for several hours.

As we age, it is easy to see the outward signs in the mirror. We can plainly see sagging skin and gray hair and a curve forming in our back. We may lose a few inches of height over time and lose some muscle each year along with strength. Slowing of memory and other cognitive functions, not so obvious in a mirror, may sneak up on us.

Cognition is our state of awareness and how we accumulate, process, and act on information coming in through our senses. Brain aging begins in our late thirties, speeds up in our fifties, and accelerates even more after age sixty. This is an exceedingly complex process in which the brain gradually shrinks, some areas more quickly than others (Fjell 2013). We may lose connections between individual brain cells, called synapses, and between the regions of the brain, called networks (Chen 2019). Brain aging leads to slowing of memory and other cognitive functions—how fast we retrieve a memory, such as a word or a face, if at all, and how well we plan, organize, and carry out each daily activity (executive functioning). Our behavior and mood may also change, along with our ability to cope with these changes.

Blood flow, which delivers oxygen and nutrients to the brain, gradually declines, and the barrier between the blood and the brain (the blood–brain barrier) weakens. The brain's ability to take up glucose as fuel for brain cells can become faulty, and the protective immune system weakens. The means of removing toxins and other waste products from the brain may become defective as well, allowing this waste to accumulate and damage delicate brain structures. When someone develops Alzheimer's disease or other type of dementia, brain deterioration is accelerated and exaggerated beyond normal aging, along with brain inflammation and accumulation of abnormal protein deposits.

While this is depressing, the good news is that we may be able to slow down the process of brain aging by adopting a healthier lifestyle—changing what and when we eat and drink, whether we exercise, how well we sleep, how much stress we have in our lives, whether our blood pressure is controlled, whether we smoke or drink too much alcohol, and many other factors. Providing ketones as an alternative fuel to the brain could fill the void left by decreased glucose uptake to help individual brain cells and the entire brain function better. Ketones are also anti-inflammatory. As you will learn, these are just two roles ketones can play in healthier aging.

THE "BRAIN-ENERGY GAP"

No one has done more to study ketones and the Alzheimer's brain than Dr. Stephen Cunnane (Photo 1) and his research associates. Cunnane's

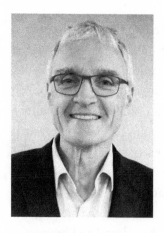

PHOTO 1.
Stephen C. Cunnane, PhD

early career focused on essential fatty acids and ketones in the developing human brain. The newborn brain represents roughly 10 percent of the baby's weight but uses about 70 percent of the total energy requirement with a substantial contribution from ketones. Cunnane and group discovered that ketones not only provide fuel but also are building blocks for lipids in the newborn brain. The chubby full-term breastfed newborn goes into ketosis soon after birth and derives ketones from burning fat and from the ketogenic medium-chain triglycerides (MCTs) in breast milk (Cunnane 1999; Cunnane 2003; Cunnane 2005).

Shifting gears to ketones and the Alzheimer's brain in 2003, access to ketone and glucose PET imaging at Sherbrooke University in Quebec allowed Cunnane to answer questions about what happens to energy in the aging brain and in Alzheimer's. Over 350 healthy young and older adults, and adults with mild cognitive impairment and Alzheimer's disease, have now been scanned and reveal that ketones provide about 3 to 5 percent of the energy requirement of the brain throughout adulthood. However, compared to younger healthy adults, healthy cognitively normal older adults have a 7 to 9 percent gap between how much energy the brain needs and how much it gets, which Cunnane calls the "brain-energy gap." This gap widens to more than 10 percent in people with mild cognitive impairment and to 20 percent or more in the early stages of Alzheimer's (Cunnane 2016). The brain is hungry for fuel and, even though it is about 2 to 3 percent of our total body weight, the brain consumes 20 to 25 percent of the calories we burn in a day. Therefore, it is important to provide the brain with all the fuel it needs to age in the healthiest possible way.

In a landmark study, Cunnane and group reported that ketones are taken up normally in the glucose-deprived areas of the brain in Alzheimer's (Castellano 2015), and that ketones produce more energy

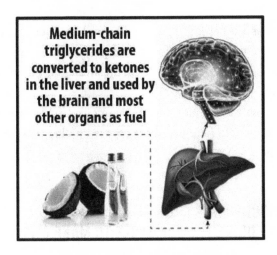

Medium-chain triglycerides are converted to ketones in the liver and used by the brain and most other organs as fuel

FIGURE 2.1. Medium-chain triglycerides are partly converted to ketones in the liver, which can be used by the brain and most other organs, except the liver, as fuel.

in the brain in direct proportion to blood ketone levels. These profound discoveries support the idea that the areas of poor glucose uptake could contain dormant dysfunctional neurons that simply lack adequate fuel to make ATP, and that increasing the ketone level could improve symptoms in people with Alzheimer's and certain other brain diseases. They also confirmed in their BENEFIC trial that medium-chain triglyceride (MCT) oil contributes energy to the brain as ketones (see figure 2.1), can bridge the "brain-energy gap" (Courchesne-Loyer 2016; Croteau 2018), and can improve cognition in people with mild cognitive impairment (MCI), a condition that can lead to Alzheimer's (Fortier 2021). Dr. Cunnane cautions that two-to-three-year-long studies of supplementation with MCT oil in people with memory impairment are needed to determine whether this strategy could prevent progression from MCI to Alzheimer's.

Cunnane and group have studied other ketogenic strategies, such as exercise (Castellano 2017) and caffeine (Vandenberghe 2016), and have demonstrated that the heart and kidneys have high uptake of ketones when taking ketone salt supplementation, suggesting that ketones could potentially be therapeutic for heart and kidney diseases (Cuenoud

2020). These and other Cunnane studies will be discussed throughout the book. Dr. Cunnane and others have published an excellent review of brain-energy rescue through ketogenic strategies in Nature Review Drug Discovery (Cunnane 2020).

Since we will be talking about energy and fuels to make energy throughout the book, here is a short course on chemistry, glucose, ketones, and the TCA cycle.

BIOCHEMISTRY 101: GLUCOSE AND KETONES DRIVE THE TCA CYCLE TO MAKE ATP

"Atoms" are the fundamental particles of matter. The basic atoms in living matter are oxygen, hydrogen, and carbon. Atoms are connected to each other by "bonds" that are much like magnetic attractions. When two or more atoms are connected, they are called "molecules." Glucose (sugar), fats, and ketones are made of different combinations of oxygen, hydrogen, and carbon. The carbon atoms line up in a chain, and the hydrogen and oxygen atoms attach to the carbon atoms or to each other. The positions of the atoms determine what a molecule does in the body. Molecules can become more complex by connecting with other atoms or molecules, such as nitrogen, sulfur, calcium, magnesium, phosphate, and many others.

Glucose has a chain of six carbons with hydrogen and oxygen atoms attached (see figure 2.2) and is the main fuel for our cells when eating a higher carbohydrate diet. Glucose is readily made in the body as needed, even while we consistently eat a very strict high-fat, low-carbohydrate ketogenic diet. Even in Alzheimer's, unaffected areas of the brain can and do use glucose.

Three ketones are made in the liver:

Glucose

H – C = O
H – C – O – H
H – O – C – H
H – C – O – H
H – C – O – H
H – C – O – H
H

| H | O | C | – | = |
| Hydrogen Atom | Oxygen Atom | Carbon Atom | Bond | Double Bond |

FIGURE 2.2. Glucose molecule.

acetoacetate, betahydroxybutyrate, and acetone (see figure 2.4). Acetoacetate converts easily to betahydroxybutyrate (see figure 2.5), and vice versa. Aceto-acetate (AcAc) also converts to acetone, which is mostly exhaled and accounts for the fruity breath that is common when in ketosis. Betahydroxybutyrate (BHB) levels steadily rise in the blood-stream over ten days or so of starvation or strict ketogenic diet, and can provide ⅔ of the fuel required by the brain. BHB is a simpler molecule than glucose—a chain of four carbons with hydrogens and oxygens attached. Fuel as glucose, fatty acids, or ketones drives the tricar-boxylic acid (TCA) cycle (also called the citric acid cycle or Krebs cycle), which feeds into the electron transport chain

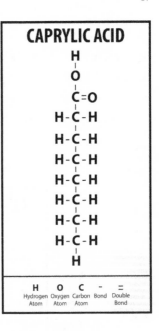

FIGURE 2.3. Caprylic acid molecule. Caprylic acid is a medium-chain fatty acid with eight carbons in the chain.

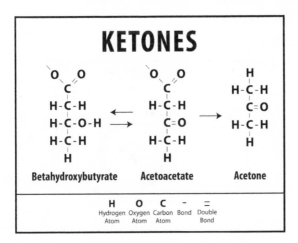

FIGURE 2.4. The ketones betahydroxybutyrate, acetoacetate, and acetone. Acetoacetate and betahydroxybutyrate can convert to each other. Acetoacetate can also convert to acetone.

to produce the energy molecule adenosine triphosphate (ATP). BHB converts back to AcAc before it enters the TCA cycle (see figure 2.6—simplified version, and figure 2.7—more complicated version of the glucose and ketone pathways to make ATP). Both glucose and ketones are involved in other biochemical processes as well.

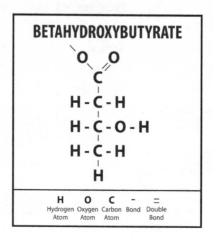

FIGURE 2.5. Betahydroxybutyrate (BHB) molecule.

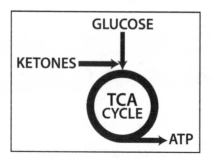

FIGURE 2.6. Glucose and ketones drive the pathway to produce ATP in the brain—simplified version. Ketones and glucose use different transporters to enter the TCA cycle, which feeds into the electron transport chain to make ATP.

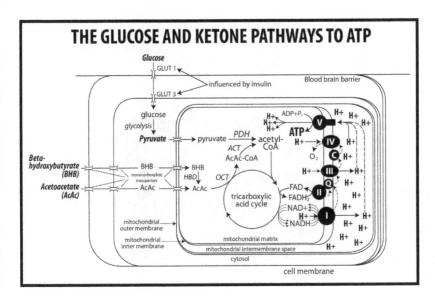

FIGURE 2.7. Glucose and ketones drive the pathway to produce ATP in the brain—a more complicated version. Glucose uses GLUT 1 (GLUT is for GLUcose Transporter) to cross the blood–brain barrier and GLUT 3 to enter neurons. GLUT 1 and GLUT 3 are influenced by insulin. A series of chemical reactions occurs in the cytosol of the neuron, called glycolysis, to convert glucose to pyruvate. Pyruvate passes through the mitochondrial membrane (see mitochondrion in figure 2.8) by way of pyruvate dehydrogenase (PDH) complex 1 and is converted to acetyl-CoA, which enters the tricarboxylic acid (TCA or Krebs) cycle, where a series of reactions feeds into the electron transport chain (oxidative phosphorylation) and ultimately lead to production of adenosine triphosphate (ATP) from addition of phosphate to adenosine diphosphate (ADP). The process requires numerous enzymes and coenzymes. The ketones betahydroxybutyrate (BHB) and acetoacetate (AcAc) can also drive the TCA cycle, leading to production of ATP. BHB and AcAc use monocarboxylate transporters to cross the blood–brain barrier, enter the neuron, and pass through the mitochondrial membrane. Insulin is not involved in the process. BHB is converted to AcAc. In a set of reactions, AcAc is converted to acetyl-CoA and continues into the TCA cycle and on to electron transport to produce ATP. Ketones can bypass the problem of insulin resistance, GLUT 1, GLUT 3, and PDH complex 1 deficiency, which occur in Alzheimer's and interfere with the entry of glucose into the brain and into neurons. Figure adapted and expanded by Joanna Newport from information in VanItallie 2008.

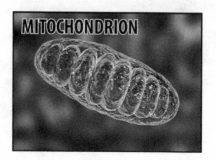

FIGURE 2.8. The mitochondrion (the singular of mitochondria) is where most ATP and many metabolites are made within all mammalian cell types, except mature red-blood cells. Most cells have hundreds of mitochondria, but energy-needy cells may have up to 1,000 mitochondria. Adapted by Joanna Newport from a figure on iStockPhoto.com.

CHAPTER THREE

DIABETES AND ALZHEIMER'S DISEASE

On low-carbohydrate diet for diabetes: "At the end of our clinic day, we go home thinking 'The clinical improvements are so large and so obvious, why don't other doctors understand?'"

—Eric Westman, MD (Feinman 2015)

Insulin resistance appears to be the early driving force behind Alzheimer's disease. If insulin resistance is not corrected, other treatments might not work very well, since the pathologies caused or aggravated by insulin resistance will continue to spread. For this reason, insulin and many factors related to insulin are at the very center of what goes wrong in Alzheimer's and in diabetes. In fact, Alzheimer's is sometimes called type 3 diabetes or diabetes of the brain.

Insulin is a critical hormone required to get glucose into most types of cells throughout the body. When blood glucose increases, the pancreas makes and secretes insulin in response. Insulin then attaches to insulin receptors on the surface of cell membranes, essentially unlocking the gate for glucose to enter the cell. The insulin signal then summons glucose transporters, called GLUTs, to the cell membrane to ferry glucose through the cell membrane (figure 3.1). Some GLUTs directly depend on insulin, and others are indirectly influenced by insulin. There are different GLUTs for different types of cells. For example,

GLUT 1 ferries glucose across the blood–brain barrier, and GLUT 3 ferries glucose into neurons, and both are influenced by insulin. We will talk more about specific GLUTs in the brain in Chapter 10.

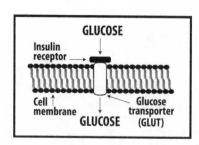

FIGURE 3.1. Glucose crosses through cell membrane when insulin attaches to insulin receptor which calls glucose transporter (GLUT) to the cell membrane to ferry glucose through. In some cell types, GLUTs are indirectly influenced by insulin, rather than directly responding to attachment of insulin to an insulin receptor.

In addition to glucose, certain amino acids, the neurotransmitter acetylcholine, and several other substances can trigger the release of insulin from the pancreas. Insulin is also a signaling (communicating) hormone that affects many other metabolic pathways in the brain and other organs. Insulin interacts with hormones, enzymes, genes, and other substances related to appetite; growth; production of cholesterol, glucose, fatty acids, and proteins; storage and release of glucose and fat; and it has many other effects not yet fully understood. Even more complicated, insulin growth factors and other insulin-related substances are also involved in these pathways. Insulin receptors are present throughout the brain and are highly concentrated in the parts of the brain involved in memory (Norwitz 2019). It is easy to see that a deficiency of insulin or resistance to insulin can have wide-ranging consequences.

Insulin resistance is a huge concern for the aging brain, since diabetes carries at least a 30 percent risk of dementia, six times higher than in the average population. The rate of diabetes has tripled to epidemic proportions over the past half-century. In the U.S. today, 10.5 percent of adults ages eighteen and above have diabetes, and 34.5 percent have prediabetes, which progresses to diabetes within five years on average. By age seventy-five, three-quarters of U.S. adults have either diabetes or prediabetes. Over the past half-century, obesity rates have also climbed while the typical U.S. diet has increased by 350 calories per day, of which 300 calories are from sugar (see figures 3.2 and 3.3).

The diabetes epidemic is rampant worldwide, in developed and developing countries. In 2017, the diabetes rate in Europe was 8.8 percent of adults ages twenty and above (with a low of 4.3 percent in Ireland and a high of 13.9 percent in Portugal); in the Middle East, 15 to 18 percent; and in Japan, 5.6 percent. The Pacific Islands have more than double the U.S. diabetes rate at 22 to 27 percent (IDF 2017).

DIABETES, TYPES 1 AND 2

Most people are familiar with type 1 and type 2 diabetes. People with type 1 diabetes have lost the ability to make insulin in the pancreas. This can happen at any age, even in infancy. Type 1 diabetes often comes on suddenly and sometimes begins after a viral infection. Early symptoms are extreme thirst, excessive urination, hunger, and weight loss; unless diagnosed and treated with insulin, it can evolve into life-threatening diabetic ketoacidosis. Since most cells can no longer use glucose without insulin, fat breaks down rapidly to provide fuel, which generates massive ketone production. In diabetic ketoacidosis, ketone levels are many times higher than the levels achieved from using a ketogenic diet and supplements. Before insulin came along in 1921, fasting was sometimes used to try to control diabetes, but people rarely lived more than a year using this approach. Restricting carbohydrate intake and increasing fat intake is a relatively new idea for controlling blood sugar in type 1 diabetes, which deserves more attention.

In the past, type 2 diabetes was called "adult onset" diabetes because it was rare in children; but, sadly, that is no longer the case. Type 2 diabetes begins with insulin resistance. The pancreas can still make insulin, but the insulin receptors on cells are no longer responding normally to insulin. It takes more and more insulin to get glucose into the affected cells, and the insulin level in the blood becomes elevated—sometimes extremely elevated. As type 2 diabetes progresses, the pancreatic cells may become exhausted and lose the ability to make insulin, necessitating insulin injection. In more advanced type 2 diabetes, it is common to be prescribed two

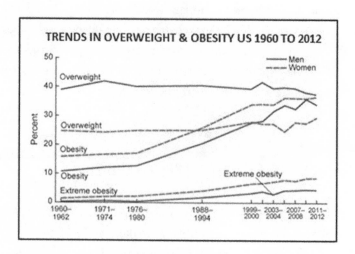

FIGURE 3.2. Trends in adult overweight, obesity, and extreme obesity among men and women aged twenty to seventy-four: United States, selected years 1960 through 2012. https://www.cdc.gov/nchs/data /hestat/obesity_adult_11_12/obesity_adult_11_12.htm.

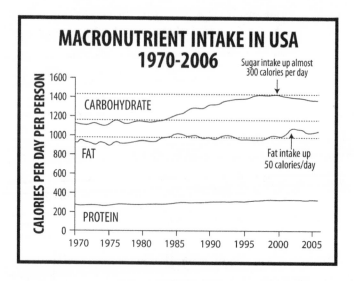

FIGURE 3.3. The increase in caloric and sugar intake in the United States since 1970 parallels the increases in overweight and obesity during the same time period, as shown in figure 3.2. Source: USDA food consumption databases, https://usda.gov.

or three oral medications and one or more forms of insulin to try to control blood sugar.

Your doctor can check for insulin resistance and diabetes with a fasting blood glucose and insulin level. A HOMA-IR calculation can help determine insulin resistance. A helpful blood test to diagnose diabetes and monitor blood glucose control is HbA1C, which approximates a three-month average of blood glucose based on the amount of glucose that is stored in red cells.

Consuming a low-carb, higher-fat diet could help people with prediabetes and diabetes type 2 achieve better blood glucose control, reduce the risk of serious complications, and extend lifespan. Physicians like Eric Westman, MD, of Duke University, and Sarah Hallberg**, DO, of Virta Health have used this approach for years to help thousands of their patients. Several sizable studies of low-carb, high-fat diets compared to standard higher-carb diets have reported excellent results in putting type 2 diabetes into remission with improvement in overall health, weight, blood pressure, lipid profiles, HbA1C, fasting glucose, and fasting insulin levels (Volek 2009; Feinman 2015; Hallberg 2018; Athinarayanan 2020). Many people with type 2 diabetes have been able to eliminate or greatly reduce their dosages of insulin and other medications with this approach.

** Dr. Sarah Hallberg is recently deceased in 2022.

Blood Tests for Insulin Resistance

To help nail down whether you have insulin resistance, ask your doctor to include these studies with your next blood work:

- **Fasting blood sugar.** Normal is less than 100 mg/dl (5.6 mmol/L), but
  less than 95 mg/dl (5.3 mmol/L) is better.

- **Fasting insulin level** (< 8 mU/ml indicates less likely insulin resistance).

- **HbA1C.** This measure roughly estimates the average glucose level
  over the previous three months. Some labs consider less than 6
  percent normal, but less than 5.6 percent is ideal.

- **HOMA-IR (Homeostatic Model Assessment of Insulin Resistance)
  Calculation.** Add fasting glucose in mg/dl plus the fasting insulin
  level in mU/ml and divide the total by 405. Or add fasting glucose
  in mmol/L plus fasting insulin level in mU/ml and divide the total by
  22.5. Less than 1.5 is normal, but less than 1.0 is optimal. Greater
  than 2.0 suggests insulin resistance. Greater than 2.9 indicates significant insulin resistance.

In chapter 9, we will discuss why excess sugar intake is so harmful and consider the role of inflammatory advanced glycation end-
products.

A ketogenic diet can also help people with type 1 diabetes who
are at great risk of serious chronic complications, including dementia.
My friend Andrew Koutnik, PhD, studies nutrition and metabolism,
focusing on the ketogenic approach to cancer and cachexia (extreme
weight loss and muscle wasting due to cancer or other late-stage diseases). Andrew has type 1 diabetes and has dramatically improved

his glucose control with a ketogenic diet. Look for my interview with Dr. Koutnik in a side box nearby.

Questions and Answers with Andrew Koutnik, PhD, on His Personal Experience with Type 1 Diabetes and the Ketogenic Diet.

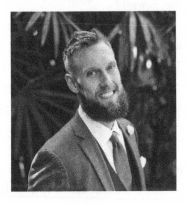

PHOTO 1. Andrew Koutnik, PhD

Newport: Is there a specific macronutrient ratio, maximum amount of carbs, and/or percent of calories as fat that you aim for?

Koutnik: For type 1 diabetes, the goal is euglycemia [staying within the normal range of blood sugar]. Thus, the formulation is specific to whatever achieves that. However, most people in the type 1 diabetes community build their diet with protein foods first, because they can match the glucose influx of protein foods with currently available insulins, then 50g or less of green fibrous veggies (no/low glycemic impact), then fat is provided as needed to substantiate caloric/energetic needs. This could look like a 15 to 30 percent calories as protein, 0 to 15 percent fibrous carbohydrate, 55 to 75 percent fat diet.

Q: What was your approximate blood-sugar range over twenty-four hours before—and then after—you started the ketogenic diet?

A: For me, I didn't have a continuous glucose monitor prior to doing my first rodeo with ketogenic diet. However, I have examples of when I tried various other diets for "fun" or sports-performance reasons in my blog on optimal blood glucose control (Koutnik 2018).

Q: Since diabetics are taught to worry so much about ketones, is there a level of ketones you aim for?

A: The word "ketones" remains a bad word in type 1 diabetes. I am trying to change this, but it will take time. People are scared that if you are on a diet that already increases ketone levels, that having type 1 diabetes, getting sick, inadvertent caloric restriction, et cetera, may push a type 1 diabetic over the edge into ketoacidosis. I feel that this is largely based on consequential thinking. Right now, the data illustrates that diabetic ketoacidosis is less common in a very-low-carb diet in type 1 diabetes. Higher HbA1c's are associated with diabetic ketoacidosis. Glycemic control shows an inverse relationship with diabetic ketoacidosis. You do not need much insulin to keep ketones under control. You just need enough. Also, the higher protein that is often consumed by type 1 diabetes on this diet (Lennerz 2018; Bernstein 2011) blunts the ketogenesis enough. Either way, it is likely safe to be anywhere below 5mm/L just based on the data in general population. However, my endocrinology friends may disagree and argue that it needs to be as low as possible. However, I am working on a review as we speak with Boston Children's, which I hope will change this narrative to better inform clinicians of this nuance, particularly on the ketogenic diet.

Q: How much were you able to reduce your insulin?

A: By 75 percent! Also, I directly considered the cost without insurance off the diet and post-diet, and it dropped from $900.00 to $150.00/ month in just insulin costs alone.

Q: Do you have any words of wisdom to address the fear of ketones?

A: Due to the clear rise in interested patients, researchers, clinicians, and the lay public on the low carbohydrate and/or ketogenic diet, the emergent evidence illustrates a number of extremely successful implementations using these dietary strategies in type 1 diabetes. It seems wise for the clinical community to become more informed on how to help guide type 1 diabetics on successfully implementing a low-carb ketogenic diet—knowing how to change the insulin regimen on this new diet, knowing how to prevent caloric restriction if needed, prioritizing particularly macronutrient intake, the patient populations, and goals, ensuring safe transition into new diet regimen, adequate hydration, et cetera. Another critical aspect is for clinicians to understand there is a clear difference between ketoacidosis (typically blood glucose >250 mg/dL, insulin absent/minimal, blood ketones >10mM) compared to nutritional ketosis (blood glucose 70 to 110 mg/dL, insulin moderate/sufficient, blood ketones 0 to 5mM). There are a number of described benefits to ketones which may actually benefit a type 1 diabetic if in the normal healthy range, and that is something currently under further critical research evaluation.

You can read more about Dr. Koutnik's experience and research on his blog (Koutnik 2018) and in a review by Koutnik and others in the Journal of Clinical Investigation (Lennerz 2021).

DIABETES TYPE 3: ALZHEIMER'S IS DIABETES OF THE BRAIN

The prevailing belief for many years was that insulin does not cross the blood–brain barrier and therefore does not play a significant role in the brain. We now know that insulin uses transporters to move through the blood–brain barrier and that insulin is also present in spinal fluid, which flows like a river through the brain and down the spinal column. Evidence suggests that insulin may be produced directly in the brain as well (Gray 2014; de la Monte 2019). In Alzheimer's, there are lower levels of insulin in the brain tissue and in the spinal fluid than in unaffected people.

In 2005, Suzanne de la Monte, PhD, and associates of Brown University studied the brains of people who died with Alzheimer's and did not have diabetes types 1 or 2. In all cases, there was insulin resistance and insulin deficiency in the brains affecting all signaling pathways involving insulin and insulin growth factor. They also found evidence that insulin is made in the brain and coined the term "diabetes type 3" to describe Alzheimer's disease (de la Monte 2005). They further learned that this process is present in the earliest stages and worsens with each stage of disease until it is widespread and severe (de la Monte 2008).

Many studies using glucose PET imaging have demonstrated that the problem of getting glucose into brain cells begins at least one to two decades before symptoms of Alzheimer's appear. This problem has also been reported in young adults in their twenties who are at risk by virtue of their family history (Reiman 2004) and in women in their mid-twenties with polycystic ovary disease, who usually have insulin resistance and often a problem with working memory (Castellano 2015).

MILD COGNITIVE IMPAIRMENT (MCI) AND DIABETES

Insulin resistance also occurs in some people with mild cognitive impairment (MCI) and various dementias other than Alzheimer's. People with prediabetes and diabetes have a much higher risk of developing dementia and pass through a stage comparable to MCI. People with diabetes or prediabetes with MCI are much more likely to progress to dementia and tend to progress more rapidly than people without diabetes or prediabetes (Xu 2010).

Chronically high blood sugar levels can lead to inflammation throughout the body and brain. Inflammation in the brain is common in people with MCI and is always present in the brains of people with Alzheimer's disease and in many other types of neurological diseases.

CAN WE PREVENT OR OVERCOME DIABETES OF THE BRAIN?

Strategies that increase ketone levels in the blood, if used consistently, might help prevent, slow down, or reverse symptoms of Alzheimer's. Many small-to-medium-size studies using the ketogenic diet, MCT oil, and coconut oil have reported promising results (see Scientific Research Articles at https://coconutketones.com). Larger studies using ketogenic diet, MCT oil, and ketone supplements are in progress at several Alzheimer's research centers in the United States and around the world.

Ketone supplements are already available to the public and are mainly used for enhancing athletic performance, fitness, and fat loss. Though they're not recognized by the FDA for use in Alzheimer's and other brain conditions yet, many people are using them for this purpose. Several studies have demonstrated that a ketone supplement could help control blood sugar (Myette-Côté 2018). Ketone supplements are discussed in chapter 5.

ALZHEIMER'S DOES NOT HAVE TO BE YOUR FATE!

I mentioned earlier that the low-carb, high-fat diet has been used for type 2 diabetics with great success. Could this diet also help people with diabetes type 3—diabetes of the brain? Kelly Gibas and associates published two case reports of people with mild Alzheimer's and insulin resistance who had excellent reversal of insulin-resistance blood markers after ten weeks on a program that included a ketogenic diet. The great news is that there was also significant improvement in their Montreal Cognitive Assessment (Stoykovich 2019; Morril 2019).

Case Report #1: A Man with Alzheimer's on 10-Week Ketogenic Diet and Program

Case #1 is a sixty-eight-year-old male ApoE4 carrier with morbid obesity and type 2 diabetes for more than fifteen years, who was taking long- and short-acting insulin injections. He had mild Alzheimer's disease with a MoCA (cognitive screening) score of 23 out of 30 points before starting the program. The patient was placed on a personalized ketogenic diet (KD) for ten weeks, with an eight-hour window of eating and a program of moderate intensity exercise three times per week, and peak brain training (language, problem-solving, mental agility, memory). The diet was designed to aim for ketone (BHB) levels > 0.5–2.0 mmol/L, and his average daily BHB ketone levels were 1.0 mmol/L (mild nutritional ketosis) per personal communication with Kelly Gibas, a co-author of the study.

Results: The patient's MoCA score improved from 23 at baseline to 29 of 30 after ten weeks of the program. Results of many blood levels improved, as shown in table 1 (Stoykovich 2019).

Table 1: Case Report #1

Key Biomarker Results (ideal range)	Before Intervention	After Intervention	Percent change
MoCA cognitive test (>26)	23 of 30	29 of 30	+26%
Fasting blood glucose mg/dL (70–90)	129	98	−24.0%
Fasting insulin mU/L (2–5)	97.2	14.3	−85.3%
HbA1C (<6.0)	7.8% (diabetic)	5.5% (normal)	−29.5%

HOMA-IR (<1.0)	31	3.5	−88.8%
Triglycerides mg/dL (<150)	137	83	−39.4%
HDL mg/dL (>50)	28	38	+35.7%
LDL mg/dL (<100)	74	61	−17.6&
VLDL mg/dL (9–13)	27.4	16.6	−39.4%
Weight (pounds)	257.2	243.0	−5.5%
Body fat (<30%)	39.8%	36.8%	−3%

Case Report #2: A Woman with Alzheimer's on 10-Week Ketogenic Diet and Program

Case #2 is a seventy-one-year-old female ApoE4 carrier, with obesity, metabolic syndrome, and mild Alzheimer's disease, with a baseline MoCA score of 21 out of 30. She was placed on a personalized ketogenic diet (KD) for ten weeks, with an eight-hour window of eating, low-impact walking on treadmill three times per week, and peak brain training (language, problem-solving, mental agility, memory). The diet was designed to aim for ketone (BHB) levels > 0.5–2.0 mmol/L.

Results: The patient's MoCA score improved from 21 at baseline to 28 of 30 after ten weeks of the program, and results of many blood levels also improved, as shown in table 2 (Morril 2019).

Table 2: Case Report #2

Key Biomarker Results	Before Intervention	After Intervention	Percent change
MoCA cognitive test (≥26)	21 of 30	28 of 30	+33.3%
Fasting blood glucose mg/dL (70–90)	116	87	−25%
Fasting insulin mU/L (2–5)	48.7	16.2	−67%
HbA1C (<6.0)	5.7	4.9	−15%
HOMA-IR (<1.0)	13.9	3.48	−75%
Triglycerides mg/dL (<150)	170	85	−50%
HDL mg/dL (>50)	64	72	+13%
LDL mg/dL (<100)	118	68	−42%
VLDL mg/dL (9–13)	34	17	−50%
Weight (pounds)	227	221	−3%
Body fat (<30%)	50	47	−6%

There is much more to Alzheimer's than what we have discussed in this chapter. There are plaques and tangles, inflammation, abnormal lipid deposits, and deficiencies in many substances. Every type of brain cell is affected. In chapter 10, you will soon notice a pattern, that each of the abnormalities in Alzheimer's has a connection to insulin and insulin resistance.

CHAPTER FOUR

CLEARLY KETO: A REASONABLE WHOLE-FOOD MEDITERRANEAN-STYLE KETOGENIC DIET

"Your life changes the moment you make a new, congruent, and committed decision."
— Tony Robbins, author and motivational speaker

Billions of dollars spent on Alzheimer's research—and more than four hundred clinical trials—have failed to turn up a drug to significantly improve the lives of the tens of millions worldwide suffering from this dreaded disease. Organizations funding Alzheimer's and dementia research are now focusing more on prevention, since modifiable lifestyle risk factors are estimated to account for 30 percent of dementia cases. In 2017, the World-Wide FINGERS Network became the first global network of multidomain dementia prevention trials, in which a combination of lifestyle interventions, such as diet, exercise, and cognitive training, are studied in people who are tested periodically for years. Poor diet tops the list of lifestyle risk factors that could impact how well our brains age. A reasonable whole-food Mediterranean-style ketogenic diet could change that.

A four-minute video from the NIH National Institute of Aging, "How Alzheimer's Changes the Brain," discusses how lifestyle changes could prevent this devastating outcome (NIA 2021).

Now, meet two people who are walking the walk.

JOE AND CAROL HENRY PRATA

*Joe holds Alzheimer's at bay with nearly ten years of
ketogenic foods and a low-glycemic-index Mediterranean diet.*

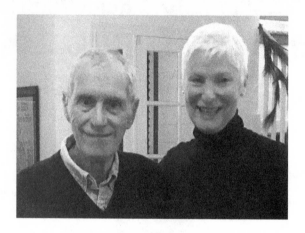

PHOTO 1. Joe and Carol Henry Prata.

Carol Henry Prata and Joe Prata have been together for fifty-two years.
When I interviewed Carol Henry Prata, her husband Joe Prata was
about to turn ninety-three years old on September 6, 2021.

Joe is not someone you would ever expect to develop dementia.
He was a world-class swimmer, narrowly missing a slot on the USA
team during the Olympic trials for the 1952 Helsinki Olympics. He
maintained a strong exercise regimen throughout his life, swimming,
and surfing, and much more. Joe believes you should do something you
enjoy every day. As a first-generation Italian-American, he has eaten a
Mediterranean diet his entire life, never smoked or used recreational
drugs, and does not drink. He sleeps well and never had a serious head
injury. Joe achieved a bachelor's degree in speech/public speaking with a

minor in social studies at Ohio State University and a master's degree in theater from San Francisco State University. He worked as an English teacher while also coaching swimming and water polo until he retired.

At age seventy-four, Carol is Joe's loving caregiver and advocate-in-chief. Carol worked in movie and television production, then became a financial planner, allowing her to be more available for Joe as he aged.

When I first interviewed Carol in 2017 for my previous book (The Complete Book of Ketones), she and Joe had just returned from seeing his neurologist with good news. Previously, in 2012, four neurologists had diagnosed Joe with early-stage dementia. Three believed it was likely or definitely Alzheimer's, and the fourth thought more likely vascular dementia. On this happy day, six years after Joe's symptoms became noticeable, the neurologist arrived at a diagnosis of amnestic mild cognitive impairment (MCI)—welcome news by comparison, since MCI does not always progress to dementia.

So, what did Joe and Carol do right? First we will talk about what went wrong.

In early 2012, when Joe was eighty-three, Carol began to recognize signs of dementia. The loss of her mother to Lewy body dementia likely heightened her awareness. Joe was much less verbal, would stare into space at times, and had personality changes. These changes evolved into periods of confusion and trouble doing everyday activities, like opening a package. His love of relaying humorous memories and anecdotes had given way to trouble speaking (aphasia) and complaints about health issues, often with agitation and frustration. He also experienced physical changes, such as difficulty with walking and balance while carrying his surfboard, and swimming freestyle with his head completely underwater, uncharacteristic of a former elite swimmer.

In April 2012, a friend alerted Carol to Steve Newport's story of improvement in his Alzheimer's symptoms while taking coconut and MCT oil. After the testing was completed and the worrisome diagnoses came in, Carol began to attend caregiver classes and workshops and decided to give Joe coconut and MCT oil in smoothies. Carol noticed obvious and dramatic improvement with each increase in the amount of coconut and MCT oil, eventually three servings per day after eight months. Joe became more verbal in the morning, and his comprehension, memory, alertness, word recall, and personality improved. Friends, neighbors, and the medical professionals who saw him regularly also noticed these changes. For Carol, the best gift of all was when his sense of humor returned. His long- and short-term memory improved dramatically after Carol added ketone salts to Joe's regimen in 2016, and he experienced another significant bump-up about three months after adding ketone ester in 2018. Considering her family history, Carol began to use coconut oil and MCT oil herself and added ketone salts to her own daily plan. Despite using coconut oil for years, Carol has experienced a dramatic improvement in her cholesterol and triglyceride levels.

Joe has done remarkably well over ten years with ketone therapy. At ninety-three, Joe deals with other health issues, but his vocabulary and conversations remain complex, and he is focused and engaged. Joe gives Carol sound advice and is quick to come up with creative solutions. Joe reads the paper and magazines and jots down notes in the margins so they can discuss politics, weather, anthropology, astronomy, and observations on everyday life, as they have for more than fifty years.

Carol and Joe both eat a Mediterranean-type low-glycemic-index diet, aiming for mild ketosis. Joe starts his day with a serving of ketone salts and MCT oil powder in water and has another half-serving in the afternoon. He also takes 10 grams of betahydroxybutyrate as ketone ester in the late morning. Carol begins her day with coconut oil and MCT oil powders added to her coffee and sometimes repeats this later in the day. She also has a half-serving of ketone salts in the morning. They eat their main meal in the early to mid-afternoon, including fish or seafood several times per week, like grilled salmon or their favorite clam chowder with canned salmon and coconut oil. Carol prepares thick stews with vegetables and legumes, like black beans, cannellini, and chickpeas, bone broth, often with fish, poultry, or meat (see Carol's Quick Minestra in the recipe section). They eat nuts, whole-grain bread, and a variety of vegetables and fruit every day. Other proteins include cheeses and lots of eggs in frittatas, a great way to use leftovers. Their meals include healthy fats like coconut oil, MCT oil, olive oil, coconut milk, and butter. They feel more satiated when coconut oil is added to stews and soups.

Joe looked out for Carol when she was young, and now she looks out for him. Carol considers herself to be a citizen scientist and activist. She has turned her personal challenges into advocacy, working hard to let others know about ketones as an alternative fuel for the brain and their anti-inflammatory properties to help them and their loved ones. She is relentless in sharing this information with neurologists and prominent Alzheimer's researchers, many of whom are resistant to the idea. Carol is grateful to those who meet her persistence with an open mind.

Joe bemoans the physical decline and ailments that come with advanced age, but remains a confident person with a positive attitude and enthusiasm for life that keep him going. In keeping with his wry humor and begrudging acceptance of ketone supplements, as he watches Carol measure out the ketone ester, Joe says, "Oh, are we going to CVS [the drug store] for dinner?" (Prata 2021)

CLEARLY KETO: A WHOLE-FOOD MEDITERRANEAN-STYLE KETOGENIC DIET

Adopting a whole-food Mediterranean-style ketogenic diet will accomplish several important goals. Eating a variety of nutrient-rich whole foods builds healthy cells throughout the brain and body that resist aging. Reducing carbohydrates and increasing healthy fats could prevent or reverse insulin resistance and provide ketones to fill the brain-energy gap that widens as we age. Consistently eating this way could get you on the path toward healthy brain aging and Alzheimer's prevention.

WHY A WHOLE-FOOD MEDITERRANEAN-STYLE DIET?

The whole-food Mediterranean-style diet is the most studied and the most hopeful diet for slowing cognitive decline and the progression of Alzheimer's disease. This is a dietary pattern consumed by populations around the Mediterranean Sea, where clusters of people age better and live longer. The basic whole-food groups are not exclusive to that part of the world, and the diet can be easily adapted to foods in other cultures.

A search on PubMed.gov in 2021 yielded more than 8,000 results for "Mediterranean diet," with more than 550 hits for "Mediterranean diet" and "cognition." Population studies report better outcomes for high compliance to the diet for cognitive performance, dementia risk, slowing dementia progress, and dementia-related death. Prospective randomized-controlled multiple-intervention trials have reported greater benefits of the Mediterranean diet for cognitive performance and other health parameters than for other diets, such as the low-fat American Heart Association diet (Aridi 2020; Chin-Yee 2018; Marcos-Pardo 2020; Neth 2020; Salas-Salvadó 2019; Scarmeas 2007; Van den Brink 2019; and many more).

The Institute for Health Metrics and Evaluation (IHME) is an independent global health-research center at the University of Washington and has created a data catalog of world population health called the Global Health Data Exchange. The data supplies a vast resource for information on risk factors for death and disease globally and in individual countries. In the IHME reports and graphs, the value assigned to each "risk factor" indicates the number of deaths that could have been prevented if that risk factor had been eliminated, for example, by diagnosing and controlling high blood pressure.

The IHME published a graph (figure 4.1) showing that of 56 million deaths in 2017, high blood pressure was the single greatest risk factor for premature death. A diet high in sugar was third and obesity fifth on the list of risk factors. The factors related to diet and nutrition add up to more than 28 million deaths, half of the total deaths, and almost triple the number of deaths from high blood pressure. Diets low in specific foods like whole grains, fruits, nuts and seeds, vegetables, seafood omega-3 fatty acids, fiber, and legumes each account for between half a million and three million premature deaths. These data provide tremendous support for eating a whole-food Mediterranean-style diet, since these food groups are all key components of the diet. This style of eating is highly adaptable to many different lifestyles and cultures.

The Mediterranean diet is not a low-fat diet, but instead emphasizes healthy fats. Of note, high intakes of fat or saturated fat do not appear on the IHME list of risk factors for premature death (figure 4.1). A high intake of red meat is near the bottom of the list, supporting moderation but not necessarily elimination of red meats. These data should allay fears of adding more healthy fat to the diet. We will discuss a few more reasons not to fear healthy fats later in this chapter and in chapter 5 on other ketogenic strategies, which include MCT oil, coconut oil, and more. Chapter 6 will focus on a few other supplements that make sense, and chapter 7 will help you put your plan together. We will discuss many other modifiable risk factors for premature death and cognitive decline in chapters 8 and 9.

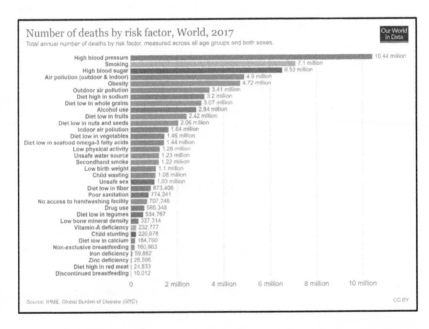

FIGURE 4.1. Number of Deaths by Risk Factor, World, 2017. Nearly 56 million people died in 2017. The data shown in the graph represent the number of lives that could be saved if the risk factor leading to the cause of death is eliminated. According to data collected by IHME, high blood pressure is the highest risk factor for preventable premature death. Factors related to diet and nutrition add up to more than 28 million deaths. High intakes of fat or saturated fat do not appear on the list, and a diet high in red meat is near the bottom. Source: Our World in Data: "Number of deaths by risk factor, World, 2017."

The IHME data have been corroborated by results of the long-term PURE (Prospective Urban Rural Epidemiology) study conducted in eighteen countries on five continents worldwide with more than 135,335 participants, which reported that sugar, but not fat or saturated fat, increased the risk of premature death. It also reported that fat and saturated fat did not increase the risk of serious cardiac events or deaths, and a higher intake of saturated fat lowered risk of stroke (Dehghan 2017).

The PURE Study is ongoing, and new reports are published periodically. In one such study, eating larger amounts of vegetables, especially raw vegetables, legumes, and fruits, was associated with reduced risk of serious cardiac events and premature death from cardiac disease and all causes (Miller 2017). Two other PURE studies reported that high intakes of refined grains and high-glycemic-index foods were associated with higher risks of premature death and serious cardiovascular diseases (Swaminathan 2020; Jenkins 2021). High-glycemic-index foods raise blood sugar rapidly to higher levels than low-glycemic-index foods. The PURE Study results clearly make the case for a Mediterranean-style diet and support a higher intake of healthy and even saturated fats, which are an important component of a ketogenic diet.

WHY WHOLE FOODS?

Eating a variety of whole foods in a Mediterranean-style diet will supply you with the macronutrients—protein, fat, and carbohydrates—as well as a wide array of the natural forms of essential micronutrients, such as vitamins and minerals, fiber, choline, and phytonutrients. Our metabolism recognizes these natural forms and processes them normally, in contrast to some synthetic forms found in fortified processed foods and supplements, which might not be digested the same or have the same metabolic fate.

Phytonutrients are chemical compounds found in plants that play a biological role in plant growth and protection of the plant from microbes and insects. There are more than one hundred thousand different phytonutrients, including pigments, polyphenols, flavonoids, antioxidants, some of which may support our metabolism. For example, unrefined cold-pressed virgin coconut oil contains many phenolic compounds, like the popular quercetin, that have anti-inflammatory and antioxidant effects. Other phenolic compounds may slow down the formation of abnormal plaques in the brain (Chatterjee 2020).

We can consume recommended intakes of the essential nutrients by choosing from each of the basic food groups, including a variety of types and colors of vegetables and fruits, eggs, meats, fish and other seafood, poultry, whole-fat dairy or goat milk, nuts, seeds, legumes, and healthy fats and oils. Herbs and spices not only add flavor and variety to meals, but many contain antioxidants and other beneficial phytonutrients. Sea salt can provide important trace elements that are removed when salt is refined, though product labels do not specify which trace elements are provided, and many brands lack important iodine (look for iodized sea salt).

A whole-food diet focuses on eating combinations of whole foods that have been mostly untouched, except perhaps to remove shells or debris, clean, and package the food. Look at the nutrition label, and avoid those with added sugar or preservatives and other chemicals you do not recognize. Whole-fat plain yogurt, for example, is technically processed, but the ingredients label may show only whole milk, cream, and active cultures, and, therefore, would be a good whole-food option.

Natural oils and fats like extra-virgin olive oil, virgin coconut oil, and butter are single-ingredient whole foods that are minimally processed for packaging purposes. Olive oil is pressed out of the olive, or coconut oil out of the coconut meat, at low heat (called cold-pressed or expeller-pressed), and debris is filtered out before packaging. Heavy cream from milk is agitated to separate the water content from the oil, then strained, leaving a clump of butter . . . simple, clean ingredients. Food manufacturers and food delivery services targeting the whole-food market are coming up with convenient and tasty combinations of whole foods: for example, a mixture of whole grain organic brown rice, red rice, and kale, cooked and ready to reheat.

While trying to feed an ever-expanding world population, foods can travel thousands of miles, and many compromises are made to reduce the need for refrigeration and extend shelf life. Taste and price are big factors in the competition for markets, so adding colors and flavors, salt, sugar, preservatives, and other ingredients to improve texture and visual appearance are common, along with processes to reduce cost of production, storage, and transportation.

Essential micronutrients are generally missing from overly processed foods. In the process of processing (pun intended), whole foods may be separated into components that are used to make processed and ultra-processed foods, often removing valuable nutrients such as vitamins, minerals, and fiber. A simple example is orange juice, which is extracted from the whole orange after cleaning, filtered to remove the pulp, and pasteurized (heated to 190° to 200°F) to kill microorganisms and inactivate enzymes that cause fermentation and degrade the juice. Then the juice may be bottled with added sugar, a flavor pack, and some synthetic vitamins and minerals to replace the natural flavor and aroma and micronutrients that were removed. Eating an orange provides better nutrition than drinking processed orange juice.

A large eight-year study of more than 22,000 people in Italy reported that the health benefits of the Mediterranean-style diet were largely erased by a diet that was also high in ultra-processed food (Bonaccio 2021).

REFINED VERSUS WHOLE GRAINS

Refined flour came along around 1870 in the United States as an idea to improve the color and texture of breads and other foods made with flour. The flour is milled to mechanically remove the outer bran layer, which contains B vitamins, minerals, and fiber, and the germ of the grain, which contains B vitamins, vitamin E, phytonutrients, and healthy fats (see figure 4.2). Grinding or sifting the grain to remove the bran and germ leaves only the starchy middle layer, which contains much less protein and vitamins than the whole grain. Thereafter, the refined middle layer is usually subjected to mixing, bleaching, and brominating.

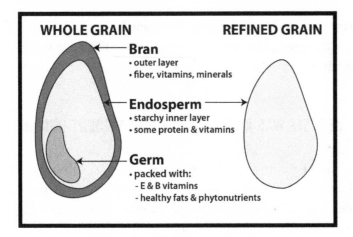

FIGURE 4.2. Whole versus refined grain.

As popularity increased, by the mid-twentieth century it was obvious that refining grains could cause serious nutrient deficiencies. This led to the public health practice of "fortifying" flours, usually with synthetic rather than the natural forms of the missing nutrients. In Asia, refining rice led to numerous cases of beriberi, a life-threatening condition caused by thiamin deficiency, until fortification of the rice with thiamin began in the 1980s. Humans were content to eat gray whole-grain breads and cereals until it occurred to someone that refined white grains might be more appealing to the eye. Rather than fortifying refined grains, encouraging people to eat whole grains would be a better public-health initiative.

WHY A REASONABLE KETOGENIC DIET?

Glucose, ketones, and fatty acids are the key fuels that drive our metabolism, an extraordinarily complex but organized intertwining of chemical reactions that are necessary to maintain life. Insulin resistance and abnormal use of glucose as fuel by the brain precede and are fundamentally connected to the other pathologies that occur in Alzheimer's and certain other neurological diseases. A ketogenic diet could help prevent or bypass the problem of poor glucose uptake by the brain and brain cells. A ketogenic lifestyle is not new, but was likely the norm for our human ancestors.

KETOSIS WAS A WAY OF LIFE FOR ANCIENT HUMANS

Since the beginning of life on earth some 3.5 billion years ago, the ketone betahydroxybutyrate (BHB) has provided fuel for the simplest one-celled organisms and many other creatures large and small, including humans. Throughout several million years of human evolution, living in a state of ketosis (elevated levels of ketones in the blood) was the natural way of life for humans, who were hunter-gatherers.

We know from studies of aboriginal peoples living today that hunter-gatherers lived along vital sources of water—creeks, lakes, rivers, and oceans—which also provided food as fish, shellfish, and other edible creatures. There were no plowed fields and orchards until 10,000 to 12,000 years ago, and domestication of animals for their meat and milk only occurred 4,000 to 9,000 years ago. Generally, humans walked miles every day, the men hunting for meat, fowl, and fish, while the women foraged for enough vegetables, nuts, tubers, grains, seasonal fruits, and sometimes insects. Their carbohydrates were whole foods with plenty of fiber, and they used animal fats to cook.

Our ancient ancestors endured periods of feast and famine, sometimes lasting days to weeks. Storing perishable food was difficult before electric refrigeration, a twentieth-century invention. Dehydration and curing techniques were used to preserve certain foods or meats, and fish might be buried in snow in colder climates. Our ancestors did not have access to large, genetically modified vegetables and fruits, much less refined grains and sugars that are prominent dietary staples of the last century. So, eating three square meals per day and raiding the refrigerator or pantry at night were simply not options.

Our ancestors suffered high mortality rates in infants, children, and women in childbirth, largely fueled by inadequate food supplies, tainted drinking water, infections, and a lack of antibiotics and vaccines to treat and prevent infections. Until the last century, the average life expectancy was about half what we enjoy today, though many earlier people lived into their seventies or beyond if they could avoid fatal infection or starvation. Those who lived longer rarely suffered from the modern-day maladies of obesity, diabetes, and dementia.

KETOGENIC DIETS FOR MODERN HUMANS

By now, you know that a low-carbohydrate high-fat diet will lead to production of ketones, an alternative fuel to glucose that the brain can use efficiently, even in areas of the Alzheimer's brain where glucose is not taken up normally due to insulin resistance and other factors. Consuming a ketogenic diet could fill in the brain-energy gap that worsens with normal aging but accelerates in mild cognitive impairment and Alzheimer's disease.

There is a wide spectrum of ketogenic diets with blood-ketone levels ranging tenfold from mild to deep ketosis (see figure 4.3). Higher ketone levels occur in direct proportion to the percent of fat in the diet relative to protein and carbohydrates. The strictest versions of the ketogenic diet are possible and can be palatable, but may be difficult for most people as a long-term strategy. A very strict ketogenic diet may be necessary to control seizures or slow cancer growth. However, studies aiming for mild nutritional ketosis report significant improvement for people with diabetes, mild cognitive impairment, and Alzheimer's. The Clearly Keto plan aims for ketone levels in the mild to moderate range (ketone levels about 0.5 to 2.0 mm/L).

Ketones are a powerful, effective, and efficient fuel, with life-extending properties, but most of us do not take full advantage of the many benefits that a state of ketosis could provide. Ketone research has exploded in the past ten years and has provided many good reasons to spend at least some of our time in ketosis. Studies detailed throughout the book report that nutritional ketosis could potentially:

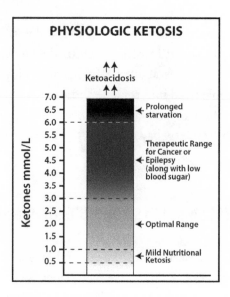

FIGURE 4.3. Physiologic ketosis: The spectrum of the ketogenic diet. Mild nutritional ketosis begins at about 0.5 mm/L, but levels can reach ten times higher on strict, very-high-fat very-low-carbohydrate classic ketogenic diets used to control seizures in drug-resistant epilepsy and as an adjunct to cancer treatment.

- Provide ketones as alternative fuel for the brain and other organs (except the liver)
- Increase your energy level
- Improve your behavior, sleep, and mood while reducing anxiety and depression
- Slow brain aging and atrophy by promoting formation of new brain cells and the connections between brain cells
- Enhance your cognitive performance, including mental focus, concentration, ability to carry out daily activities, more skillful use of language, learning, and memory
- Enhance your physical performance by preserving muscle mass which in turn improves strength and coordination
- Slow aging by removing damaged cells, promoting growth of new cells, and repairing DNA

- Protect your brain and other cells from damage by free radicals/reactive oxygen species
- Reduce effects of inflammation on the brain and other tissues, such as in walls of arteries and joints, potentially reducing aches and pain
- Lower resting heart rate and blood pressure
- Help you lose body fat by decreasing appetite and increasing use of fat as fuel
- Help you overcome obesity, insulin resistance, prediabetes, diabetes type 2, and the long-term complications of these conditions
- Prevent, improve symptoms, or slow or reverse progression of Alzheimer's, Parkinson's, and other neurodegenerative diseases
- Slow growth of cancer cells and enhance effectiveness of standard-of-care treatments.

The idea of using a ketogenic diet to treat neurological diseases is steadily gaining momentum, with reviews (Rusek 2019; Taylor 2019) and results of clinical trials of the ketogenic diet appearing in the scientific literature for Alzheimer's (Taylor 2017; Neth 2020; Phillips 2021), Parkinson's (VanItallie 2008; Phillips 2018), and autism (Li 2021; Varesio 2021). At present, there are dozens of clinical trials in progress or beginning soon for ketogenic diet and ketone supplements for a variety of neurological and other conditions.

Clearly, adopting a reasonable diet and lifestyle that results in mild ketosis in combination with a whole-food Mediterranean-style diet could provide a foundation for healthy brain-aging and Alzheimer's prevention.

A Mediterranean-Style Keto Diet Improves Cognition, Brain Blood Flow, and Energy Uptake in the Brain from Ketones

Twenty people with subjective memory complaints or mild cognitive impairment (MCI) consumed either a modified Mediterranean-ketogenic diet (5 percent to 10 percent carbohydrate, 60 percent to 65 percent fat, and 30 percent protein) or an American Heart Association (AHA) Diet (55 percent to 65 percent carbohydrate, 15 percent to 20 percent fat, and 20 percent to 30 percent protein) for six weeks. They resumed their usual diet for six weeks, then switched to the other diet for six more weeks. While on the Mediterranean Keto diet, everyone had elevated ketone levels and significantly improved HbA1c, fasting glucose, fasting insulin, triglycerides, and very-low-density lipoprotein (VLDL) cholesterol. There was a trend toward higher HDL cholesterol ("good cholesterol"), and total cholesterol was unchanged. For people on the Mediterranean Keto diet, brain blood flow and uptake of ketone bodies increased. Cerebrospinal fluid Aβ42 increased (usually decreased in Alzheimer's) and tau protein decreased (usually increased in Alzheimer's). The AHA diet did not increase brain blood flow, ketone uptake, or blood ketone levels, or change fasting glucose, fasting insulin, HbA1c, total cholesterol, VLDL cholesterol, or triglyceride levels, and HDL cholesterol levels were lower. Memory performance improved after both diets. (Neth 2020).

100 Years of the Classic Ketogenic Diet

Fasting was used for at least two millennia to stop seizures. Then, in 1921, Dr. Russel Wilder reported that a very-high-fat, very-low-carbohydrate diet could increase ketones, as in starvation, and stop or reduce the frequency of seizures. Interest in the "classic ketogenic diet" waned after effective anti-seizure medications came along, but Johns Hopkins University and a few other centers still used it in the most drug-resistant cases. Awareness of the diet has steadily increased since the early 1990s due to the advocacy of Jim Abrahams, whose one-year-old son Charlie responded dramatically to the diet. Jim founded The Charlie Foundation (https://charliefoundation.org), which has helped train dietitians and other clinicians at hundreds of ketogenic diet centers around the world. Use of the classic ketogenic diet and modifications of the diet have expanded to provide nutritional support for people with cancer (to slow down tumor growth), autism, rare metabolic disorders, diabetes, migraines, and certain neurological, psychiatric, and neurodegenerative disease.

THE MACRONUTRIENTS

There are long-held misconceptions that the ketogenic diet is an "unpalatable" diet, lacking flavor and variety, and is all about eating unlimited bacon and beef. Nothing could be further from the truth. With knowledge and careful planning, the ketogenic diet can embrace an endless variety of foods and flavors. The key to ketosis is how you combine the foods.

PROTEINS IN THE CLEARLY KETO DIET

A healthy diet will include protein equaling at least 0.5 gm/lb (1.1 gm/kg) of body weight, representing about 10 to 15 percent of total calories. For an average-size person of 150 pounds (68 kg), this equates to 75 grams of protein per day. Physically active people, especially bodybuilders and elite athletes, could easily consume up to double that amount of protein to build and maintain muscle mass. Unlimited protein could thwart ketosis since amino acids in excess protein can be converted to glucose.

One controversy in "keto world" is whether the grams of protein consumed per day should be based on current weight or ideal weight. I lean toward using current weight, because more muscle and other lean body mass is needed to support extra body weight (Bouxsein 2005). For someone weighing 200 pounds instead of 150 pounds, this would add only ⅓ more protein from the baseline amount. Eating 75 grams of protein can easily be reached with five ounces of salmon or poultry, one cup of cottage cheese, two ounces of nuts, and some vegetables. Look for charts on dairy and eggs (table 4.7), fish and seafood (table 4.8), poultry and meats (table 4.9), and legumes (table 4.3) for the macronutrient breakdown of many higher-protein foods. Proteins are also listed on charts for the other food groups.

PROTEIN AND MUSCLE MASS

Muscle mass and function tend to gradually decline as we age and can become quite severe, called age-related sarcopenia. That is why, compared to physically active counterparts with more muscle mass, frail elderly people walk more slowly and have more difficulty climbing steps, getting up from a chair, and lifting a heavy bag of groceries. Muscle fibers are gradually replaced by fat as muscle mass is lost, and weakness can become problematic. Therefore, eating adequate protein is important to build and maintain as much muscle mass as possible. Exercise can also help slow down loss of muscle with aging (Chambers 2020), allowing us to maintain strength and functionality (see figure 4.4). We will discuss more on this in chapter 8.

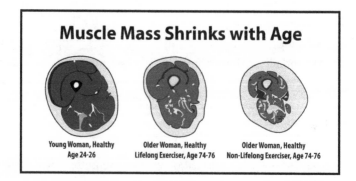

FIGURE 4.4. Muscle mass shrinks as we age, especially in people who do not exercise routinely. The muscle becomes surrounded and infiltrated by fat tissue. Drawing by Joanna Newport based on MRI photo in Chambers 2020.

A ketogenic diet with adequate protein can help maintain muscle mass. For example, when someone tries to lose a large amount of weight by reducing calories with a high-carbohydrate low-fat diet, glucose is the predominant fuel. Due to the deficit in total calories, in glucose-burning mode muscle breakdown may occur to provide amino acids that can be converted to glucose. In a ketogenic diet, fat is the main source of fuel, with less need to break down muscle.

People who do not eat enough protein and eat a high-carb weight-loss diet will lose fat but may also lose important muscle, which is a major factor in the basal metabolic rate. Basal metabolic rate (BMR) is the number of calories burned per unit of time to maintain vital bodily functions while at complete rest. The BMR can be measured in a lab with special equipment, but you can get a rough estimate of your BMR at BMR Calculator (https://bmi-calories.com/bmr-calculator.html). With less muscle to burn calories, the BMR will become lower and, therefore, the number of calories to maintain the new lower weight will also decrease. For example, a 200-pound (90-kg) seventy-year-old female with a BMR of 1,480 calories/day loses 60 pounds and wants to maintain her body weight at 140 pounds. The BMR is now down to 1,230 calories per day. If she returns to her pre-weight-loss daily intake of food, she will either need to increase her level of activity by 250 calories per day, such as adding a 45-minute walk to her daily regimen, or expect to regain one pound (0.45 kg) about every fourteen days.

Loss of muscle mass and lower BMR at least partly explain the phenomenon of "yo-yo" dieting (to which I am no stranger). Also, it takes more calories per day to maintain bodily functions with a higher body weight, as well as larger muscle and other lean body mass to support the extra weight on the skeleton (Bouxsein 2005). During weight loss, to avoid a plateau, the total calories consumed per day will need to be adjusted downward and/or activity increased incrementally to adjust to the lower BMR. A ketogenic diet with adequate protein can help maintain muscle mass, especially when combined with weight or resistance training, even during weight loss (Jabekk 2010). Medium-chain triglycerides and exogenous ketone supplements can temporarily cause a metabolic switch from glucose to ketones and may also help to conserve muscle mass, so long as there is adequate protein in the diet.

OILS AND FATS IN THE CLEARLY KETO DIET

In the Clearly Keto diet, you will aim for at least 60 percent of your total daily calories as fat to support ketosis and fight insulin resistance. Virtually all diets are composed of fat, protein, and carbohydrate. How you tweak the ratios of fat, protein, and carbohydrate will determine whether you are eating a ketogenic diet; a high-carb, low-fat diet; or somewhere in between (see figure 4.5). There are two good reasons why fat is an important part of the Clearly Keto diet. It is difficult to get into mild sustained ketosis unless the

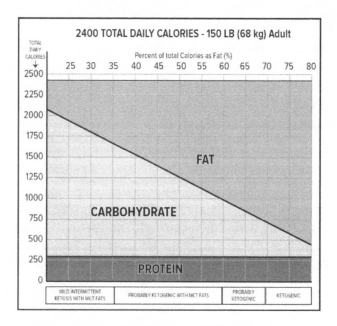

FIGURE 4.5. Ketosis and macronutrients as percent of total calories. At 2,400 calories per day, while keeping protein at about 12.5 percent, increasing fat beyond 60 percent and reducing carbohydrates to not more than 27.5 percent of calories may support ketosis. Including some MCT oil in the diet may allow for a lower percent of fat to get into and sustain ketosis.

percent of fat in the diet is at least 60 to 65 percent and the combined intake of protein and carbohydrate is no more than 35 percent of calories. While keeping protein at about 10 to 15 percent of calories, the higher the percent of fat you aim for while tweaking down the carbohydrates, the deeper into ketosis you will go. Adding ketogenic oils like MCT oil and coconut oil can make getting into ketosis easier (see more on these oils in chapter 5).

The second reason that fat is so important in the Clearly Keto diet is that eating more fat calories than carbohydrate and protein calories combined can help prevent or overcome insulin resistance, as discussed in chapter 3.

EATING HEALTHY FATS AND OILS NEED NOT BE SO SCARY

The Mediterranean-style diet has never been a low-fat diet, but rather emphasizes eating healthy fats as a mainstay of the diet, with olive oil as the centerpiece. The centenarians in the Mediterranean regions did not get so old by eating fat-free and low-fat dairy and leaving the olives on the vine. In many European countries, traditional eating centered on olives and olive oil, as well as milk from cows and goats, butter, cheeses, cream, and yogurt.

Eating a diet that is low-fat, low-saturated fat, with low-fat dairy, and lean meats is a modern-day twist that began to appear in dietary guidelines in the early 1960s. This has not changed sixty years later. In a recent advisory on dietary cholesterol, the American Heart Association promoted a hybrid low-fat Mediterranean diet emphasizing polyunsaturated fat and without mention of olive oil (Carson, 2020). This may be a "plant-based" diet, but it is not a true Mediterranean diet. A big unanswered question that deserves more study is how much polyunsaturated fat is too much (more on this in chapter 9).

To further illustrate these points, in population studies of fat consumption in the United States and European countries completed in the 1950s (discussed in chapter 9), France had the lowest death rate from heart disease despite the highest fat and saturated-fat intake, eating a lot of butter, full-fat cheeses, yogurts, and other animal fats. This "French paradox" did not support the proposed "lipid-heart hypothesis," and the data from France were excluded from the results. In addition, many households in the United States and Europe were using substantial amounts of the new, cheap high-trans-fat shortenings and margarines, which were later found to be harmful, in place of animal fats in their cooking. The consumption of dietary trans fat was not factored into the data due to a lack of awareness of the potential harm and inability to analyze fatty acid composition, both of which may have muddied up the results.

Nevertheless, based on the flawed 1950s studies, in 1961 the American Heart Association began to discourage us from eating saturated fat and later promoted limiting fat overall, launching an onslaught of "reduced-fat," high-carbohydrate foods in the United States and other markets in the 1980s and beyond. The AHA encouraged us to eat trans fat margarines and shortenings (the real "artery-clogging fat"). The AHA has continued to rely on these same old flawed studies as "core studies" in its current advice on dietary fats and cholesterol (Sacks 2017; Carson 2020). The AHA has also spent decades demonizing coconut oil, even though its consumption was virtually nil in the United States and Europe throughout the twentieth century when rates of heart attacks and deaths from heart attacks skyrocketed (see figure 4.6).

As the twentieth century unfolded, lard, beef tallow, chicken fat, and butter were substantially replaced in the U.S. diet with shortenings and margarines high in trans fats. Soybean oil, which is high in polyunsaturated fatty acids, has become the dominant edible oil in the U.S. diet, climbing from about two pounds (about 1 kg) per person per year in 1950 to about 26 pounds (12 kg) per person per year by 2000. Soybean oil stands at 67 percent of total edible oil consumption in the U.S. in 2020 (per USDA data), while coconut oil at 3 percent and olive oil at 2 percent are barely blips on the radar. Deep-frying potatoes and other foods also became common practices as fast-food restaurants popped up in the United States and then globally.

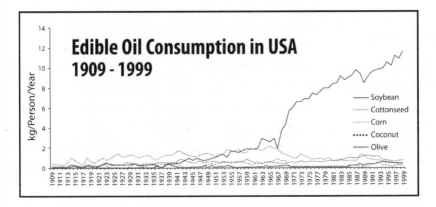

FIGURE 4.6. U.S. consumption of soybean, coconut, and palm oils, 1965 to 2011. Source: Chart prepared by Dr. Fabian Dayrit using data from USDA ERS https://www.ers.usda.gov/.

It is a common practice for restaurants to keep the same batch of oil hot for hours on end and reuse the oil repeatedly for days, which can produce numerous toxic lipids that our metabolism and cell membranes might not know how to handle.

In 2002, the USDA began to require food manufacturers and restaurants to disclose trans fat content of >0.5 grams per serving on nutrient labels. For some products, serving sizes were adjusted accordingly. More importantly, a huge shift occurred in the types of fats and oils used in processed and fast foods. Trans fats were phased out and finally banned from foods in the United States in 2018, based on evidence that trans fats were responsible for more than 30,000 annual cardiac deaths in the country. In the process, much of the fats used in restaurants and manufactured foods has been replaced with palm oil or new hydrogenated fats with most of the trans fat removed. Time will tell if these new processed oils affect our health.

Could the major changes in the types of fat we ate over the past sixty years explain the abnormalities in lipid metabolism that occur in Alzheimer's, Parkinson's, and other brain diseases? The story is still unfolding, but it is reasonable to think this diversion from our evolutionary diet, along with a massive increase in sugar and high-fructose corn syrup consumption and synthetic additives in our diet, could play a role.

Eating a low-fat diet leads to eating much more sugar to make up the difference in the total calories a person needs to maintain weight, or for an infant or child to grow and develop. As discussed in chapters 2 and 3, eating too much sugar is a setup for obesity, insulin resistance (prediabetes and diabetes), inflammation, many chronic diseases related to excessive sugar consumption, and dementia, which have become epidemic since these low-fat dietary guidelines first appeared.

For people who hesitate to flout the AHA and DGA low-fat guidelines, chapter 5 considers why fat, and especially saturated fat, does not deserve such a bad reputation. The problem with animal fat may have more to do with what is stored in the fat—fertilizers, pesticides, hormones, antibiotics, other toxins—than the fat itself, and can be largely avoided by choosing meat, milk, milk products, and eggs from pasture-raised animals raised without exposure to these harmful substances. We will discuss specifics of healthy fats and oils under the food groups of the Mediterranean-style diet.

CARBOHYDRATES IN THE CLEARLY KETO DIET

It is not unusual for Americans to eat 400 or more grams of carbohydrate per day, and sometimes double that much. For many years, the American Diabetes Association (ADA) espoused eating a low-fat diet with 65 percent of total calories as carbohydrate, which equates to 390 grams, or 1,560 calories as carbohydrate on a 2,400-calorie-per-day diet. It is no wonder that type 2 diabetics following these guidelines tend to need more medication over time and eventually require insulin. Since sugar is the problem, why not simply cut down on the sugar? As discussed in chapter 3, many diabetics have been able to go into remission and reduce, or even eliminate, their insulin and other diabetes medications by switching over to a low-carbohydrate, higher-fat diet.

In its Dietary Reference Intakes, the Institute of Medicine (IOM 2006) recommends a daily allowance of 130 grams of carbohydrates, which is certainly more reasonable than 390 grams for a diabetic or someone who hopes to prevent diabetes. Under the question "How many carbs should I eat?" the ADA's obscure answer is "As for the ideal number of carbs per meal, there's no magic number. How much carbohydrate each person needs is in large part determined by your body size and activity level" (ADA 2021). True, but not very helpful.

Let us consider the IOM recommendations of 130 grams carbohydrate and 0.8 grams protein per kg body weight, equal to 75 grams for an average 150-pound person. At about 4 calories per gram, this amount of protein and carbohydrate would provide 820 calories. This would allow 1,580 calories for fat which would provide 65.8 percent of calories in a 2,400-calorie diet. This is intriguing, since this is clearly not a low-fat diet and is in the ketogenic range. The IOM guidelines state elsewhere that "A Tolerable Upper Intake Limit (UL) was not set for total fat because of the lack of a defined level at which an adverse effect, such as obesity, can occur" (IOM). Perhaps the AHA, ADA, and USDA should heed that statement in their own guidelines.

A 2,400-calorie-per-day diet is probably too generous to maintain a healthy weight for most of us, especially older adults. The overall percent of fat will drop as the calories drop if you stick with 130 grams of carbohydrate and the recommended amount of protein. How much carbohydrate you eat will also have a big effect on how ketogenic your diet will be. There is no minimum amount of carbohydrate that is considered essential, since glucose can be manufactured in the body.

It is relatively easy to stay under 60 grams of total carbs with good planning. Elderly people and those who are accustomed to a very high carbohydrate intake might start with—and even stick to—130 grams of carbohydrate per day. If eating under 60 grams of carbohydrate is too difficult, a happy medium could be achieved between 60 and 130 grams per day by adding ketogenic MCT oil or coconut oil to meals and eating naturally ketogenic foods for snacks. I strongly advise people who are older and/or have other medical conditions to discuss planned dietary changes with their doctor before getting started.

With a doctor's approval and close monitoring of blood sugar, people with diabetes, prediabetes, or metabolic syndrome could start with 60 grams of carbohydrate per day and gradually work down to as low as

15 to 20 grams. Those who want to get a jump-start on losing weight or controlling blood sugar could just "rip the Band-Aid off" and start directly with 15 to 20 grams of carbs per day. People taking insulin or other diabetes medications should monitor blood sugar very closely and consult their doctors about adjusting or stopping medications. When glucose blood markers (fasting glucose, fasting insulin, and HbA1C) reach the normal range and/or weight-loss goals are achieved, a good strategy is to add back 5 grams of carbohydrate per day every couple of weeks. If the blood sugar sneaks back up or lost pounds are regained, then return to a lower amount of carbohydrates that will help you maintain your weight and blood sugar.

Generally, fish, seafood, meats, eggs, hard cheeses, poultry, and fats and oils used for cooking do not contain carbohydrates. Carbohydrates in the Clearly Keto diet will come from vegetables and fruits, milk, yogurt, soft cheeses, legumes, nuts, seeds, and whole grains. Look at tables for individual food groups to find the carbohydrate, fiber, fat, and protein gram counts.

Cups of vegetables allow more bulk for the same amount of carbohydrate as much smaller portions of legumes, nuts, seeds, and whole grains. Leafy greens and sprouts have less than 2 grams of carbohydrate and no protein in two cups. A cup of raw chopped broccoli contains 4 to 6 grams carbohydrate with just 2 grams of protein, while a tiny quarter cup of adzuki or black beans contains more than 30 grams of carbs but also provides 10 grams of protein. With careful planning, it is possible to stay under 60 grams of carbohydrates per day by making low-carb vegetable and fruit choices on days that you consume high-carb legumes.

Some fruits like apples, pears, and bananas are quite high in carbohydrate, at 28 grams for a medium fruit, so dividing the fruit into halves or quarters and sharing or freezing the rest will allow more room for carbs from other food groups. Low-sugar fruits like small servings of berries, an apricot, or a tomato are good choices.

You can "keto-up" carbohydrates by including foods that are high in fat with the meal or snack. Look for ideas in the Recipes section.

TOTAL CARBS OR NET CARBS?

One controversy in keto world is whether to count total carbs, or to subtract fiber and sugar alcohols from the total carb content to arrive at "net carbs." Fiber contains about two calories per gram, but is undigested and does not increase insulin or blood sugar. Fiber is important because it serves as food for the important bacteria in your gut (intestinal tract). The effects of the gut microbiome and gut inflammation on other organs, especially the brain, have become an intense focus of research. Providing adequate fiber can help maintain a healthier gut microbiome. Sugar alcohols (erythritol, sucralose, maltitol) do not have calories, but limited research suggests sugar alcohols could increase glucose and insulin levels.

If you choose to use net carbs in your calculations but do not achieve the desired results, consider counting total carbs.

SPEAKING OF SWEETENERS

Stevia is a natural intense sweetener brewed from the stevia plant, forming glycosides in the process which are not metabolized and provide no calories. Stevia may have a slightly bitter aftertaste when used in coffee or tea, but it works very well in many other foods. Monkfruit (Luo Han Guo) is a traditional natural sweetener used for centuries in China and other countries. An extract from monkfruit naturally contains some sucrose and fructose but also intensely sweet mogrosides, allowing small amounts to be used in food and drink without adding calories. Stevia and monkfruit are sometimes combined with erythritol. Powdered, granular, and liquid forms of natural sweeteners are available for different cooking applications or to add to coffee or tea. I use a few drops of stevia in my coffee but also in yogurt, ricotta, and "keto" pancakes, and I add monkfruit to my delicious nut and seed granola recipe (see Recipes section).

OTHER TIPS FOR SUCCESS WITH THE CLEARLY KETO PLAN

Drink Plenty of Fluids

At the start of a ketogenic diet, muscles tend to release water, explaining the large weight loss that many report. It is important to drink plenty of fluids to avoid dehydration. I recommend eight to ten 8-ounce (240 ml) glasses daily of water, tea, coffee, or other clear calorie-free fluids without added sugar.

Ketogenic Diet and Weight Loss

If you are happy with your weight, the ketogenic diet can be calibrated to help you maintain your weight. To lose weight, a ketogenic diet with adequate protein can be worked out with fewer calories. Adding exercise can speed the process up and help maintain muscle mass.

It is especially tough for people with type 2 diabetes and high insulin levels to lose weight if they continue to eat a high-carb diet, since a function of insulin is to put fat into storage as adipose tissue and keep it there. Mild to moderate ketosis tends to do the opposite, since ketones stimulate fat breakdown with release of fatty acids. A consistent ketogenic diet can help overcome insulin resistance by lowering glucose and insulin levels while increasing ketone levels, all of which will allow fat to burn more easily. Two more bonuses of eating a ketogenic diet for weight loss are reduced craving for sweets and appetite suppression.

Low versus High Glycemic Index

The glycemic index was originally developed by David J. A. Jenkins, D.M. and associates in 1981 (Jenkins 1981) to help diabetes patients make healthier food choices to avoid the marked increases in blood sugar levels that occur after eating certain types of carbohydrates. A calculation using the rise in blood-glucose levels over two hours after consumption and the area under the curve after eating many different foods were compared to glucose, which was assigned a value of 100. Foods less than 56 are considered low-glycemic, 56 to 70 are medium, and greater than 70 are high-glycemic-index foods.

Fortunately, the whole foods of the Clearly Keto Mediterranean-style diet naturally fall into the low to low-medium glycemic index ranges at the recommended serving sizes, including high-carb legumes and fruits. The fiber these foods contain likely plays an important role in blunting the glucose response.

What about GMO?

Genetically modified organism (GMO) foods began to appear in the 1970s and are quite prevalent now. GMO foods have had their genetic material altered through genetic engineering, not by natural selection. The engineering occurs in bacteria, yeast, and viruses that may be inserted into cells of the organism or transferred through tissue cultures. The impetus for GMO foods stems from trying to feed the growing population. Genetic engineering can enhance the size, color, and appearance of fruits and vegetables, provide greater nutritional value (though sometimes less), create crops that are resistant to herbicides, diseases, and pests, and have greater yields in much less space. A successful GMO food can significantly extend shelf life, allowing more time from harvest to the table.

GMO foods include many types of vegetables, fruits, grains, and other plant foods, and animals can also be GMO. More recently, plant proteins have been created in bacteria that are intended to have the look and taste of animal proteins, such as ground beef, as in the "Impossible Burger," which was launched in 2016. In the process of creating this "meat analogue," the inventors use yeast to produce a "heme" protein that gives meat its red color and is also found in legumes, and the product is made using a fermentation process. Meat analogs may be engineered to contain more protein and less fat than the meat they are mimicking. They take up much less space to create and contribute much less to greenhouse gases than raising animals. On the other hand, it is unlikely that an engineered meat substitute will contain the many other nutrients beyond protein that animal meat provides.

Wheat has been greatly modified over the years, and eating it substantially raises insulin levels, whether refined or whole-grain. According to Dr. William Davis in his book *Wheat Belly*, wheat contributes to accumulation of excessive fat around abdominal organs.

It is unclear whether GMO foods could be harmful; and whether to eat them is definitely controversial. For example, virtually no wheat or corn exists anymore in the United States that has not been genetically engineered. GMO labeling is inconsistent, and many companies label their produce as non-GMO to reach the market of people who worry about this. Local small farmers are less likely to grow GMO foods, explaining the growing popularity of farmer's markets. Hopefully, governments will require GMO labeling soon, at least from larger food manufacturers, so we can make informed choices.

What about Gluten-Free?

Another consideration is whether to eat a gluten-free diet. Eliminating gluten could reduce the amount of carbohydrate in the diet. More importantly, there appears to be a strong gut-brain connection, and there is some evidence that diets high in gluten may contribute to the development of insulin resistance and ultimately Alzheimer's or other neurologic diseases. In his book *Grain Brain*, David Perlmutter, MD, a Florida neurologist whose own neurosurgeon father suffered from Alzheimer's, discusses this in detail. Wheat is the most obvious source of gluten, but gluten turns up in many other grains and in unexpected places, such as additives, to provide a certain consistency to processed foods, such as cereals, ice cream, and condiments like mayonnaise and ketchup. Dr. Perlmutter joins a growing number of experts who agree that a diet higher in healthy fats and lower in carbohydrates is healthier than the alternative.

If gluten is contributing to brain fog or more serious symptoms, it may take just a few weeks of a gluten-free diet to feel the difference, according to Perlmutter. There are many whole grains available that are not wheat and have no gluten, including rice, rolled or steel-cut oats (if labeled gluten-free), corn, potato, buckwheat, tapioca, soy, quinoa, millet, chia, amaranth, arrowroot, sorghum, and teff. Gluten-free flours made from those grains, as well as coconut flour and flours made from almonds or other nuts, can be used to make breads, pancakes, and other tasty gluten-free, lower-carb foods. Look for ideas in the recipe section.

What about Alcohol?

Alcohol itself does not contribute to calories and is not considered a "macronutrient," but beer and wine, and liquids mixed with hard liquors, often contain sugar. Beer and wine manufacturers are not required to label nutrient content like other food and drink, but you may be able to get this information from the manufacturer.

Though wine is a traditional part of the Mediterranean diet in some locales, I do not encourage daily consumption of wine for a few reasons. Some proponents of the Mediterranean diet justify drinking a glass of red wine each day, because it contains resveratrol, a phenolic antioxidant substance found in the skins of grapes. Some studies suggest that drinking red wine may be "heart-healthy" due to its effect on cholesterol, though other studies do not confirm this. In a well-rounded Mediterranean diet, you can choose plenty of other foods that contain antioxidants, including grapes with the skin, and not worry about the effects of alcohol on the brain.

While some studies suggest that a small amount of alcohol intake may possibly be protective of the brain, excessive intake is clearly harmful. It increases brain inflammation and promotes brain shrinkage with loss of neurons. Excessive alcohol intake can lead to depression, episodes of hypoglycemia, and even seizures. Alcohol in small doses is a stimulant that can interfere with sleep, but at higher doses has a sedative effect which may increase risk of falling, which can be quite serious, especially as you get older. Alcohol can also interfere with absorption of important nutrients like the vitamin thiamin and temporarily upset the balance of neurotransmitters in the brain. People who are alcohol-dependent, especially over age sixty-five, are three to four times more likely to develop Alzheimer's (Zilkens 2014). Excess alcohol intake can also indirectly increase the risk of dementia by causing damage to the liver and kidneys, coronary artery disease, diabetes, high blood pressure, abnormal heart rhythms, and stroke (Kivimäki 2020). In addition to the alcohol, some beers and scotch contain nitrosamine compounds that may promote brain insulin resistance (de la Monte 2009). For more on excessive alcohol intake and nitrosamine compounds, see chapter 9.

Is this to say that you should not drink wine or beer at all? The answer may be yes if you have trouble controlling how much you drink, if you take certain prescription and over-the-counter medications, or if you have chronic medical conditions. I would add to that list people who have memory or other cognitive impairment, because having a glass of wine may not be worth the harm the alcohol could do and could contribute to greater confusion and brain fog. Not long after his Alzheimer's diagnosis, my husband Steve decided to forgo alcohol because he sensed greater confusion and memory impairment when he consumed it. Why add more trouble to a brain that is already compromised?

For otherwise healthy people, I suggest you not use the Mediterranean diet as an excuse to start drinking alcohol if you have not been. If you decide to include one serving of an alcoholic beverage occasionally, it probably will not harm you permanently. How much you drink is your personal choice. The National Institutes of Health/National Institute on Alcohol Abuse and Alcoholism (NIH/NIAAA) recommends intake of no more than one serving per day for women and men over age sixty-five, and no more than two servings for younger men. A serving is defined as 12 ounces of beer, 5 ounces of wine, or 1.5 ounces of distilled spirits.

In addition, some people on a ketogenic diet report feeling the effects of alcohol with smaller amounts. The ketogenic diet has a diuretic effect early on, and so does alcohol, especially beer. It is important to drink plenty of non-alcohol clear fluids while consuming a ketogenic diet for this reason. I have not included red-wine intake in the Clearly Keto plan for these and the many other reasons discussed above.

FOOD GROUPS OF THE WHOLE-FOOD MEDITERRANEAN-STYLE DIET

One of the many great things about eating a healthy whole-food Mediterranean-style diet is the wide range of foods to choose from. Foods that were not a regular part of your diet before could add new interest to your meals.

WHY ARE NUTS, SEEDS, LEGUMES, AND WHOLE GRAINS SO IMPORTANT?

For 2017, the IHME ranked low intakes of some foods among the highest risk factors leading to 56 million deaths worldwide, including legumes (>500,000 deaths), nuts and seeds (>2 million deaths), and whole grains (>3 million deaths) (see figure 4.1 at the beginning of this chapter). Nuts, seeds, legumes, and whole grains fit very well into a whole-food Mediterranean-style diet and are packed with a variety of vitamins, minerals, choline, fiber, and many phytonutrients.

Nuts and seeds are composed of fat, protein, and carbohydrates, and most types have more calories as fat than carbohydrate and protein combined, so they fit very well into a ketogenic diet and make great ketogenic snacks. The natural fats in plant and animal foods are various ratios of saturated (SFA), monounsaturated (MUFA), and polyunsaturated (PUFA) fatty acids, and nuts and seeds lean toward MUFAs and PUFAs. MUFAs are considered healthy fats in the Mediterranean-style diet.

I must mention cacao and cocoa powder, since chocolate is loved and contains its own special antioxidants and other phytonutrients. Cacao comes from crushing the unroasted cacao bean (which is really a seed). When the cacao bean is roasted and the fat pressed out of it, the remainder is cocoa powder. For some chocolates, the cocoa comes from fermented dried cacao beans.

The meat, milk, and water of the coconut are not parts of a nut, but come from the seed at the center of the coconut fruit. Coconut is currently included in the list of tree nuts that may cause an allergic reaction. The designation of coconut as a tree nut is required on packaging, but the coconut is not a "tree nut." Like nearly every other food, an occasional person may be allergic to coconut. Coconut milk, which contains much of the oil, is pressed from the meat. Grated coconut is high in oil, and most of the carbohydrate is fiber.

Look for Mary's Nut and Seed Granola (with grated coconut) in the recipe section for an enjoyable way to get many vitamins, minerals, fibers, and phytonutrients packed into a great snack or grain-free "cereal." See tables 4.1 and 4.2 for a breakdown of the macronutrient and fiber content of nuts and seeds.

NUTS - Naturally Ketogenic

1 OUNCE (28 gm)	FAT (gm)	PROTEIN (gm)	CARB (gm)	FIBER (gm)
Almond	14	6.0	6.0	3.5
Brazil	19	3.3	3.3	2.1
Cashew	13	4.3	9.3	0.8
Macademia	21.5	2.2	3.9	2.4
Pecan	20.4	2.6	4.0	2.7
Pistachio	12.8	5.7	7.7	3.0
Walnut	18.5	4.3	3.9	1.9

Note: Fiber is part of total carbohydrate (carb)
Source: USDA FoodData Central - https://fdc.nal.usda.gov/

TABLE 4.1. Nuts, macronutrient breakdown.

SEEDS - Naturally Ketogenic

1 OUNCE (28 gm)	FAT (gm)	PROTEIN (gm)	CARB (gm)	FIBER (gm)
Cacao/Cocoa	14	4.0	8.0	6.0
Chia	11.8	5.1	8.1	7.6
Coconut meat	10.0	1.0	4.5	2.6
Flax	11.8	5.1	8.1	7.6
Hemp	14.6	9.5	2.6	1.2
Pepitas/Pumpkin	14.0	9.0	5.0	3.0
Sesame	14.0	5.0	6.5	3.3
Sunflower	14.0	5.5	6.8	3.1

Note: Fiber is part of total carbohydrate (carb)
Source: USDA FoodData Central - https://fdc.nal.usda.gov/

TABLE 4.2. Seeds, macronutrient breakdown.

Legumes include beans, lentils, soybeans, peanuts, and dried peas and are a great source of protein with some fat but tend to be heavy in carbohydrates. So legumes are not particularly "keto-friendly." Popular tofu is made from soybean curd, so would fit into the legume category. Kidney beans contain about 39 grams of carbohydrate for an average cup cooked, compared to 15 grams of protein and 13 grams of fat (from https://fdc.nal.usda.gov/). About ⅓ to ½ of the carbohydrate in legumes is fiber, which is fermented by gut bacteria and explains the gassiness many people experience after eating legumes. Except for peanuts, which are high in fat, legumes are more difficult to fit into a ketogenic diet in servings large enough to meet protein requirements for a vegan diet, though this is possible with good planning. Like nuts, the fats in legumes lean more toward MUFAs and PUFAs. See table 4.3 of legumes for the breakdown of macronutrient and fiber content.

Like legumes, whole grains are relatively low in fat and high in carbohydrate, with small to moderate amounts of protein, and are rich in vitamins, minerals, fiber, choline, and phytonutrients. Whole grains include foods like rice, wheat, maize, barley, oats,

LEGUMES - Not Keto Friendly
Eat small portions with oils & fats

1/4 CUP 50 gm	FAT (gm)	PROTEIN (gm)	CARB (gm)	FIBER (gm)
Adzuki beans	< 0.5	10.0	31.5	6.3
Black beans	0.7	10.8	31.2	7.7
Black-eyed peas	3.5	3.6	9.6	3.0
Chickpeas	4.5	4.1	12.7	3.5
Edamame	3.8	5.8	4.3	2.5
Kidney Beans	3.5	4.0	10.6	3.5
Lentils	3.4	4.2	9.3	7.3
Lima Beans	3.4	3.6	9.7	3.2
Mung Beans	3.4	3.2	8.9	3.5
Peanuts (1/3 cup)	25.0	12.2	10.6	4.2
Pinto beans	3.6	4.2	12.2	4.2
Soybeans	7.4	8.4	3.8	2.8
Split peas	< 0.5	4.1	11.0	4.1
Tofu	1.8	3.5	0.9	< 0.2

Note: Fiber is part of total carbohydrate (carb)
Source: USDA FoodData Central - https://fdc.nal.usda.gov/

TABLE 4.3. Legumes, macronutrient breakdown.

and quinoa that is typically cooked. Whole grains found in breads, crackers, pastas, and cereals provide more texture and color, as well as essential nutrients, compared to refined versions of these foods, which can be bland and relatively tasteless. Whole grains have little fat and small to moderate amounts of protein, and are heavy on carbohydrate, of which 10 percent or so is fiber. Like legumes, whole grains are not very "keto-friendly," but small portions can be worked into a ketogenic meal. Instead of putting a big dollop of white rice on your plate, consider eating whole-grain rice, and cut your usual portion in half. When you are used to that, cut the portion in half again. See table 4.4 of whole grains for the breakdown of macronutrient and fiber content.

WHOLE GRAINS - Not Keto Friendly
Eat small portions with oils & fats

COOKED WITH WATER	GM	CUPS	FAT (gm)	PROTEIN (gm)	CARB (gm)	FIBER (gm)
Amaranth	60	1/4	1.0	2.3	11.2	1.3
Barley groats	42	1/4	< 0.5	1.6	20.0	2.7
Buckwheat	42	1/4	< 0.5	2.4	14.2	1.9
Couscous	40	1/4	< 0.2	2.4	14.8	0.9
Maize as masa harina	60	1/4	< 0.5	1.4	12.8	1.0
Oats, steel cut	90	1/2	1.7	2.0	10.5	2.0
Quinoa	46	1/4	1.4	3.1	15.1	2.0
Rice, brown	50	1/4	< 0.3	0.7	6.4	0.4
Rice, wild	40	1/4	< 0.2	1.6	8.5	0.7
Rye grain	120	1/2	0.5	3.7	25.6	4.0
Whole wheat cereal	120	1/2	0.8	4.5	29.9	3.7
Whole wheat bread	1 slice	-	1.5	5.3	18.5	2.6

Note: Fiber is part of total carbohydrate (carb)
Source: USDA FoodData Central - https://fdc.nal.usda.gov/

TABLE 4.4. Whole grains, macronutrient breakdown.

There are many creative ways to change up old favorite recipes to replace pasta or pizza crust, such as slices of roasted eggplant in place of lasagna, spaghetti squash or spiralized zucchini to replace spaghetti, and riced cauliflower to substitute for rice. One innovative company uses chicken and mozzarella to make pizza crust and enchilada wraps, swapping out the refined grains for protein and fat. Konjac flour noodles and rice are incredibly low-calorie options with 3 grams of carbs, including 2 grams of fiber totaling 12 calories in 3 ounces, though they have a chewy and unique taste and texture.

It is worthwhile to eat one or two ounces of nuts and/or seeds routinely, perhaps as a snack or to "keto-up" a meal. I often have 1.5 ounces of nut and seed granola (see recipe section) with a small amount of coconut milk as a dessert or snack. You could also plan for a small serving of legumes or whole grains in a meal each day that contains enough oil or fat to offset the combination of protein and carbohydrates. Including these foods in your everyday diet could lead to healthier aging and lower your risk of premature death.

VEGETABLES AND FRUITS: WHY ARE A VARIETY OF TYPES AND COLORS OF VEGETABLES AND FRUITS IMPORTANT?

In its risk-factor analysis for premature death, IHME reported that (see figure 4.1 earlier in chapter) almost 4 million of the more than 56 million deaths globally were attributed to diets low in vegetables (1.46 million) and fruits (2.4 million). Eating a variety of types and colors of vegetables and fruits provides a vast array of essential vitamins, minerals, fiber, non-fiber carbohydrates, proteins, and substances that act as antioxidants, anti-inflammatory agents, as well as support for normal blood clotting and immunity. Some vegetables and fruits, like olives and avocados, contain fat as well. There is considerable overlap in the types of nutrients in vegetables and fruits, but there are also important differences. For example, the greens of turnips and beets have many different nutrients than the actual turnip and beet.

Vegetables come in much color and variety. To get a broad combination of nutrients, it is important to mix it up and eat leafy greens, other types of more solid green vegetables, brightly colored vegetables and fruits, and sulfur-rich vegetables. Sulfur is used metabolically to synthesize many proteins needed in various tissues and organs, such as in the hair, nails, and skin, and collagen in cartilage. Cartilage with collagen lines joints and supports the skin on your nose and ears, and collagen is an important component of tendons and ligaments that connect muscle to bone and bone to bone, respectively. Most vegetables, nuts, seeds, legumes, and animal foods contain sulfur, but certain vegetables are especially rich in sulfur, including asparagus, garlic, mushrooms, cabbage, leeks, shallots, scallions, and other onions.

Aim for at least two cups of leafy greens and a mixture of other types and colors of vegetables totaling at least one cup per day, preferably two or more cups if your "carbohydrate allowance" can accommodate them. The specific vegetables can vary from day to day. Fresh vegetables and fruits are ideal, but nutrients can deteriorate if the time between harvest and consumption is prolonged. Frozen vegetables are a great alternative, since nutrients are for the most part locked in. Cooking can affect certain nutrients either positively by activating nutrients (biotin in eggs is an example), or negatively when the nutrient is degraded or lost in cooking water that is tossed away. For this reason, it may be beneficial to eat some raw and some cooked vegetables. Good practices to cook vegetables and retain nutrients are steaming, roasting, using vegetables in stews and soups, and lightly sautéing vegetables at lower heat and consuming the sauce. See table 4.5 of vegetables for some guidelines and carbohydrate content.

I disliked vegetables during my first half century of life, due to growing up with mostly mushy, salty canned vegetables, but now a

VEGETABLES
Choose variety of types and green, white, and bright colors
Make at least 10 grams per day of carbohydrates (carbs) as vegetables. Aim for:
- **At least 2 cups per day** leafy greens and/or sprouts up to 1.5 grams total carbs per cup, raw
- **At least 1 cup per day** with variety of types and colors between 2 to 9 grams per cup, raw.
- **Limit servings** of vegetables with more than 10 gm/serving to 2 or 3 times per week (if at all).
- Choose from **sulfur-rich** vegetables* several times per week.
- **Add flavor** with 1 teaspoon or more of garlic, shallots, banana or jalapeno peppers, chives.

FOOD	SERVING SIZE	CARBS (gm)	FIBER (gm)
Alfalfa or broccoli sprouts, arugula, endive, kale, lettuces (red and green), spinach, water cress	1 cup	0-1.5	0-1
Seaweeds, sauerkraut, kimchi	½ cup	1-3	0-2
Bok choy, celery, Chinese cabbage, cucumber, mushrooms (Portabella, white)*, zucchini	1 cup	2-3	1-3
Asparagus*, broccoli, cabbage*, cauliflower, peppers (sweet and bell), mushrooms (enoki, maitake, shitake, oyster)*, radishes, yellow squash	1 cup	4-6	1-3
Beets, Brussels sprouts, onions, snap green beans, scallions, spaghetti squash, string beans, turnips	1 cup	7-9	1-3
Acorn squash, carrots, leeks, rutabaga	½ cup	7-9	1-3
Corn, green peas, sweet potato, white potato, or ¼ cup yams	½ cup	10-14	1-2

NOTE: Most servings of vegetables listed here have minimal fat, and less than 2 grams of protein.
*The values are rounded and based on average sizes.
Source: These and other choices can be found at
USDA FoodDataCentral at https://fdc.nal.usda.gov/

TABLE 4.5. Vegetables, macronutrient breakdown.

FRUIT

Choose various colors and lower-sugar fruits like apricot, berries, olives, or tomato

Include fruits in total daily carbohydrate allowance.
Choose at least **one serving of fruit per day.** Split a higher-carb whole fruit to lower carb count.
Add flavor to water and other foods with a teaspoon or more lemon or lime juice.
Note: Most fruits have minimal protein or fat, except olives have about 5 grams fat per quarter cup and minimal protein; Florida avocados (1/2 fruit) have 15 grams fat and 3.5 grams protein; California avocados have 10 grams fat and 1.3 grams protein per serving.

FOOD	SERVING SIZE	CARBS (gm)	FIBER (gm)
Cherry or grape tomato	1 fruit	0.3 – 0.7	< 0.5
Olives, green, black, or kalamata (pitted)	¼ cup	1.5 -2	< 0.5-1
Italian or plum tomato, grape	1 medium fruit		
Blackberries, raspberries, loquat (cubed)	¼ cup	3-4	2-4
Tomato	1 medium fruit	5-7	1-2
Apricot, lemon, lime, plum	1 fruit		
Blueberries, cherries (pitted), elderberries	¼ cup		
Strawberries	½ cup		
Red or green grapes	10 fruits	9	< 1
Kiwi, peach	1 medium fruit	10	2
Avocado, Florida or California	½ medium fruit	11-12	8-9
Nectarine, tangerine	1 medium fruit	12-15	2
Cantaloupe, honeydew, watermelon	1 cup cubed	12-15	< 1-2
Grapefruit	½ medium fruit	16-17	1
Orange	1 medium fruit	18	4
Apple, banana, pear	1 medium fruit	28	4-5

NOTE: Most servings of vegetables listed here have minimal fat, and less than 2 grams of protein.

*The values are rounded and based on average sizes.

Source: These and other choices can be found at
USDA FoodDataCentral at https://fdc.nal.usda.gov/

TABLE 4.6. Fruit, macronutrient breakdown.

variety of fresh raw and cooked vegetables is an enjoyable and valued part of my everyday diet.

Low-sugar fruits like apricots, berries (in small servings), olives, or tomatoes can easily work with a ketogenic diet. For example, a half cup of cut fresh strawberries (about 75 gm) has less than 6 grams of carbohydrate, including 1 to 2 grams of fiber. My personal favorites are olives and blueberries. I often enjoy five or six olives (<2 grams carbs) with salad, or ten to twelve blueberries (3 to 4 grams carbs) with Greek yogurt or ricotta. A whole medium apple or banana has about 28 grams of carbohydrate and therefore can take up half of the daily carbohydrate allowance if you are aiming for 60 grams or less. Small portions of other fruits can be worked into a ketogenic diet, such as a few grapes or slices of apple or pear, or half of a medium banana (about 60 grams), which has 14 carbs. There are other creative ways to tackle the problem, such as breaking up a banana into quarters, eating one, and freezing the other pieces to use another day in a smoothie or mix into yogurt.

Many people do not realize that avocados and olives are fruits, since they are not sweet. Avocados and olives are naturally ketogenic, since their fat content is higher than protein and carbohydrate content combined. Most other fruits have minimal fat and protein. Look at table 4.6 for the macronutrient breakdown of various fruits.

ANIMAL PROTEINS

The food groups we have discussed so far, except most fruits, all contain some protein. However, fish, seafood, animal meats, eggs, and dairy provide the most efficient sources in terms of the quality of the protein as well as essential fatty acids, vitamins, minerals, choline, and other micronutrients that are important to human metabolism. It is possible to provide adequate protein with combinations of plant sources, like legumes, nuts, seeds, whole grains, and certain vegetables, but plant foods do not supply certain essential micronutrients, notably vital vitamin B12, which can only come from animal sources.

Eggs and Dairy

Eggs contain everything needed to grow a baby chicken: protein, fat, and carbohydrate, as well as a wide array of micronutrients. The protein in eggs is about as close to perfect that a food can get for humans. For decades, eggs were vilified for their potential to increase total cholesterol before HDL- and LDL-cholesterol were routinely measured. It turns out that eggs mostly raise desirable HDL-cholesterol. I see no good reason for most people to limit eggs unless your doctor advises you to due to a medical condition.

DAIRY AND EGGS
Use in moderate amounts

WHOLE FAT, PLAIN	SERVING SIZE (GM)		FAT (gm)	PROTEIN (gm)	CARB (gm)
Cow milk	½ cup	122	3.9	4.0	5.7
Goat milk	½ cup	122	5.0	4.3	5.9
Buttermilk	½ cup	122	4.0	3.8	6.0
Kefir	½ cup	122	4.0	4.0	6.5
Mozzarella cheese	1 oz	28	6.3	6.3	0.7
Cheddar cheese	1 oz	28	9.6	6.6	0.7
Goat cheese	1 oz	28	6.0	6.0	1.0
Feta cheese	1 oz	28	7.0	5.0	0
Cream cheese	1 oz	28	9.8	1.7	1.6
Cottage cheese	1 cup	225	9.7	25.0	7.6
Ricotta cheese	½ cup	123	11.8	11.3	7.4
Greek yogurt	½ cup	112	5.6	10.0	4.5
Cow milk yogurt	½ cup	122	4.0	4.2	5.7
Goat milk yogurt	½ cup	121	5.0	5.5	6.0
Heavy cream	1 oz	30	10.8	0.8	0.8
Butter	1 tbsp	14	11.4	0.1	0
Egg, whole, raw	1 large	50	4.8	6.3	0.4

Note: Dairy and eggs contain no fiber.
Source: These and other choices can be found at
USDA FoodDataCentral at https://fdc.nal.usda.gov/

TABLE 4.7. Dairy and eggs, macronutrient breakdown.

In the traditional Mediterranean-style diet, dairy is used in moderation and includes not only dairy from cows but also from goats and sheep. The milk fat from mammals, including humans, contains some ketogenic medium-chain triglycerides (MCTs). The MCT composition of goat milk is close to human milk and much higher than cow milk. Cheeses also contain MCTs. Cream and butter are mostly fat, contain MCTs, and can be used to bring up the percent of fat into the ketogenic range in meals and snacks. Hard and softer cheeses, like feta, goat cheese, and cream cheese can provide substantial protein and fat in a small portion with minimal carbohydrate.

The percent of calories from fat in most hard and softer cheeses is at least 65 percent, and is about 87 percent for cream cheese. Cottage and ricotta cheeses are very high in protein, with a moderate amount of fat and carbohydrate, and adding an oil or coconut milk brings the fat content into the ketogenic range. Nuts and grated coconut can add more fat, fiber, and flavor.

Look for eggs and dairy from pasture-raised animals that have not been fed antibiotics, hormones, or pesticides. Also, please look at table 4.7 of dairy and eggs for information on the macronutrients and general guidelines.

Fish, Seafood, Poultry, and Meat

In general, fish, seafood, poultry, and meats contain the largest amounts of quality protein for a typical serving, with all the essential amino acids humans need to make their own proteins and an abundance of other nutrients needed for our metabolism to run smoothly. Broths from cooking fish and meats, especially bone broth, may contain vitamins and minerals with small amounts of protein, fat, and calories that have been cooked out of the meat or poultry so are well worth eating. The drippings from cooking meats can be saved to make beef broth soup, or stew.

In the IHME risk-factor analysis for premature death (figure 4.1), high intake of red meat was low on the list, with just over 10,000 of more than 56 million deaths in 2017. Therefore, sticking with the standard Mediterranean-style diet guidelines of limiting red meat to once per week or less may seem prudent at first glance; however, the risk factor for red meats does not differentiate between overly processed meats (like many bacons, sausages, hot dogs, and deli meats) and minimally processed meats. The long-held belief that dietary cholesterol and saturated fat increase the risk of cardiac disease has come under intense scrutiny, as more recent research suggests otherwise. A more compelling reason to limit intake of red meat might be the effects on climate change of raising so many animals for human consumption. Personally, I eat much less red meat more because I have increased my intake of fish than out of fear of dietary cholesterol and saturated fat.

Pasture-raised animals are fed very differently from their caged mass-produced cousins. The natural diet for cows is mainly grass, some leaves, and bark. Wild or pasture-raised pigs are omnivores, like humans, and eat vegetation like cows, but also tubers, nuts, berries, insects, small reptiles, amphibians, eggs, worms, young birds, and small mammals. Chickens naturally like fruit, seeds, leaves, tubers, and other plants, worms, and insects. Animals raised for mass production purposes are mainly fed grains to fatten them up quickly with added vitamins and minerals, but they may also receive antibiotics, hormones, herbicides, and pesticides with the grain. Eating pasture-raised animals, as well as their dairy and eggs, seems like a better idea for humans.

The IHME attributed 1.44 million deaths to a low intake of seafood omega-3 fatty acids, supporting the higher fish intake of the Mediterranean diet. If you are worried about mercury in fish, please look at chapter 9. Also, please look at table 4.8 of fish and seafood and table 4.9 of poultry and meat for information on the macronutrients and general guidelines.

ANIMAL PROTEINS ARE IMPORTANT, BUT WHAT ARE THE ALTERNATIVES?

While the fat-soluble vitamins A, E, and K, as well as vitamin C and most of the B vitamins, can be provided by plant sources, vitamin B12 is not essential for plants nor contained in plants but is found in animal meats and fish, and, to a lesser degree, in eggs, milk, and milk products. Therefore, supplementation with vitamin B12 is important for a vegetarian or vegan who avoids animal meats and fish. Most vegetables, nuts, seeds, legumes, and whole grains do not contain vitamin D except for certain mushrooms exposed to UV light. An oil-based vitamin D supplement and/or exposure to sunlight for perhaps fifteen minutes per day could solve the problem, but use caution with sun exposure if you are at risk for skin cancer.

Many people do not efficiently convert alpha-linolenic acid, the plant form of omega-3, to the biologically important omega-3 fatty acid docosahexaenoic acid (DHA). DHA is not found in vegetables and other plants, except algae and some seaweeds in small amounts, but vegan DHA supplements from algae are available. Population studies have shown that countries where pregnant women have the highest fish intake have the highest DHA blood levels and the lowest rates of preterm birth and infant mortality. Studies have also shown that pregnant women who eat at least 12 ounces of fish and seafood per week had the best developmental outcomes in their children. A big difference between a DHA supplement and fish is that many supplements contain only free DHA, but much of the DHA in fish is bound to phospholipids which may be treated differently metabolically and reach the brain by a different transport mechanism. See more discussion on this and references in chapter 6.

Getting enough choline is critically important, and about half of the US population does not meet the daily recommended intake. Choline is richer in animal than in plant sources, but taking soy or sunflower lecithin as a supplement is an easy way to get enough choline. We will discuss each of the vitamins, choline, and DHA in more detail, including how much is recommended, and rich food sources, in chapter 6 on supplements that make sense.

In general, animal sources provide more complete proteins for humans than plants, since they contain the full complement of the nine essential amino acids required to make our own proteins. It is important for vegans to eat a variety of plants that will provide a good balance of essential amino acids. Soy is one of a few plant-based foods that can be eaten in quantity and contains all essential amino acids; chia and hemp seeds also contain the full complement but are not usually eaten in large quantities. Animal meat and fish/seafood contain a significant amount of protein per serving without much if any carbohydrate. However, high-protein plants, like whole grains and legumes, tend to be much higher in carbohydrate than protein without much lipid content and therefore are more difficult to work into a ketogenic diet, though it's possible, if you are willing to eat enough fat with the meal.

The bottom line for vegetarians and vegans is to eat a variety of plant foods that will provide adequate protein and the full complement of amino acids, add enough fat to the diet to support ketosis (using MCT and coconut oil could help with that), fast overnight, and supplement

FISH AND SEAFOOD

Aim for at least 12 ounces of fish and other seafood. Choose fattier fish at least once per week.

Fresh, raw 3 oz (85 gm)	FAT (gm)	PROTEIN (gm)	CARBS (gm)
Caviar, sturgeon roe	15.2	20.9	3.4
Eel	9.9	15.6	0
Herring, Atlantic, wild	7.7	15.3	0
Salmon, sockeye, wild	4.0	19	0
Bass, freshwater, wild	3.1	16.1	0
Trout, wild	2.9	18.7	0
Mackerel	1.7	17.3	0
Seabass	1.7	15.6	0
Herring eggs, Pacific	1.6	16.1	3.8
Halibut	1.1	18.7	0
Tuna, skipjack	0.9	18.7	0
Catfish, wild	0.9	13.9	0
Clams	0.8	12.5	0
Lobster	0.6	14.0	0
Crab	0.5	15.6	0
Shrimp	0.4	17.1	0
Scallops, mollusks	0.4	10.3	0

Source: These and other choices can be found at
USDA FoodDataCentral at https://fdc.nal.usda.gov/

TABLE 4.8. Fish and Seafood, macronutrient breakdown.

POULTRY AND MEAT

Look for pasture-raised poultry and meats, organically fed without antibiotics, hormones, or pesticides
Poultry, no limit
Beef, pork, lamb, game meats consider ≤1 per week

Raw 4 oz (113 gm)	FAT (gm)	PROTEIN (gm)	CARBS (gm)
Chicken, breast, skinless	2.96	25.4	0
Chicken, dark meat with skin	5.6	22.6	0
Turkey, breast, skinless	1.7	26.8	0
Turkey, dark meat with skin	7.6	22.0	0
Veal, breast	16.7	19.8	0
Beef, ground, grass-fed	14.4	21.9	0
Beef, retail cuts, meat with fat	80.1	9.3	0
Beef, sirloin strip, lean meat	3.0	26.1	0
Beef liver, grass-fed	4.0	23.0	4.0
Pork, ground	29.0	19.1	0
Pork, belly with fat	59.9	10.6	0
Lamb, ground	26.4	18.8	0
Lamb, whole shank with fat	19.3	20.2	0

Source: These and other choices can be found at
USDA FoodDataCentral at https://fdc.nal.usda.gov/

TABLE 4.9. Poultry and Meat, macronutrient breakdown.

with important nutrients like choline, DHA, vitamin D, vitamin B12, and possibly exogenous ketone supplements. A low-fat, plant-based diet will not fit very well into the Clearly Keto plan, although striving for a whole-food Mediterranean-style diet will have its own benefits.

Healthy Fats and Oils

In the Clearly Keto diet, you will aim for at least 60 percent of your total daily calories as fat to support ketosis and fight insulin resistance. Fats as a group include more than just cooking oils, since many different types of foods in the Mediterranean-style diet are high in fat, like nuts, seeds, avocados, eggs, cheese and other dairy, fatty fish like salmon, as well as untrimmed animal meats.

Oils from almond, avocado, hazelnut, macadamia, sesame, walnut, sometimes infused with garlic or other herbs and spices, can enhance the flavor of cooked foods and salads. Canola oil is a high-oleic oil, like olive oil in that regard. Some versions of canola oil have been highly hybridized to increase the oleic acid content, but this reduces the linoleic acid content, which may be a good trade-off (see linoleic acid in chapter 9).

When planning your meals and snacks, choose oils and fats that are organic and cold-pressed or expeller-pressed whenever available; these oils have not been subjected to high heat during processing, which could change the structures of some of the fatty acids. Also, look for virgin coconut oil and for extra-virgin olive oil since they have been subjected to less processing and will retain maximum nutritional value. It is also possible to find organic expeller-pressed canola oil. Organic MCT oil is also available, as are most plant oils, organic chicken fat, lard, and beef tallow from organically fed animals. Also, look for butters, cheeses, yogurt, and other dairy products from pasture-raised animals. For information on oils, look at table 4.10 of Naturally Ketogenic Foods, for oils, which are usually 100 percent fat, and the fat content for other food groups on their respective tables.

Naturally Ketogenic Foods

Foods that are high in fat (more than 60 percent) are naturally keto-genic and work very well in meals (and especially well as snacks). If the food is packaged, be sure to double-check the nutrition label to make sure the manufacturer has not added surprise ingredients like sugar. Looking at the label, you can add the total grams of protein and total grams of carbohydrate; if the results are less than the total grams of fat, the food is at least 70 percent fat. Fat has nine calories per gram, whereas protein and carbs each have about 4 calories per gram. If the food label shows 10 grams total fat, 4 grams carbohydrate, and 6 grams protein, this food has 90 calories as fat and 40 calories as protein plus carbs, making fat about 69 percent of the total calories. Look for table 4.10 of Naturally Ketogenic Foods for ideas.

NATURALLY KETOGENIC FOODS
At least 60% fat

Naturally ketogenic foods contain at least 60% fat and fit nicely into a ketogenic meal or snack.
Avoid lite or reduce-fat versions of coconut milk, mayonnaise, salad dressings, sour cream, and cheeses.

HIGH-FAT FOOD	% OF TOTAL CALORIES AS FAT
Any pure natural oil, MCT oil, beef tallow, ghee, lard, mayonnaise	99-100% fat
Butter, cream, many salad dressings	≥ 90% fat
Coconut meat, coconut milk, heavy cream, cream cheese, olives, sour cream, macadamia nuts, pecans, walnuts	≥ 80% fat
Avocado, almonds, cheddar cheese, feta cheese, sunflower seeds, sesame seeds, hemp seeds, pumpkin seeds	≥70% fat
Cashews, eggs, mozzarella cheese	≥ 60% fat

Source: These and other protein choices can be found at
USDA FoodDataCentral at https://fdc.nal.usda.gov/

TABLE 4.10. Naturally ketogenic foods.

Make It Keto

You can easily make many foods "keto" by simply adding one-half to one tablespoon (7 to 14 grams) of oil, butter, cream, mayonnaise, or a high-fat salad dressing. Foods that come to mind are yogurt, ricotta, cottage cheese, milk, salads, any vegetable side dish, soup, chili, rice, and hot cereals. While writing this book, I used a food service for a few weeks that provides whole food Mediterranean-style "keto-friendly" heat-and-eat meals. I would add enough of my MCT/coconut oil mixture, a tablespoon or so, to push the fat into the "keto" range. Look for examples of how to "keto-up" meals and snacks in the recipes section. Also, the amounts of fat in foods are included in the charts for each food group.

Fiber Is a Friend to Your Gut Bacteria

Getting adequate fiber is important to our gut health, which also affects our brains, heart, and other organs. In their risk-factor analysis for premature death (figure 4.1), the IHME attributed more than 873,000 deaths of 56 million globally to a low intake of fiber.

The recommended daily intakes for fiber (IOM 2006) are 38 grams for men and 25 grams for women between ages nineteen and fifty, and 30 grams for men and 21 grams for women over age fifty. The Mediterranean-style diet easily supports getting enough fiber, which is present in nearly all vegetables and fruits, legumes, nuts, seeds, and whole grains. There is no fiber in animal meats, dairy, eggs, or natural oils and fats. Chapter 5 offers more discussion of fiber and the gut microbiome. Look for the fiber content on the charts for each food group.

Spices and Herbs

Spices and herbs not only provide color, flavor, and aroma to foods, but they may contain bioactive phytonutrients that convey health benefits as well. At least two groups have published a review searching PubMed.gov

SPICES AND HERBS
With special properties

ANTIOXIDANTS/ANTI-INFLAMMATORY
Allspice, anise, basil, bay leaf, capers, caraway, cardamom, cayenne pepper, celery seeds, chili pepper, cinnamon, cloves, coriander (cilantro), dill ginger, fennel/flower fennel, fenugreek, garlic, horseradish, lavender, marjoram, mustard, myrtle, nutmeg, onion, oregano, parsley, peppermint, red & black pepper, rosemary, saffron, sage, tea, thyme, turmeric (curcumin), wormwood

CARDIOVASCULAR BENEFIT
Cinnamon, fenugreek, garlic, ginger, onion, red pepper, tumeric (curcumin)

ANTI-DIABETIC
Bay leaf, cinnamon, fenugreek, mustard, pomegranate, wormwood

ANTI-CANCER
Bay leaf, garlic, mustard & mustard seeds, onion, turmeric (curcumin), saffron

NEUROPROTECTIVE
Mint, onion

OBESITY
Saffron, tumeric (curcumin)

Source: Yashin, et al. *Antioxidants* V.6 No. 3 (2017)

TABLE 4.11. Spices and herbs with beneficial effects.
Source: Yashin, 2017.

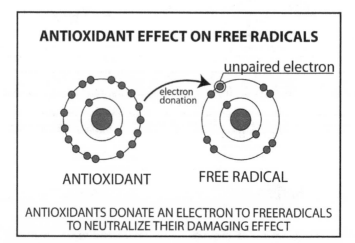

ANTIOXIDANT EFFECT ON FREE RADICALS

unpaired electron

electron donation

ANTIOXIDANT   FREE RADICAL

ANTIOXIDANTS DONATE AN ELECTRON TO FREERADICALS TO NEUTRALIZE THEIR DAMAGING EFFECT

FIGURE 4.7. Antioxidants donate an electron to free radicals to neutralize their damaging effect.

and several large food databases for articles on positive and negative associations of biomedical effects with culinary spices and herbs, which included 188 different spices. They found thousands of laboratory, animal, and human studies reporting that certain spices have anti-inflammatory and antioxidant properties (see figure 4.7) and may have both positive therapeutic effects for specific disorders like obesity and diabetes, and anti-cancer activity (breast, colorectal, prostate, and liver). Studies of turmeric (curcumin), garlic, and ginger, and nearly all other spices, reported many more positive than negative biomedical effects. Notably, licorice and celery had equal numbers of positive and negative associations reported. Common negative effects of spices were the triggering of allergic reactions and dermatitis, or worsening of high blood pressure (Rahki 2018; Yashin 2017). See table 4.11 for a listing of some spices and herbs and their beneficial effects.

Herbal supplements like ashwagandha and St. John's wort may have positive but also serious negative effects related to interactions with prescribed and over-the-counter medications (see chapter 6 for more details and references).

THE CLEARLY KETO WHOLE-FOOD MEDITERRANEAN-STYLE DIET PLAN

Here are the guidelines for what to eat on the Clearly Keto whole-food Mediterranean-style diet plan. Look for charts for each food group for the macronutrient breakdown. Also, look for a quick reference chart for the Clearly Keto Whole-Food Mediterranean-Style Diet Plan.

CLEARLY KETO DIET PLAN

Basic Macronutrient Ratios: The less carbohydrate and the more fat in the diet, the higher ketone levels will become. Consider monitoring ketone and blood sugar levels (see chapter 6).

- Aim for carbohydrate intake of no more than 130 grams, and, ideally, 60 grams or less per day. May start at 20 to 25 grams per day to kickstart weight loss or to control blood sugar (with close blood-glucose monitoring).
- Keep daily protein intake at around 0.5 gram per pound (1.1 gm/ kg) of body weight. Athletes and body-builders may be able to double this amount and maintain ketosis.
- Gradually adjust fat intake to at least 60 percent of total calories. Increase percent of fat and lower carbohydrates if you're having trouble getting into ketosis.

Animal proteins: Preferably pasture-raised animals.
- Ideal: 12 ounces (336 grams) of fish and seafood, with fatty fish at least weekly.
- No limit on poultry or eggs.
- Moderate amounts of dairy.
- Consider limiting to once per week or less: red meats (beef, pork, lamb, game animals).

Plant proteins (for vegans and vegetarians): Eat a variety of legumes, tofu, nuts, seeds, whole grains, and vegetables. Soybeans are an especially efficient source of plant protein.

Vegetables: At least 10 carb grams per day of a variety of types and colors.
- Daily: At least 2 cups leafy greens and sprouts, and at least 1 cup of other vegetables.
- Choose from sulfur-rich vegetables a few times per week.
- Limit choices with more than 10 grams per serving to two or three times per week or less.

Fruits: At least one serving per day of low-sugar or small portions of higher-sugar fruits with a variety of colors.

Nuts and seeds: At least one 1-ounce serving daily.

Clearly Keto | WHOLE FOOD MEDITERRANEAN-STYLE DIET PLAN

BASIC MACRONUTRIENT RATIOS:

CARBS: 60 gm or less per day. 20-25 gm per day to kickstart weight loss or control blood sugar with close blood glucose monitoring.
- Optional: 130 gm carb per day for elderly or for moderate carb diet

PROTEIN
- **Minimum** 0.5 gm/pound (1.1 gm/kg) of body weight
- **Maximum**: up to 1 gm/pound (2.2 gm/kg) of body weight

FAT: Begin at ≥ 60% of total calories
- Use higher % fat and lower carbs to increase ketosis

ANIMAL PROTEINS: (Preferably pasture-raised organically fed animals)
- **Fish and seafood:** ≥12 oz (336 gm) weekly, include fatty fish.
- **Dairy:** Moderate amount | • **Poultry or eggs:** No weekly limit
- **Red meats:** Consider weekly or less often (beef, pork, lamb, game).

PLANT PROTEINS: Vegans & vegetarians: To get adequate protein, increase legumes, tofu, nuts, seeds, whole grains, and vegetables.

VEGETABLES: ≥10 gm carb daily, use variety of types and colors.
- **Daily:** ≥ 2 cups leafy greens & sprouts, and ≥ 1 cup of other vegetables.
- Choose **sulfur-rich vegetables** a few times per week.
- **Limit** choices with ≥10 gm/serving to 2-3 times per week.

FRUIT: ≥1 serving per day | **NUTS/SEEDS:** ≥1 oz(28 gm) per day

WHOLE GRAINS: ≥ 1 small serving per day

LEGUMES: 2-3 small servings per week, more for vegan/vegetarians

HEALTHY FATS:
Extra virgin olive oil, virgin coconut oil, olives, avocados, butter, nuts, nut butters, seeds, whole-fat dairy. MCT oil to enhance ketogenic effect.
Ideal: Organic cold-pressed or expeller-pressed oils

OTHER TIPS:
- Drink at least 8-10 cups of water and clear liquids per day.
- Limit sodium to 2300 mg per day (1500 mg for high blood pressure).
- Write down plans for meals and snacks, be patient and persistent.
- **Optional:** Check ketone and blood sugar levels.

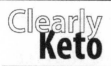 **QUICK REFERENCE CHART FOR DAILY PLANNING**

Step 1: Calculate daily protein gm's = 0.5 gm x body weight in pounds OR 1.1 gm body weight in kg
Step 2: Select heading with desired # calories per day. |
Step 3: Choose your selected % fat in left column to find your daily allowance for "fat" and "protein & carbs"

% CALORIES AS FAT	1400 CALORIES/DAY		1600 CALORIES/DAY		1800 CALORIES/DAY	
	FAT (gm)	PROTEIN & CARBS (gm)	FAT (gm)	PROTEIN & CARBS (gm)	FAT (gm)	PROTEIN & CARBS (gm)
40%	62	209	71	240	80	270
45%	70	192	80	220	90	247
50%	78	175	89	200	100	225
55%	86	156	98	180	110	203
60%	93	140	106	160	120	180
65%	101	123	115	140	130	157
70%	109	105	124	120	140	135
75%	117	88	133	100	150	113
80%	124	67	142	80	160	90
85%	132	52	151	60	170	68

% CALORIES AS FAT	2000 CALORIES/DAY		2400 CALORIES/DAY		2800 CALORIES/DAY	
	FAT (gm)	PROTEIN & CARBS (gm)	FAT (gm)	PROTEIN & CARBS (gm)	FAT (gm)	PROTEIN & CARBS (gm)
40%	89	300	107	360	124	420
45%	100	275	120	330	140	385
50%	111	250	133	300	156	350
55%	122	225	147	270	171	315
60%	133	200	160	240	187	280
65%	144	175	173	210	202	245
70%	155	150	187	180	218	210
75%	166	125	200	150	233	175
80%	177	100	213	120	249	140
85%	189	75	227	90	264	105

Shaded boxes: May not allow for adequate protein for adult if any carbohydrates are in diet.

Clearly Keto | QUICK REFERENCE CHART FOR MEAL PLANNING

Step 1: Select desired number of calories per meal.
Step 2: Choose desired % fat to find "fat" and "protein & carbs" for the meal.

% CALORIES AS FAT	400 CALORIE MEAL		500 CALORIE MEAL		600 CALORIE MEAL	
	FAT (gm)	PROTEIN & CARBS (gm)	FAT (gm)	PROTEIN & CARBS (gm)	FAT (gm)	PROTEIN & CARBS (gm)
50%	22	50	28	63	33	74
60%	27	39	33	50	40	60
70%	31	30	39	37	47	44
80%	35	21	44	26	53	30
90%	40	10	50	13	60	15

% CALORIES AS FAT	700 CALORIE MEAL		800 CALORIE MEAL	
	FAT (gm)	PROTEIN & CARBS (gm)	FAT (gm)	PROTEIN & CARBS (gm)
50%	39	87	44	100
60%	47	70	53	80
70%	54	53	62	60
80%	62	35	71	40
90%	70	18	80	20

Legumes: About two or three small servings per week if eating animal proteins. More for vegans.

Whole grains: At least one small serving per day.

Healthy fats: Emphasis on foods high in monounsaturated fatty acids—extra-virgin olive oil, olives, avocados, nuts, nut butters, and seeds. You may also include butter and other whole-fat dairy, virgin coconut oil, and MCT oil to enhance ketogenic effect. Look for organic cold-pressed or expeller-pressed vegetable oils and fats from grass-fed, pasture-raised animals.

Other tips:
- Stay well hydrated. Drink at least 8 to 10 cups of water and clear liquids per day.
- Limit sodium to about 2,300 mg if healthy, or about 1,500 mg per day if you have high blood pressure.

PLANNING, PATIENCE, AND PERSISTENCE WILL PAY OFF—AND BE KIND TO YOURSELF

The time and effort you put into planning meals and snacks up front, and writing them down, will save you much more time later. Most people gravitate toward one or two typical breakfasts, lunches, and snacks, and perhaps seven main meals. Therefore, you can build a collection of meal and snack plans to fit your needs within a couple of weeks. Don't beat yourself up if you deviate on occasion. You can get right back on the plan with your next meal. You deserve kudos for each step you take toward eating a healthier diet, and each step will add up on the road to healthier aging.

A digital kitchen scale that can display ounces or grams, and a set of measuring cups and measuring spoons, can help you figure out appropriate portions. I have used a digital scale every day for many years to keep me on track. I have gotten used to servings in grams and find it easy to use the scale to add anything and everything when I am putting meals and snacks together. Weighing and measuring every gram and calculating macronutrient ratios is very strict and important for success in the classic form of the ketogenic diet for drug-resistant epilepsy and cancer support. I strongly recommend that anyone with those issues work closely with a ketogenic-certified dietitian.

You can also make your life easier by finding recipes with macronutrients calculated for you on the many keto websites out there. I have found great recipes at The Charlie Foundation, Matthews Friends, Ketogenic.com, Aaron Day's Fat for Weight Loss, and on TikTok (see Resources for website information).

It takes years to develop insulin resistance, but you could see good results within six to ten weeks. For people with severe insulin resistance, it could take twelve to eighteen months or longer to see fasting glucose, fasting insulin, and HbA1C levels back in the normal range; but these values should begin to trend in the right direction not long after beginning a low-carb, higher-fat diet. Patience, persistence, and consistency will pay off. It is important to think of this diet plan as a lifestyle choice that you will keep from this point on, to enjoy healthier brain aging. Steps you take to slow down or prevent dementia will be very beneficial to your overall health as well, since your brain and body are intricately intertwined.

THE "MEDITERRANEAN" DIET IN JAPAN

The Japanese are known to have one of the longest life spans and lowest rates in the world of preterm birth, newborn mortality, and chronic diseases like diabetes. This has been attributed to the healthy diet in Japan, which also has one of the highest intakes of fish and other seafood. In a world of historical cultural parallels, the centuries-old traditional diets in Japan and in populations around the Mediterranean contain the same basic food groups, even though the specific foods on the plate may look very different. Exemplified in both the Japanese and Mediterranean diets are animal proteins, highlighting fish and seafood, with some dairy and egg, and limited red meats, along with legumes; seeds; nuts; whole grains; a variety of seasonal vegetables and fruits; oils for cooking and finishing foods; teas; other herbs; and spices.

I have had the great privilege of visiting Japan three times since 2013 to give presentations and attend conferences, the first time with my daughter Julie, a great adventure for both of us. When an American (like me!) visits Japan for the first time, it is immediately obvious that a traditional meal in Japan could not look more different from what appears on our plates in the United States. Unless you go into a Westernized or fast-food restaurant, you will not see big bowls of sugary cereal, a sandwich of processed meats between two slices of white bread, or a large dollop of mashed potatoes or French fries on the plate. Portion sizes are much smaller, often cut into small, perfect rectangles, and are carefully positioned in small bowls or in a bento box with dividers.

Some differences between Mediterranean and Japanese cuisine, though still within the same basic food groups, are seaweeds, fermented soybeans (natto), and fermented vegetables (called pickles), which are staples in Japanese homes. Eating various types of raw fish cut into strips (sashimi) is common in Japan, as well as sushi, which may consist of raw or cooked fish, eel, or other seafood and vegetables, rolled in vinegared rice, and wrapped in seaweed or coated with sesame seeds. Sushi and sashimi are becoming more popular elsewhere in the world, including the United States. Sake, fermented rice wine, is a traditional Japanese drink, usually consumed in small portions, cold or warm.

On one of my trips to Japan, we visited a restaurant that mainly served eel cooked various ways, which was quite good grilled with a sort of barbecue sauce. Another restaurant specialized in delicious sukiyaki prepared at the table, consisting of thinly sliced beef cooked in a shallow iron pot with soy sauce, rice wine, a little sugar, and vegetables cooked together in a larger pot. After cooking, the meat and vegetables are dipped into a bowl of raw egg and eaten . . . unexpectedly yummy.

Most meals, including breakfast, are accompanied by a many-centuries-old Japanese tradition, miso soup, which consists of fish-bone broth and miso, a fermented soybean paste made with salt and kōji fungus. Miso soup may also contain various seaweeds; tofu (bean curd); barley; brown rice or other whole grain; onion and other vegetables; sesame oil; and seasonings. The miso-and-broth mixture contains a good amount of protein (about 4 to 5 grams in 8 ounces) before adding the other ingredients and is loaded with vitamins and minerals. Clear broths are mainly made from dried bonito and kelp and are consumed alone or used in cooking.

Like the U.S. shift from whole-grain to white bread, over the last half-century or so many in Japan, especially younger people, have shifted from eating whole-grain rice to refined white rice; sweets, fast foods, and other Westernized foods have also become much more common. Alzheimer's is a growing problem in Japan. Public awareness of Alzheimer's disease and dementia became a social issue with the publication of The Twilight Years by Sawako Ariyoshi in 1972.

INTERVIEW WITH KAORI NAKAJIMA ON THE JAPANESE DIET

One of the most wonderful experiences of my life was a trip to Japan in 2013 with my daughter Julie at the invitation of The Nisshin OilliO

Group, Ltd., the largest edible oil company in Japan, to give a presentation on coconut oil, MCT oil, and ketones for Alzheimer's disease. We were surprised with a special sightseeing visit to beautiful Kyoto, where there are many temples and shrines, such as the beautiful Golden Pavilion surrounded by a serene lake. We were treated to a night at a traditional Japanese inn, eating traditional cuisine, wearing kimonos and traditional footwear, and sleeping on futons. Since 2013, Kaori and I have become good friends, meeting up at many symposiums and conferences in the United States, Canada, UK, Europe, Asia, Australia, and New Zealand.

I asked Kaori many questions about the typical Japanese diet, and here are her answers:

Q: What types of vegetables are eaten in Japan, and which vegetables would be considered "leafy greens"? Are vegetables with sulfur, such as mushrooms, onions, and cabbage, eaten much in Japan?

A: In Japan, we are keen on vegetables of the season. The Japanese are known to be "agricultural" from the olden days, not so much as hunters. And we have an abundance of veggies all year round. We eat lots of mushrooms (all kinds, but especially shiitake, raw or dried and then cooked), onions (very sweet in the beginning of summer), and cabbage (so soft in the spring!). Leafy greens are the different types of lettuce, spinach, and others that are original here or originated in China.

Q: Are seaweeds a routine part of the diet in Japan, and how many times per week are seaweeds part of a meal in a healthy diet?

A: Seaweeds are very much a routine part of the diet in Japan. I think we eat some in different formats almost every day! Either dried and tasty with rice (or just munchies), or soft seaweed in miso soups. They are a staple. Seaweeds (especially kelps) are an important part of Japanese cuisine, since they become the source of typical Japanese "broth." We use dried kelp (which is harvested usually in Hokkaido, the northern island of Japan) to make the basic soup broth for all kinds of dishes in "pots," like Shabu-shabu. Kelp is also used to give a nice "umami" for fish. Ah, "umami." That is what kelps are for, to provide a savory flavor to food.

Q: Do most people include some fermented vegetables (pickles) in their diet routinely?

A: Yes, most people do. We love pickled vegetables. But they tend to be very salty, so people use them more moderately nowadays, or buy or make their own with less salt. Pickled vegetables are eaten with cooked rice. Again, many of us eat fermented soybeans ("natto"), mainly those living in the eastern half of Japan. Maybe that's a stereotype nowadays! People from the western half are said not to be very fond of natto.

Q: What fruits are popular in Japan?

A: Fruits! Peaches, watermelons, oranges (from the United States, Australia, Mexico), figs, apples, pears, and bananas all year round. Strawberries starting in the fall. Tangerines and Japanese oranges (many types and brands). Most fruits are seasonal, so we eat/enjoy "the season" with the fruits. Right now [in August] it is peaches as big as your fist—so juicy and sweet! And figs and watermelon.

Q: Do many people eat whole-grain rice these days?

A: People do eat whole-grain rice, yes. I don't, because Mom doesn't like it. She says it reminds her of the days during and after the Second World War. Many people eat it because it reminds them of those days, too, I am sure. I don't know if young people like whole-grain rice. It is recognized to be "healthy," I think. There is also an "image" for its being "organic." Organic is considered to be good in Japan, but there is no strong advocacy.

Q: Besides soybeans and edamame, what other legumes are eaten in Japan? How does tofu and other soy fit into the diet in Japan?

A: Beans: All sorts! Red beans ("azuki" beans) are the basis of Japanese sweets. We eat peas and broad beans (in the spring) a lot. We also eat lots of roots. We get our fiber and vitamins from them. Tofu, we eat almost every day. Other soy foods—edamame in the summer and fermented soybeans all year long. Also, many people drink soy milk.

Q: How are oils and fats used in Japan? For example, what types of cooking oils and fats are typically used for deep-frying eggplant or tempura or cooking in a skillet, and do you add oil to soups or broths or other foods, like vegetables?

A: The Japanese people love deep-frying and frying in general. We use canola, soybean, blended oils (e.g., palm and soybean for frying). For tempura, many of us use rice oil, since it gives a nice toasty aroma. We use lots of sesame oil too, but again to give a nice aroma right before turning the heat off. Nowadays we eat a lot of olive oil for frying, deep-frying, and salads; it is almost as popular as any other oil. I think it originated from our love of Italian food! We also have other oils like flaxseed and perilla, which come from their "functional" origins. I do not know if many people know that we must use oil/fat in order to absorb the nutrients of food inside the body. . . . Bioavailability is so important! A carrot is just a carrot without the oil to get the Vitamin E working in the body!

I will never forget my wonderful trips to Japan, my time with Kaori, or the many wonderful meals we shared there.

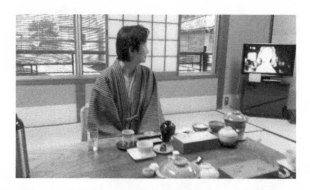

PHOTO 2. Kaori Nakajima at a traditional Japanese Inn, Kyoto, Japan, 2013.

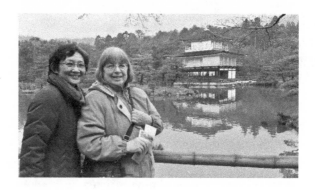

PHOTO 3. Kaori Nakajima and Mary Newport visit the Golden Pavilion in Kyoto, Japan, 2013.

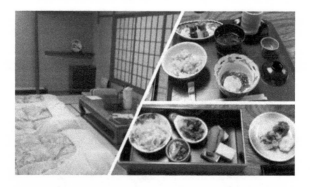

PHOTO 4. Foods and futons at the traditional inn, Kyoto, Japan, 2013.

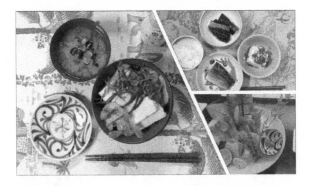

PHOTO 5. Sashimi plate (bottom right) and two dinners at Kaori's home. Upper right, grilled mackerel; eggplants deep-fried, then cooked with Japanese soup stock, based on dried fish (bonito), soy sauce, sake, and a hint of sugar; cold tofu with spring-onion topping and soy sauce; and a small bowl of rice, eaten with iced green tea and a sweet juicy peach for dessert. Left, miso soup with small clams; sushi rice in a bowl topped with raw tuna, raw amberjack, raw northern shrimp, cucumber, thick-baked egg, and sprinkled perilla leaves with soy sauce and wasabi on the side, prepared by Kaori's mother.

Japan is just one of many countries around the world that have populations that live longer and healthier by eating a diet that emphasizes the nutrient-packed food groups of the Mediterranean-style diet.

CHAPTER FIVE

OTHER KETOGENIC STRATEGIES AND KETONE SUPPLEMENTS

"Ketones are a primitive fuel for the brain."
—Richard L. Veech, MD, D.Phil.

We discussed the many good reasons to adopt a whole-food Mediterranean-style ketogenic diet and some basics about what ketones can do in chapter 4. There are other ketogenic strategies you can use to build on the foundation of a healthy diet—adding coconut oil and/or MCT oil to your diet, intermittent or overnight fasting, exercise, caffeine, branched-chain amino acids, and exogenous ketone supplements. William Curtis's experience with ketogenic strategies perfectly illustrates what is possible with this approach.

WILLIAM CURTIS GETS THE UPPER HAND ON PARKINSON'S WITH OVERNIGHT FASTING, COCONUT OIL, A LOW-CARB CONTROLLED-PROTEIN DIET, AND MORNING EXERCISE

William "Bill" Curtis, sixty-six years old, was the proverbial "professional student," earning a B.S. in agriculture but also taking undergraduate and graduate-level courses in math, chemistry, physics, and other sciences. He found his niche in computer programming and creating software while working for a large financial institution.

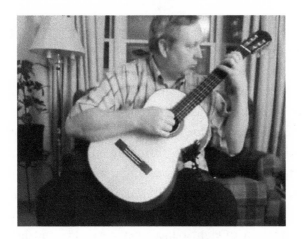

PHOTO 1. William Curtis.

In 2000, Bill began to develop symptoms of cognitive impairment like difficulty remembering phone numbers, organizing, and carrying out everyday activities, and his administrative and executive-type work deteriorated. He developed a "pill-rolling" movement between his thumb and index finger. His right arm stopped swinging normally when he walked, and he had trouble doing things that had been easy before. At just forty-nine years old, Bill was diagnosed with Parkinson's disease. The prescribed medications made him too drowsy to drive safely. He worked longer hours to compensate for his disabilities, which worsened his condition and left little time for his family.

In 2006, Bill read about a pilot study of the positive results of ketogenic diet in five people with Parkinson's disease (Vanitallie 2005) and hypothesis papers by Dr. Richard Veech on ketones as alternative fuel for the brain in Alzheimer's, Parkinson's, and other diseases (Veech 2001) but he was in the earlier stages and passed on trying the ketogenic approach at that time. Despite great medical care and the latest medications, Bill's tremors worsened; he developed involuntary muscle contractions called dystonia; he would "freeze" while starting to walk; he lost his sense of smell; and he suffered from hallucinations. Bill recalls staring at a blank computer screen at work, which did not go unnoticed, and by 2012 Bill made the difficult decision to stop working.

As Bill's condition continued to deteriorate, he became completely disabled and spent most of his days in a chair having tremors.

While researching Parkinson's in the NIH library in 2013, Bill called Dr. Veech, who invited him to his lab—the first of many visits. With Dr. Veech's guidance, Bill tried various ketogenic strategies. The regimen that works for Bill begins with an overnight fast from dinner until lunch the next day, drinking only coffee in the morning with two tablespoons each of coconut oil and heavy cream, plus one tablespoon of grass-fed butter. Bill avoids carbs with a high glycemic index (which spike blood-sugar and insulin levels) like sugary cereals, and limits protein to eight ounces per meal. He and his wife take advantage of a ketogenic-meal food-delivery service several times per week. Bill also takes a brisk thirty-minute walk up and down hills each morning.

This regimen has allowed Bill to get up out of the chair and become more involved in life again for the past nine years. None of his six Parkinson's medications has been increased since 2013—quite unusual. Bill's symptoms come roaring back if he deviates from the plan, such as eating birthday cake or pizza crust. Nighttime eating, even a good protein like chicken, worsens his symptoms for the day, likely because excess protein can convert to glucose and interfere with ketosis.

In 2021, Bill says he is the same as or better than when I interviewed him in 2017 for my previous book, *The Complete Book of Ketones*. He is not cured of Parkinson's, but his symptoms are controlled and stable. Bill points out that "the body makes ketones for free" and ketogenic strategies provide "mitochondrial quality control." Mitochondrial dysfunction is a key feature of Parkinson's and other neurodegenerative conditions like Alzheimer's.

Bill shares what he has learned about the benefits of the ketogenic lifestyle with other people with Parkinson's. For reasons unknown, the ketogenic lifestyle does not help everyone, but it does seem to help most people who have severe symptoms. He advises people that there is "no rush" with this type of diet—there are "plenty of days to get it right." Bill strongly recommends coordinating with a Parkinson's specialist and working closely with a dietitian certified in the ketogenic diet.

That fateful telephone call Bill made to Dr. Veech in 2013 took him on a new pathway toward a ketogenic lifestyle and a new lease on life. His background and extensive education in the sciences has made it possible for Bill to understand, explain, and coauthor scientific papers on ketones (Curtis 2021).

To increase awareness, Bill has posted videos on YouTube.com showing his symptoms while off and on ketones (Curtis, YouTube Videos). The difference is obvious and truly remarkable.

THE "KETO" LIFESTYLE IS MORE THAN A DIET

The ketogenic strategies discussed in this chapter will boost ketones regardless of what you eat, but will be more effective if combined with a low-carb, higher-fat diet. Ketone levels tend to fluctuate throughout the day, depending on how long you fast overnight, whether you exercise, and what you eat with each meal and snack (see figure 5.1).

KETOGENIC STRATEGY:	KETONE LEVELS mmol/L:
Caffeine ➤	0.2 to 0.3
Coconut Oil ➤	0.3 to 0.5
Vigorous Exercise ➤	0.3 to 0.5
Overnight Fast ➤	0.3 to 0.5
MCT Oil ➤	0.3 to 1.0
Branched Chain Amino Acids ➤	0.3 to 1.0
Ketone Mineral Salts ➤	0.5 to 1.0
Classic Ketogenic Diet ➤	2 to 6
Starvation ➤	2 to 7
Ketone Esters (Oral or IV) ➤	2 to 7 or higher
Diabetic Ketoacidosis ➤	10 to 25

FIGURE 5.1. Strategies to increase ketone levels. The values for the ketone level are for each strategy alone. Combining strategies could boost ketone levels higher.

OVERNIGHT FASTING

Fasting is a centuries-old tradition used by various cultures for religious reasons or health benefits. Our ancestors almost certainly fasted overnight since they did not have access to a bulging pantry or refrigerator. Fasting was used successfully to stop seizures until the ketogenic diet was found to similarly increase ketone levels and stop seizures in 1921. Fasting was also used as a strategy to delay death in type 1 diabetes before insulin was available as a treatment just one century ago. Numerous studies have supported the potential of fasting to benefit health and extend life (Mattson 2018, two articles). During prolonged fasting and starvation, ketones can supply up to two-thirds of the fuel the brain needs (Owen 1967) (see figure 5.2).

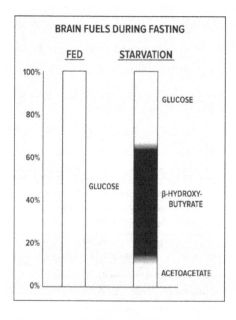

FIGURE 5.2. Brain fuels during fasting. A "metabolic switch" from using glucose to ketones as fuel occurs during prolonged starvation or fasting, but also with a low-carbohydrate, high-fat ketogenic diet. The percent of energy in the brain derived from ketones increases in direct proportion to the blood ketone level. Blood ketone levels increase steadily as fasting continues, leveling off at around ten days. Likewise, as the percent of fat in the diet increases beyond 60 percent of calories, ketone levels increase in direct proportion. Figure adapted by Joanna Newport from information in Owen 1967.

The average person at rest uses up the glucose stored in the liver as glycogen after ten hours or so without food, and stored fat begins to break down to provide fuel as fatty acids, which are partly converted to ketones to fuel the brain. Overnight fasting with no solid food for at least ten hours is an easy way for adults of any age to enjoy the health benefits of fasting. Many people fast for eighteen hours or more, considered an extended overnight fast.

Breaking the fast ("breakfast") with fat (called a fat fast), such as coconut oil and/or MCT oil in coffee or tea, or a ketogenic meal, can build on the ketone level achieved during the fast. Narrowing the window of eating may also help with weight loss. Exercise during the fast will use up glycogen stores sooner, to kickstart ketosis. After ten hours or so of overnight fasting, the ketone level could be at least 0.3 mmol/L and will tend to increase as the duration of the fast is extended.

There are numerous other ways to fast, such as reducing intake to 500 to 1000 calories two or three times a week or drinking only liquids for 24 hours. During any fast, it is important to drink plenty of water or other sugar-free, calorie-free fluids to prevent dehydration. Use of fluids with caffeine, like coffee and tea, could give an additional small bump in ketone levels (Vandenberghe 2017).

Prolonged fasts may result in loss of muscle mass and carry more risks than benefits to health. During a fast of twenty-four hours or longer, you could lose important electrolytes, including sodium, potassium, chloride, calcium, and magnesium from your body. This problem can be avoided by drinking water infused with electrolytes or broth, adding sea salt or Himalayan pink sea salt to water, or using an electrolyte supplement. Some people enjoy adding a teaspoon or two of lemon or lime juice to plain water, or using sparkling water.

People who are diabetic or prone to hypoglycemia need to know that blood sugar and insulin levels will almost certainly drop, possibly substantially. You may need to monitor blood sugar closely and adjust medications in consultation with your doctor.

EXERCISE

Making the "metabolic switch" from burning glucose to ketones with fasting and exercise positively impacts many signaling pathways (Mattson 2018).

In 1909, a researcher named G. Forssner noticed that the levels of ketones in his urine always increased after he took a brisk four-kilometer walk lasting at least thirty minutes. In 1911, ketones were elevated in the urine of a patient of L. Preti who walked up and down steps until exhausted. Beginning in 1936, a two-decade flurry of research studied the phenomenon called the "Courtice Douglas effect" or "post-exercise ketosis" (Forssner 1909; Preti 1911; Courtice 1936).

More recently, using ketone PET imaging, Dr. Stephen Cunnane and associates found that in people with mild Alzheimer's, moderately vigorous exercise for forty minutes using a treadmill nearly tripled ketone uptake in the brain (Castellano 2017). Cunnane and group also found that taking 15 ml (about 1 tablespoon) of MCT oil about one hour before the start of a thirty-minute session of aerobic exercise (exercise that increases heart rate) increased the ketone level 69 percent higher than when the same participants either took MCT oil alone or exercised without taking MCT oil first. This effect was greater in women who were not prediabetic than in women who were prediabetic, but both groups had higher ketone levels (Vandenberghe 2019). These and other studies on exercise and its many benefits are discussed in much more detail in chapter 8.

More intense and/or prolonged exercise could increase ketone levels even more and sustain them longer. Eating a ketogenic meal, perhaps containing coconut and/or MCT oil prior to the exercise, or combining an overnight fast with morning exercise, could further enhance ketosis.

CAFFEINE

It is well known that caffeine increases the basal metabolic rate and stimulates breakdown of fat (lipolysis), which may explain the caffeine-related boost in ketones. Coffee is also known to have antioxidant, anti-inflammatory, and anti-diabetic properties (Baumeister 2021). Drinking coffee with added coconut oil, MCT oil, and/or butter has become a popular way to begin the day with a boost in ketones.

Cunnane and group reported that the caffeine equivalent of one or two cups of coffee results in a slight bump in ketone levels. Two men and eight women (average age thirty-three) were given caffeine, dosed at either 2.5 mg/kg or 5 mg/kg of body weight (about 150 or 300 mg for the average participant). Between two and four hours after the caffeine dose, the ketone betahydroxybutyrate increased by 88 percent for the lower caffeine dose and by 116 percent for the higher caffeine dose. The increase in ketone levels is equivalent to levels following an overnight fast of about 0.2 to 0.3 mmol/L (Vandenberghe 2017).

Adding MCT oil to your coffee or tea with caffeine could increase ketones more than either alone. Baumeister and group studied seven young female adults in their twenties who each received ten different combinations of decaffeinated coffee with or without 150 mg caffeine added and with or without 10 grams of one of four different oils (three types of MCT oil—C8:0 alone, C10:0 alone, C8:0/C10:0, or coconut oil). The participants fasted overnight before each test with a twenty-four-hour washout period between tests. Blood betahydroxybutyrate (BHB) was tested before and every 40 minutes for 240 minutes. Adding caffeine without oil increased ketones from just over 0.20 mm/L for decaffeinated coffee, to just over 0.40 mm/L. Adding caffeine to coffee with each type of oil consistently led to higher BHB levels than oils with no caffeine. Adding C8:0 and caffeine to the coffee was the clear winner, peaking at 0.8 mm/L BHB on average at about two hours; and C8:0/C10:0 with caffeine peaked at about 0.5 mm/L BHB, also at two hours. None of the interventions affected blood glucose (Baumeister 2021). See figure 5.3.

BRANCHED-CHAIN AMINO ACIDS

Certain amino acids, the building blocks of protein, are converted to glucose or to ketones when they are metabolized. However, three branched-chain amino acids—leucine, isoleucine, and valine—are

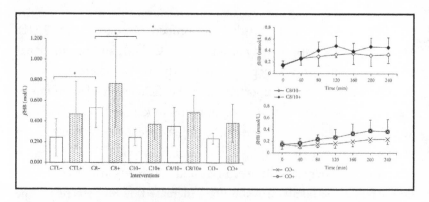

FIGURE 5.3. Effects on betahydroxybutyrate levels of MCT oils and coconut oil with and without caffeine. Acetoacetate levels were not measured. CTL = decaffeinated coffee, CO = coconut oil, + = with 150 mg caffeine, – = no added caffeine, C8:0 = tricaprylic acid, C10:0 = capric acid. Open access article with permission under the Creative Commons Attribution License with citation: Baumeister A, J Gardemann, M Fobker M, et al. "Short-term influence of caffeine and medium-chain triglycerides on ketogenesis: A controlled double-blind intervention study." J Nutr Metab (2021):1861567.

ketogenic and have been used as supplements by bodybuilders for many years to build and maintain lean body mass.

Due to their ketogenic propensity, branched-chain amino acids have been used in studies of childhood epilepsy and autism. Adding branched-chain amino acids to the ketogenic diet in seventeen children with seizures who did not respond well to the diet alone led to seizure-freedom in three children and a 50 to 90 percent reduction in seizures in five other children. Adding branched-chain amino acids decreased the overall percent of fat in the diet without lowering the ketone level, thus allowing for a more satisfying, versatile diet (Evangeliou 2009).

Like lauric acid in coconut oil, leucine rapidly stimulated production of ketones in astrocyte cultures, even with glucose present (Bixel 1995). Therefore, adding the branched-chain amino acids leucine, isoleucine, and valine as one of your strategies could help increase ketone levels, not only in the plasma but potentially in brain astrocytes as well.

Branched-chain amino acids are widely available in health-food stores and on internet sites which suggest doses of 5 to 15 grams per day for an average-size person. However, high blood levels of branched-chain amino acids may interfere with brain uptake of tryptophan, a precursor for serotonin, which regulates mood and sleep. Therefore, taking too much branch-chained amino acids could have a negative impact on mood and sleep. Tryptophan is also a precursor for the important vitamin niacin. This speaks to how complex metabolism is and how upsetting the balance with too much of a good thing could have negative consequences. So, if you decide to try branched-chain amino acids, I suggest a small amount, such as 1 or 2 grams.

MEDIUM-CHAIN TRIGLYCERIDES

If you are eating a standard high-carbohydrate diet, incorporating oils with medium-chain triglycerides (MCTs) into your meals and snacks could get you into mild nutritional ketosis and sustain ketone levels if taken several times per day and regardless of what you eat. Adding MCTs to a low-carbohydrate high-fat diet could help sustain even higher levels of ketones.

MCTs are naturally produced in the mammary glands of lactating women, making up 10 to 17 percent of the lipids in breast milk (Hamosh 1985). After weaning, MCTs must come from foods. Coconut oil, the richest natural source of MCTs (about 60 percent), is widely available in stores and online. Palm-kernel oil, about 53 percent MCTs, is extracted from the seed of the palm fruit, has a dry flaky texture compared to coconut oil, and is mainly used in the U.S. in processed foods and for soap-making and moisturizing. The orange pulp of the palm fruit surrounding the seed is used to extract red palm oil, which contains many other beneficial nutrients but almost no MCTs. A few other less available natural oils contain MCTs, such as babassu oil (55 percent MCTs) and ucuhuba butter (13 percent MCTs).

In addition to human milk, the full-fat milk of other mammals, such as goats, cows, and sheep, contains MCTs, as do butters, creams, full-fat yogurts, kefirs, and cheeses made from these milks. Most commercial infant formulas worldwide contain coconut and/or palm-kernel along with soybean and other oils to try to mimic the fats in human breast milk. Many formulas also contain MCTs, particularly those made for premature newborns, as well as children and adults with fat-malabsorption disorders. Some commercial fitness shakes and nutritional drinks for elders contain MCTs. Vitamins and medications are incorporated into MCT oil to promote better absorption. See table 5.1 for a list of some foods containing MCTs.

FOODS WITH MEDIUM-CHAIN AND SHORT-CHAIN FATTY ACIDS

Note: The following commonly eaten fats and oils contain no short- and medium-chain fatty acids: Canola, cod liver, corn, fish, flaxseed, olive, peanut, safflower, soybean, and sunflower oils. Some margarines and mayonnaises contain medium-chain triglycerides.

FATS AND OILS	Grams per 0.5 oz (~ 3 tsp/15 ml)
Medium-chain triglyceride oil	14.0
Coconut oil	8.3
Babassu oil	7.7
Palm kernel oil	7.5
Goat butter	2.4
Ucuhuba butter	1.8
Cow butter	1.6
Nutmeg butter	0.4
Shea nut butter	0.24
Lard	0.04
CREAM AND CHEESE	Grams per oz (~6 tsp/30 ml)
Goat cheese	2.0
Feta cheese	1.4
Cream (heavy)	1.3
Cream cheese	1.0
American cheese	0.85
Mozzarella	0.78
Milks and Cottage Cheese	Grams per 8 oz (~1 cup/240 ml)
Goat milk	1.7
Infant formula	1.0
Cow milk (full-fat)	0.9
Human breast milk	0.78
Cottage cheese	0.78

Note: Fiber is part of total carbohydrate (carb)
Source: USDA FoodData Central - https://fdc.nal.usda.gov/

TABLE 5.1. Foods with medium-chain and short-chain fatty acids. Medium-chain and short-chain fatty acids are ketogenic.

COCONUT OIL

Coconut Oil Is Not Animal Fat!

Coconut oil has an enticing fragrance and is a soft white creamy solid at room temperature and below, and a clear liquid above room temperature.

Coconut oil has gotten a bad rap for decades because it is high in saturated fat, though no study has ever proven that coconut oil directly causes cardiovascular disease (AHA 2017). More than 70 percent of the saturated fats in coconut oil are MCTs. Saturated fats are often equated to solid fat, but MCT oil is 100 percent saturated fat and is liquid above 23°F (−5°C). Coconut oil melts at 76°F (24.4°C), well below body temperature, and contains about 11 percent long-chain saturated fats, in the same range as other plant oils like soybean (15 percent), corn (12 percent), sunflower (10 percent), and olive oil (13 percent). Animal fats, like beef tallow and lard, are less than half saturated fat (37 to 44 percent), almost entirely long-chain saturated fatty acids with less than 1 percent MCTs. Even though animal fats have much less total saturated fat than coconut oil, lard melts at about 86°F (30°C) and beef tallow at more than 100°F (38°C). The MCT content most likely explains the difference.

From 1911 until about 2007, Crisco Oil, a hydrogenated shelf-stable vegetable oil, contained substantial trans fat and was used for cooking in a great many American households, mainly replacing lard. The pre-2007 formulation of Crisco had a melting point between 117°F and 119°F (47°C and 48°C).

Around 1984, the soybean oil industry, together with the Center for Science in the Public Interest (CSPI), launched a media-and-letter-writing campaign targeting competing "artery-clogging" saturated fats. CSPI declared hydrogenated oils "healthy," which we now know is not accurate, and promoted replacement of coconut oil, lard, beef tallow, and butter with partially hydrogenated soybean oil to major fast-food chains and movie theaters. Coconut oil became known as "the artery-clogging fat" and, unfortunately, this undeserved nickname stuck (Fife 2005). Trans fats were slowly phased out by the FDA in the U.S. between 2013 and 2018 due to their harmful effects on the heart, leading to an estimated 30,000 heart attacks in the United States annually. As it turns out, shortenings like Crisco and margarines with trans fats were the true "artery-clogging fats." There is more extensive discussion of trans fats in chapters 4 and 9.

Coconut Oil Has Many Special Properties That Support Health

The misconception that coconut oil has no health benefits has been perpetuated for decades by the American Heart Association (AHA) and promoted by the media. However, hundreds of studies supporting its health benefits can be found by conducting a simple search on PubMed.gov. Detractors of coconut oil tend to ignore studies that are favorable to coconut oil. For example, in an early observational study of the entire adult population of a Polynesian island who consumed 60 percent of total calories as coconut, including 20 percent as coconut oil, there was no evidence of heart disease, and rates of obesity and high blood pressure were very low (Prior 1981). This should perhaps merit as much attention as the olive oil–based Mediterranean diet and could provide some reassurance that virgin coconut oil is a healthy oil.

Throughout human evolution, billions of humans in tropical parts of the world have eaten coconut meat, which is about 35 percent oil, its water at the center, and milk pressed out of the meat. Coconut is often part of the diet of domesticated animals raised where coconuts are plentiful. The coconut palm is called the "tree of life" for many reasons: the tree provides food and drink; coconut sugar is made from sap tapped from the blossoms; the trunk and fronds provide wood and roofing for shelter; and parts of the shell are used to make mulch and activated charcoal (Adkins 2010).

Coconut oil does not contain cholesterol, and virgin coconut oil (VCO) raises desirable HDL-cholesterol without increasing LDL. Like all other hydrogenated fats, hydrogenated coconut oil will increase total and LDL cholesterol. Early studies of the effects of coconut oil on cholesterol levels in animals and humans used hydrogenated or highly processed coconut oil. However, four studies conducted between 2009 and 2018 with a total of 354 participants found that virgin coconut oil increased desirable

HDL-cholesterol (Forouhi 2018) and either decreased or did not significantly change LDL-cholesterol levels. Higher total cholesterol levels were attributable to higher HDL-cholesterol levels (Assunção 2009; Khaw 2018; Oliveira-de-Lira 2018; Vijayakumar 2016).

Virgin coconut oil is rich in phenolic compounds such as caffeic acid, p-coumaric acid, ferulic acid, methyl catechin, dihydrokaempferol, gallic acid, quercetin, and myricetin glycoside, which have anti-inflammatory and antioxidant properties that could be beneficial to healthy brain aging and Alzheimer's prevention (Chatterjee 2020). Studies have shown that the antioxidant polyphenols and fatty acids in coconut oil can repair the skin barrier, reduce inflammation, protect skin exposed to UVB radiation, promote wound healing, reduce skin aging related to environmental effects, and kill skin pathogens such as Staphylococcus aureus, S. epidermidis, and Propionibacterium acne (Lin 2018). Oral application of whole coconut oil through the practice of oil pulling has been demonstrated to reduce gingivitis (Peedikayil 2015; Thaweboon 2011).

Lauric acid (C12:0) makes up about 50 percent of the fats in coconut oil and about 7 percent of the fats in human breast milk, providing antiviral protection to the human newborn (Dodge 1991; Hamosh 1998). Lauric acid and, to some degree, capric acid (C10:0) have known antimicrobial effects to a variety of pathogenic bacteria, viruses, fungi, and protozoa, including herpes viruses, candida, chlamydia, Lyme (Borrelia burgdorferi), dental pathogens, and many other organisms (Kabara 1972; Thormar 1987). There are numerous commercial uses for C12:0 and its monoglyceride monolaurin, which is also found in coconut oil and released from the triglycerides when coconut oil is eaten. Lauric acid and monolaurin are used as antimicrobial agents in animal feed and for other medical and veterinary applications. Other derivatives of lauric acid, such as sodium lauryl sulfate, are used in antiviral/antibacterial sprays and wipes, and in oral, hair, and skin-care products.

We have already discussed the ketogenic nature of the MCTs in coconut oil. The most ketogenic MCTs in coconut oil, caproic acid (C6:0) and caprylic acid (C8:0), make up only about 0.5 percent and 6.8 percent, respectively, of the fats in coconut oil (https://fdc.nal.usda.gov). Therefore, much more coconut oil than MCT oil would be required if the only goal were to consume those specific fatty acids. Capric acid (C10:0) and lauric acid (C12:0) are metabolized much more slowly and are not as ketogenic in the liver as C6:0 and C8:0. However, after coconut oil is consumed, the level of C12:0 remains much more elevated for much longer than the other medium-chain fatty acids. Nonaka and others reported that C8:0, C10:0, and C12:0 all potently stimulate ketone production in cultured astrocytes (astrocytes nourish neurons) and, if confirmed, the prolonged elevation of C12:0 in the blood could allow more time for this ketogenic process to occur in brain astrocytes (Nonaka 2016). A direct ketogenic effect of C12:0 in the brain could explain how someone with Alzheimer's, like my husband Steve and many others, could improve so much simply from taking coconut oil.

A large, respected Alzheimer's research group in Sydney, Australia, at Macquarie University headed by Dr. Ralph Martins published extensive, highly referenced reviews in 2015 and updated them in 2020, examining the potential for the fatty acids and other compounds in virgin coconut oil to ameliorate and possibly prevent Alzheimer's. The review includes numerous studies of virgin coconut oil related to ketogenic MCTs, antioxidant, and anti-inflammatory cytokinin and polyphenolic compounds, and compounds that inhibit formation of beta amyloid plaques and protect mitochondria from damage related to beta amyloid. These studies also discuss the evidence that virgin coconut oil may be beneficial in the treatment of obesity, dyslipidemia, elevated LDL, insulin resistance, and hypertension, which are known risk factors for heart disease, type 2 diabetes, and Alzheimer's (Chatterjee 2020; Fernando 2015).

The same Alzheimer's research group at Macquarie also conducted a promising pilot study of a high lauric acid MCT oil (see side box).

Macquarie University Alzheimer's Research Group Studies Lauric Acid and MCT Oil

An Alzheimer's research group at Macquarie University in Sydney, Australia, led by Ralph Martins, PhD, studies many facets of Alzheimer's pathology, biomarkers, and treatments. At the Alzheimer's Association International Conference 2021 (AAIC 2021), the group reported clinical trial results of a high-lauric-acid MCT oil:

- Ketone levels were measured in twenty healthy adults ages 50 to 77, who were given a high lauric acid MCT oil (40 percent caprylic acid (C8:0), 28 percent capric acid (C10:0), 32 percent lauric acid (C12:0) beginning with 5 ml three times daily (15 ml/day total) and increased weekly by that amount for seven weeks to 30 ml three times per day (total 90 ml, equivalent to six tablespoons, per day). At baseline and weekly, measurements were taken and blood drawn. The levels of ketones increased proportionately with each increase in high lauric acid MCT oil, and there were no significant changes in body mass index (BMI), fasting triglycerides, total, LDL cholesterol, and HDL cholesterol (Hillenbrandt 2021).

- Nineteen participants also had cognitive and motor testing at baseline, midway, and final appointments using the National Institutes of Health (NIH) Executive Abilities: Measures and Instruments for Neurobehavioral Evaluation and Research (EXAMINER). Despite lack of diagnosed memory issues, they showed improvements in working memory, inhibitory processing, problem-solving, and motor control (Hillebrandt 2021).

- The high lauric acid MCT oil used in this study is quite inexpensive, and an identical product is available in the United States as Carrington Farms Liquid Coconut Cooking Oil. I like the idea of a high-lauric-acid MCT oil because of the antimicrobial properties of lauric acid and its potential to stimulate ketone production in astrocytes (Nonaka 2016), as discussed elsewhere in this section.

Lauric acid also appears to have cancer cell–killing properties. Dr. Rosamaria Lappano and her associates published study results demonstrating that lauric acid caused the death (called apoptosis) of breast and endometrial cell cancers and found metabolic and gene expression changes in the cells to explain this phenomenon. Other studies have reported similar results for colon cancer. A study of women with breast cancer who ate coconut oil during chemotherapy experienced improved "global quality of life" (Lappano 2017; Fauser 2013; Law 2014).

The medium-chain triglyceride capric acid (C10:0) has its own special properties. In addition to the antimicrobial effects, it has anticonvulsant effects and stimulates mitochondria to multiply, which means more ATP available to carry out the cell's work (Augustin 2018; Schoeler 2021). A high C10:0 medical food has been developed (K. Vita) for use in epilepsy to take advantage of the special properties of C10:0.

I recommend reading a comprehensive review of the biochemistry of the fats in coconut oil and lauric acid, in particular by Fabian Dayrit, PhD, a biochemist in the Philippines who has studied coconut oil extensively (Dayrit 2015)

A Diet with Coconut Oil Improves Cognition in People with Alzheimer's

A group in Spain studied forty-four people with various stages of Alzheimer's whose diet was changed to a Mediterranean diet for twenty-one days, half with and half without coconut oil 20 ml added to meals twice per day (total 40 ml). The people who had coconut oil in their meals experienced cognitive improvement in the orientation and language-construction areas of the Mini-Mental Status Exam, compared to those who did not (de la Rubia Ortí 2018).

SATURATED FAT MAY NOT BE SO BAD AFTER ALL

Is saturated fat as bad as its reputation? Saturated fat is demonized mainly because it is purported to increase LDL-cholesterol, and high levels of LDL-cholesterol have been linked to higher risk of cardiovascular disease. It is uncertain whether LDL-cholesterol causes heart disease or is merely at the scene of the crime. It is conceivable that other conditions present in cardiovascular diseases, such as inflammation and high blood pressure, promote elevation of LDL-cholesterol, since LDL-cholesterol is part of the patch used to repair damaged artery walls. Also, oxidized cholesterol in the artery wall (Nielsen 1999) and LDL particle size (Forouhi 2018) may be more important to heart disease risk.

While a high intake of long-chain saturated fat can increase LDL-cholesterol, medium-chain triglyceride oil—which is 100 percent saturated fat—does not (Fortier 2021).

Saturated fat is critical for our very survival. Even if you do not eat saturated fat, your body and brain will make it. There is little connection between the types of fats and saturated fats we consume in the diet and blood levels of saturated fat (Volk 2014). Cells, including brain cells, store fat in vesicles and can shorten, elongate, and make new fatty acids that are saturated or unsaturated to provide whatever fatty acids are needed, wherever they are needed. The only exceptions are the essential omega-3 and omega-6 fatty acids, which we must get in our diet.

Saturated fatty acids (SFAs) are a major component (about 22 to 26 percent) of our adipose tissue, which is a source of fuel, heat, and insulation for our organs as well as hormones and signaling molecules. Like other fatty acids, glucose, and ketones, SFAs can drive the TCA cycle to make ATP and can be converted to ketones during fasting or on a ketogenic diet. SFAs are a critical component of lung surfactants that keep alveoli (air sacs) open. Long-chain SFAs do not cross the blood–brain barrier but are made in the brain, where they are a major component of gray matter, white matter, and myelin and are incorporated into more complex lipids (Rioux 2007; Legrand 2010). In other words, saturated fat is necessary and important to our health, and our body and brain will use other fatty acids to make SFAs in whatever tissues need them.

As mentioned in chapter 4, the enormous long-term PURE Study reported that sugar, but not fat or saturated fat, increased the risk of premature death. The authors also reported that higher fat and saturated fat intake did not increase risk of serious cardiac events or deaths, and higher intakes of saturated fat lowered the risk of stroke (Dehghan 2017). Also, none of the IHME nutrition risk factors that accounted for 28 million of 56 million deaths in 2017 were a diet high in fat or saturated fat (Our World in Data 2017).

The AHA position on coconut oil and cholesterol is confusing. Their recommendation to avoid coconut oil ignores the minimal overlap in fatty acid composition between coconut oil and animal fat. In a 2017 Presidential Advisory, the AHA admitted that "Clinical trials that compared direct effects on cardiovascular disease of coconut oil and other dietary oils have not been reported" (Sacks 2017). In a 2020 scientific report, the AHA further admitted that studies conducted in several countries failed to show any impact of dietary cholesterol on cardiovascular disease. Confusingly, in the same report, the AHA committee also advised avoiding or limiting foods that are high in cholesterol because they are the same types of foods that are high in saturated fat, like animal fat and eggs.

Coconut oil contains no cholesterol and no more long-chain saturated fat than other common plant oils, and therefore should not be on the "bad-for-you" foods list put out by the WHO, AHA, and other organizations, which instead promote oils that are high in polyunsaturated fatty acids (PUFA) without providing guidance on how much is too much (Carson 2020). We will discuss the potential problems of consuming too much omega-6 fatty acids, like linoleic acid (a PUFA), in chapter 9.

MEDIUM-CHAIN TRIGLYCERIDE (MCT) OIL

MCT oil is a man-made product usually extracted from coconut or palm-kernel oil and was first produced and studied around the late

1950s. MCT oil is a clear, colorless, odorless oil, and it can be found in liquid and powder forms as well as with organic certification. Coconut oil is the richest natural source of MCTs at 60 percent, with palm-kernel oil a close second at about 54 percent. MCT oil is made by separating the fatty acids through distillation or another extraction process from the oil in coconut meat, or from the white kernel in the center of the palm fruit. See table 5.2 on the structure and names of the MCTs. MCT oil can contain caprylic (C8:0) triglyceride alone, in various ratios with capric acid (C10:0), and sometimes with a significant proportion of lauric acid (C12:0). Caproic acid (C6:0) is very ketogenic but quite bitter, and is usually just a tiny percent of MCT oil products. MCT oil increases blood ketone levels regardless of what else someone eats. Many good brands of MCT oil as liquid, as powder, in capsules, and as ingredients in foods are available in grocery stores, health-food stores, and online, including organic-certified MCT oil.

MCT oil is easily absorbed from the digestive system and enhances absorption of other substances such as calcium, magnesium, and amino acids. MCT oil has been used medically since the late 1960s for premature infants with immature bowel and for children and adults with

MEDIUM-CHAIN FATTY ACIDS

ABBREVIATION # CARBON ATOMS IN CHAIN	CHEMICAL STRUCTURE	COMMON NAMES
C6:0	$CH_3(CH_2)_4COOH$	caproic acid hexanoic acid
C8:0	$CH_3(CH_2)_6COOH$	caprylic acid octanoic acid
C10:0	$CH_3(CH_2)_8COOH$	capric acid decanoic acid
C12:0	$CH_3(CH_2)_{10}COOH$	lauric acid dodecanoic acid

Source: USDA FoodData Central - https://fdc.nal.usda.gov/

TABLE 5.2. Medium-chain fatty acids, chemical structure, and abbreviated and common names.

impaired fat metabolism and malabsorption syndromes, such as biliary cirrhosis, Crohn's disease, regional enteritis, celiac disease, or pancreatitis. MCT oil has also been used for fifty years (Huttenlocher 1971) in a less-restrictive ketogenic diet for epilepsy. In the "MCT-modified ketogenic diet," MCT oil ranges from 30 to 60 percent of total daily calories. Smaller amounts of MCT and coconut oil are used in other versions of the diet to help support and maintain ketosis.

Biochemistry 102: Triglycerides and Fatty Acids

Most of the fats in natural oils are in the form of triglycerides but also contain monoglycerides, diglycerides, and free fatty acids. A triglyceride consists of a glycerol backbone with three fatty acids in various combinations attached (see figure 5.4). Fatty acids are composed of a chain of carbon atoms attached to each other and to hydrogen and oxygen atoms by single bonds (like a magnetic force) or stronger double bonds. The carbon chain length and the presence or absence of, and numbers of, double bonds greatly influence physical properties such as the melting and smoke points and the biological activity of an individual fatty acid. See figure 5.5 and another side box for more on the classification of fatty acids.

Classification of Fatty Acids by Chain Length and Saturation (see figure 5)

Short-chain fatty acids have fewer than six carbons, are produced from fermentation of undigestible food such as fiber or by bacteria in the human gut, and are ketogenic. Medium-chain fatty acids (MCFAs) have six to twelve carbon atoms in the chain and are also ketogenic

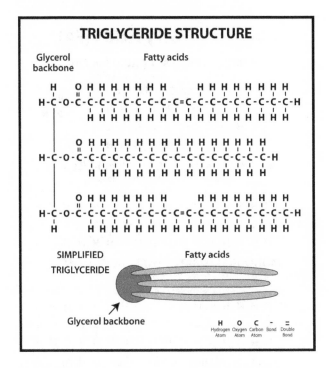

FIGURE 5.4. Triglyceride structure. A triglyceride consists of three fatty acids attached to a glycerol backbone. The fatty acids can be different, and the position of the fatty acids (sn-1, sn-2, sn-3) can affect the biological function of the triglyceride.

(see example of a medium-chain fatty acid in figure 5.6). All short- and medium-chain fatty acids are fully saturated, meaning that all docking sites that hydrogen atoms can occupy are occupied, and there are no double bonds. Long-chain fatty acids (LCFAs) have fourteen or more carbons in the chain, and very long-chain fatty acids have twenty-two or more carbons. LCFAs can be saturated, monounsaturated, or polyunsaturated. In an "unsaturated" fatty acid, one or more stronger double bonds form between two carbons, replacing two hydrogen atoms. A monounsaturated fatty acid has one double bond, and a polyunsaturated fatty acid has two or more double bonds. There are tiny amounts of odd-numbered fatty acids such as C7:0 in some foods, like milk fat.

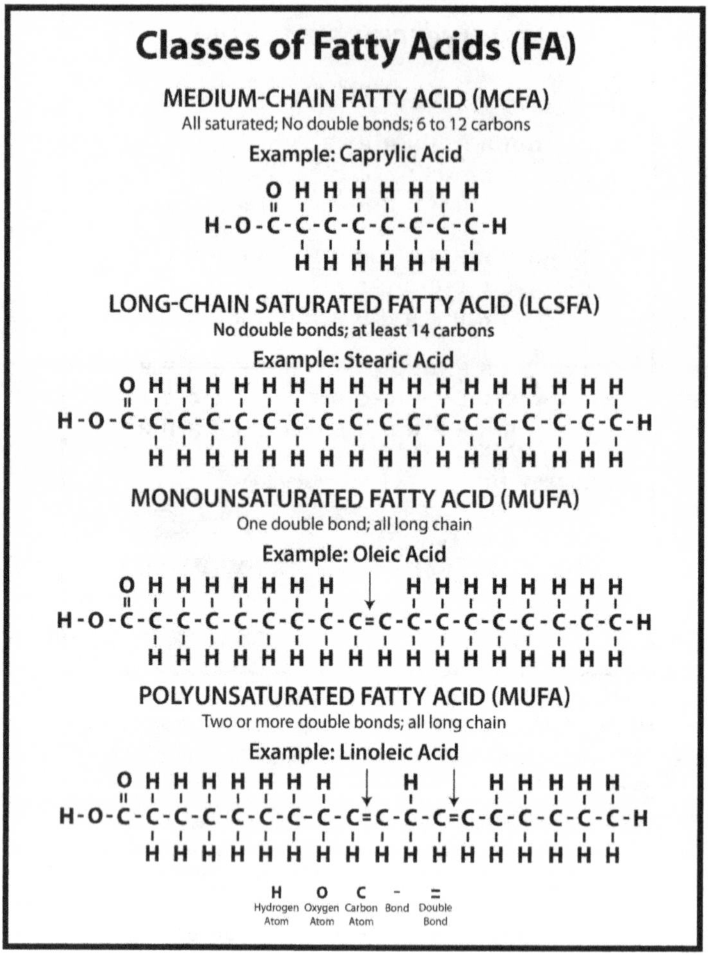

FIGURE 5.5. Classification of fatty acids by chain length and saturation. Fatty acids can be classified by the number of carbons in the chain and by whether they are saturated (no double bonds), monounsaturated (one double bond), or polyunsaturated (two or more double bonds).

There are many differences between MCTs and the long-chain triglycerides (LCTs) that account for their efficiency in conversion to fuel for immediate use by the brain, muscles, and other organs with related health advantages. During digestion, LCTs are broken apart into long-chain fatty acids (LCFAs) and then absorbed and packaged into chylomicrons that enter the general bloodstream. LCFAs are not converted to

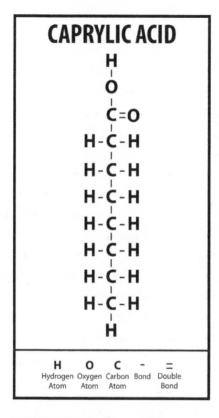

FIGURE 5.6. Caprylic acid, a medium-chain triglyceride with eight carbons.

ketones unless a person is fasting or eating a high-fat, low-carbohydrate ketogenic diet. Unlike LCTs, MCTs do not require digestive enzymes to be broken down into medium-chain fatty acids (MCFAs) and are absorbed from the bowel into the portal vein and taken directly to the liver. MCFAs are partly converted in the liver to ketones, which can be taken up by the brain and most other organs, except the liver, to use as fuel to make ATP (see figure 5.7). The remaining MCFAs are released into the bloodstream and used immediately as energy. MCFAs do not require carnitine to cross the mitochondrial membrane. MCFAs can be used in mitochondria of the brain and other tissues to produce acetyl-CoA, which can feed the TCA cycle to make ATP and can be used to make ketones or, alternatively, to build long-chain fatty acids. MCTs provide about 8.3 kcals per gram compared with 9.0 kcals for LCTs and are not usually stored as fat. For these reasons, MCTs are useful for people who have increased energy needs, such as those recovering from surgery, healing from severe injuries or burns, or dealing with cancer. MCTs could also be useful to those who want to enhance their athletic performance, as well as the elderly or frail who, very literally, wish to have more energy.

In addition, compared to LCTs, MCTs are relatively thermogenic, meaning that they increase the metabolic rate and therefore more calories are burned over twenty-four hours. Studies in animals and people have shown that when equivalent amounts of either MCTs or LCTs are added to the diet, or when a high-fat diet rich in MCTs is eaten compared to a low-fat diet, significantly less fat is deposited by those consuming the diet with MCT oil. MCTs appear to suppress appetite, resulting in fewer calories consumed. The net result is that a diet rich in MCTs could be useful as a weight-loss or weight-maintenance strategy, if MCTs are substituted for other fats and carbohydrates in the diet and are not simply added to the existing diet.

In recent years, MCT oil and coconut oil have come into popular use for people with Alzheimer's disease, other dementias, Parkinson's disease, ALS, and other neurodegenerative diseases in which there is decreased glucose metabolism in the affected areas of the brain and/or peripheral nervous system. Nutritional ketosis through consumption of MCTs could effectively bypass the problem of insulin resistance and improve function and survival of the affected cells.

Relatively small- to medium-size studies of MCT oil in Alzheimer's disease and mild cognitive impairment (MCI), which can precede Alzheimer's, have shown improved memory and cognitive performance, and that MCT oil can help fill in the brain-energy gap as discussed in chapter 2 (Courchesne-Loyer 2016; Croteau 2018). In the larger randomized controlled BENEFIC Trial, sixty-five people with mild cognitive impairment (MCI) were given a supplement with 1 tablespoon (15 ml) of MCT oil (versus

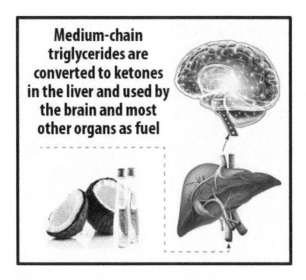

Medium-chain triglycerides are converted to ketones in the liver and used by the brain and most other organs as fuel

FIGURE 5.7. Medium-chain triglycerides (MCTs) are partly converted to ketones in the liver, which are used by the brain and most other organs as fuel, except in the liver where they are produced.

sunflower oil in controls) twice per day with meals for six months. The people taking MCT oil experienced improvement in three of five cognitive domains—memory, executive function, and attention (Fortier 2021). Improvement in information-processing speed from taking MCT oil correlated with higher ketone levels in white-matter nerve tracts in the related brain network, called the "dorsal attention network." This finding implies that ketones could help maintain the quality of myelin, the insulation that protects nerves, in white matter (Roy 2020).

In addition, MCT oil has been shown to protect cognition in people with brittle type 1 insulin-dependent diabetes during severe hypoglycemic episodes (Page 2009). This and other MCT oil studies for cognition are detailed in other chapters throughout the book.

BEGIN MCT OIL AND COCONUT OIL SLOWLY

If you have not used MCT oil, coconut oil, or palm-kernel oil before, and especially if you have been eating a low-fat diet or no longer have a gallbladder, adding oils to the diet too quickly can have intestinal consequences, such as diarrhea (sometimes explosive), gassiness and bloating, and possibly nausea and vomiting. Begin coconut or MCT oil slowly with one-half to one teaspoon (2.5 to 5 grams) two or three times a day with food, or less if you find you are overly sensitive. If you can tolerate this amount without a problem, increase by this same amount every two to three days as tolerated. If there is some diarrhea, back off to the previous level, wait for at least a few days, and increase more gradually.

Adding coconut oil and/or MCT oil to meals and snacks can provide a baseline level of ketones to build on with other ketogenic strategies like overnight fasting, exercise, caffeine, and exogenous ketone supplements.

Adding MCT Oil to the Diet Gets to Ketosis Sooner and Maintains Higher Levels than Ketogenic Diet Alone

Harvey and group studied the effect of adding 30 ml three times per day of medium-chain triglyceride (MCT) oil (C8:0/C10:0 in a 65/35 ratio) versus long-chain triglyceride (LCT) oil as sunflower oil to a ketogenic diet with a 4:1 ratio of fat grams to combined carbohydrate and protein grams for twenty days. Twelve people taking MCT oil and eleven taking LCT oil completed the study. Compared to LCT oil, the participants taking MCT oil had higher betahydroxybutyrate (BHB) levels on the first day and arrived at the cutoff for nutritional ketosis of BHB level >0.5 mm/L on average two days sooner (see figure 5.8). By day 9, BHB levels were at least double for the MCT group compared to the LCT group. Also, higher BHB levels in both groups correlated strongly with lower blood-glucose levels. Unexpectedly,

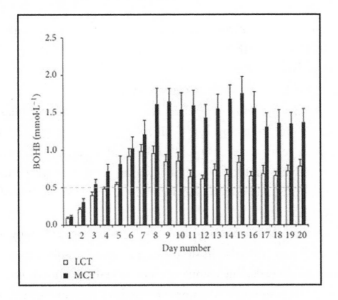

FIGURE 5.8. MCT oil shortens time to ketosis and increases ketone levels higher than ketogenic diet alone. Open access article permission under Creative Commons Attribution License: Harvey CJ DC, GM Schofield, M Williden, JA McQuillan. "The effect of medium chain triglycerides on time to nutritional ketosis and symptoms of keto-induction in healthy adults: A randomized-controlled clinical trial." J Nutr Metab (2018):2630565.

symptom scores were higher for the LCT oil than the MCT oil groups (Harvey 2018). Blood BHB levels correlate strongly with the percent of energy provided by ketones in the brain on ketones PET studies (Cunnane 2020).

WHAT TYPES OF MCT FOODS ARE ON THE MARKET?

In addition to MCT oils and powders with various combinations of medium-chain fatty acids, many foods also contain MCTs, including instant coffees, creamers, chocolates, cookies, protein bars, shakes, margarines, and shortenings. Some companies market "keto" flour, often a combination of coconut flour and almond flour, to make pan-cakes, waffles, and other bread-like foods. At the Metabolic Health Summit in January 2020, I counted more than forty companies with ketogenic foods, most of which contained MCT oil.

The Nisshin OilliO Group, Ltd., in Japan (see Resources) has been researching and producing MCT oil for about fifty years, and it has developed several tasty easy-to-swallow-and-digest MCT products for the elderly population. These include small sachets with a creamy MCT gel, called Memorion, and Ene puddings with a variety of fruit and savory flavors.

Dr. Schär (see Resources) is a leading gluten-free company with a global reach and expertise in developing innovative solutions for special nutritional needs. The company markets ketogenic foods under the brand name Kanso and has a product portfolio of modulars and foods enhanced by MCTs such as creamy cocoa bars, cocoa biscuits, tomato, champignon, chocolate spreads, and an MCT fiber drink. Dr. Schär also makes foods, powders, and formulas intended for use in the keto-genic diet for specific medical purposes, such as drug-resistant epilepsy or rare enzyme disorders such as glucose transporter protein 1 (GLUT 1) deficiency syndrome and pyruvate dehydrogenase (PDH) deficiency.

The sky is the limit on how MCT and coconut oils and powders can be used in foods prepared at home and in commercially available products. For more information on studies and reviews related to ke-tones, coconut oil, and MCT oil, please see Scientific Research Articles at https://coconutketones.com.

MIXING COCONUT AND MCT OIL

About two months after starting Steve on coconut oil, after receiving results of his ketone levels from Dr. Veech, I began to mix MCT oil and coconut oil. After Steve took coconut oil in the morning, his ke-tone levels peaked at about three hours and were nearly gone after eight to nine hours, just before dinner time. Steve's ketone levels with just MCT oil were higher and peaked at about ninety minutes but were gone within three hours. I reasoned that a mixture of MCT and co-coconut oils would result in steadier, higher, longer-lasting ketone levels overall and, by giving him this mixture three or four times a day, ketones would always be circulating and available to his brain.

Why Not Use Just MCT Oil?

If you use just MCT oil alone several times a day, the ketone levels may fluctuate up and down more than with coconut oil alone or with a mixture of coconut and MCT oils. Also, some fatty acids in whole coconut oil that could be beneficial are not found in standard MCT oil. As previously mentioned, the lauric acid in coconut oil kills certain types of viruses, such as those that cause fever blisters. Several groups of researchers have found the presence of the DNA of herpes simplex virus type 1, which causes fever blisters, in the beta-amyloid plaques in the brains of people with Alzheimer's, especially those with the ApoE4 gene like my husband Steve (Itzhaki 2016). Taking coconut oil seemed to be helpful in this way for Steve, who was constantly fighting fever blisters, sometimes for several weeks at a time, and had less severe and much less frequent outbreaks, with just four episodes over six years. These fever-blister outbreaks coincided with other infections and set-backs, adding more weight to the idea that this virus may have contrib-uted to Alzheimer's disease progression, at least for Steve.

Why Not Use Just Coconut Oil?

Many people have reported to me that they have seen improvements in their loved ones with Alzheimer's using just coconut oil. Steve had a dramatic improvement using just coconut oil for the first two months. Adding MCT oil to coconut oil would achieve higher ketone levels. In the Axona (MCT oil) studies, people with higher levels tended to have more improvement in cognitive function. Higher blood levels of ke-tones also correlate strongly with higher uptake of ketones in the brain on ketone PET imaging studies (Cunnane 2020). Only part of MCT oil is converted to ketones, so the remaining medium-chain fatty acids might also be used by neurons (and other tissues) as an alternative fuel. So, the more MCT oil one can tolerate, the more ketones and MCTs will be available to the brain. We need to learn much more about exactly what medium-chain fatty acids do.

Mixing MCT and coconut oil in a four-to-three ratio reduces the long-chain saturated fatty acids to well below 10 percent of the total fat. Recent studies are finding less and less evidence that saturated fat and cholesterol are the culprits in heart disease; but for those who are still worried about the possible health issues related to saturated fats, this mixture of MCT and coconut oil offers an alternative to using an equivalent amount of just coconut oil. Another alternative is to use a high-lauric-acid MCT oil from which all the long-chain fatty acids have been removed.

A MIXTURE OF MCT AND COCONUT OIL IS A VERSATILE ADDITION TO FOODS

A mixture of coconut and MCT oil that is at least half MCT oil stays liquid at room temperature and can safely be stored at room temperature. Typical shelf life for coconut oil and for MCT oil is at least two years, and the oil rarely becomes rancid. This oil mixture is clear, light, creamy, tasteless, and nearly odorless and works well when added to many different foods, hot, warm, and cold, unlike coconut oil which chunks when added to cold foods. The oil mixture can be used to cook on the stove at low to low-medium heat and in the oven when mixed into foods at up to 350°F (177°C). The mixture can be added to coffee, tea, milk, smoothies, soup, stew, cottage cheese, or ricotta, or drizzled on vegetables or salad. Like coconut oil and MCT oil separately, the oil mixture may also have a laxative effect. Therefore, it is a good idea to start with a small amount, such as ½ to 1 level teaspoon with food once or twice a day, and increase every two or three days as tolerated to lessen the chances of intestinal distress. If a problem occurs, cut back to the previous level for one or two weeks before trying to increase again, and do so more gradually.

Are There Any Commercially Prepared Mixtures of MCT and Coconut Oil on the Market?

In 2017, the Pruvit company approached me about producing the 4:3 mixture of MCT and coconut oil that helped Steve so much. In my homemade formulation for Steve, I also added soy lecithin to provide Steve with important brain phospholipids, specifically phosphatidylcholine. My formulation for Pruvit called MCT//143 is a proprietary blend of organic virgin coconut oil, medium-chain triglycerides (MCTs) from virgin coconut oil, and pure concentrated phosphatidylcholine extracted from lecithin. This formula contains more than 85 percent medium-chain triglycerides (C6:0 through C12:0) and less than 10 percent long-chain saturated fats.

Exogenous Ketone Supplements

Endogenous ketones are ketones produced naturally inside the body, and exogenous ketones are those that originate outside the body (see figure 5.9). When you fast, exercise, eat a low-carbohydrate diet, or eat coconut or MCT oil, your body produces endogenous ketones. On the other hand, exogenous ketone supplements contain the ketones used by our bodies, usually betahydroxybutyrate. There are many other ketones in nature that do not have such effects in our metabolism. For example, a fad supplement called raspberry ketones was promoted for weight loss; but while it is a component of the raspberry's fragrance, it does nothing to produce ATP or affect pathways in our metabolism.

Exogenous ketone supplements first appeared on the market as ketone salts in early 2016 and, in 2021, include ketone salts, ketone esters, and hybrids of the two, some with added MCT oil. Other types of exogenous ketone supplements are available, such as buffered "free" betahydroxybutyrate, unattached to a salt or other molecule.

Exogenous supplements provide a rapid increase in ketone levels, sometimes called "instant ketosis." The ketone level usually peaks by thirty to sixty minutes after consumption, and drops steadily over

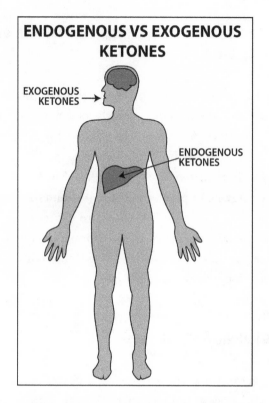

FIGURE 5.9. Endogenous ketones are produced within the body, and exogenous ketones are supplements that usually contain betahydroxybutyrate.

several hours back to baseline. In my opinion, a sustained-release form of ketone supplements could be more beneficial by providing a steadier level of ketones and could be more effective even with a lower peak level. For now, an alternative is to make up a serving or two of the ketone supplement and take sips throughout the day, or divide the total into four to six smaller doses.

Ketone Salts

Ketone salts "have not been evaluated or approved by the FDA to treat any medical condition" as of 2021. On the other hand, there is plenty of scientific evidence that raising ketones can provide alternative fuel to the brain, reduce inflammation, and burn fat. Countless people taking ketone salts have reported increased energy, endurance, focus, mental clarity, improved mood and sleep, fewer aches and pains, less hunger, and fat loss.

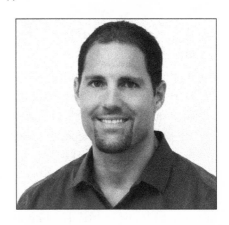

PHOTO 2. Dominic D'Agostino, PhD

Betahydroxybutyrate ketone salts were developed and tested at the University of South Florida in the labs of Dominic D'Agostino, PhD (see photo 2). Ketone salts first appeared on the scene in January 2016 from Pruvit Ventures, a U.S. multi-level marketing company, which has been the leader in increasing awareness and education on ketones and the use of ketone salts. Many other companies now market racemic ketone salts, and just a couple of companies (including Pruvit) sell exclusively non-racemic ketone salts (explained shortly). Ketone salts are "salty," as might be expected, slightly bitter, though flavoring helps, and contain various combinations of betahydroxybutyrate combined with sodium, potassium, calcium, and/or magnesium. Ketone salts are widely available online and in grocery stores, drugstores, and health-food stores with a wide range of flavors and prices. Some ketone-salts products are combined with MCT oil and/or whey protein, branched-chain amino acids like leucine, vitamins, antioxidants, and other supplements.

The natural form of betahydroxybutyrate found in the bloodstream is called D-betahydroxybutyrate (D-BHB), but there is a mirror-image form called L-betahydroxybutyrate (L-BHB) that is found mainly within mitochondria (see figure 5.10). L-BHB takes a different enzyme pathway and has a different metabolic fate than D-BHB (see figure 5.11) and does not appear to contribute as much to the production of ATP, but it may have other metabolic effects, largely unknown at present. Non-racemic BHB salts are at least 90 percent D-BHB, whereas racemic BHB salts are roughly 50/50 D-BHB and L-BHB. So there could be considerable differences in how these exogenous ketone salts are utilized in the body. Please see figure 5.10 and caption for further explanation of "non-racemic" or "racemic" mixture.

A typical suggested serving of 5 to 12 grams of D-BHB ketone salts can quickly increase BHB levels from the baseline by about 0.5 to 1.5 mmol/L or more, depending on the individual. Blood ketone testing strips measure only D-BHB at present and might underestimate the total BHB present in the blood as both the D- and L-forms.

In 2021, the Cunnane group at Sherbrooke University is moving forward with clinical trials using ketone salts and a low-carbohydrate

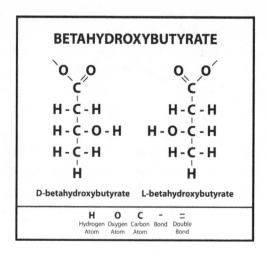

FIGURE 5.10. Betahydroxybutyrate comes in two forms: racemic versus non-racemic ketone salts. There are two mirror-image forms of betahydroxybutyrate (BHB), D-betahydroxybutyrate (D-BHB), which is the main form in the bloodstream, and L-betahydroxybutyrate (L-BHB), which is found mainly in mitochondria where ATP is produced. A "racemic mixture" of ketone salts contains about half D-BHB and half L-BHB. A "non-racemic" mixture is almost all D-BHB.

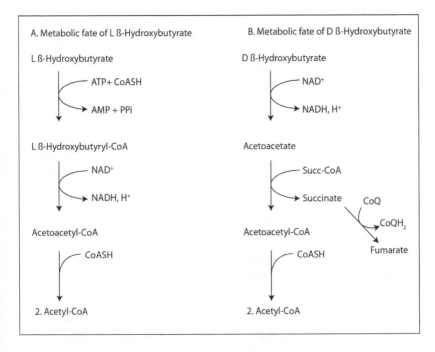

FIGURE 5.11. Metabolic fates of L-betahydroxybutyrate (A) and D-betahydroxybutyrate (B). The "metabolic fates" of the D- and L- forms of betahydroxybutyrate are different and could potentially have different effects. Reproduced with permission from Todd King.

diet and has already done preliminary pharmacokinetic studies (blood levels) of racemic versus non-racemic ketone salts. See side boxes for the results of these interesting studies (see side box on Cuenoud study, Part II) (Cuenoud 2021).

Cuenoud et al., Part 1: D-Betahydroxybutyrate Salts Outperform Racemic Salts and MCT Oil in a Head-to-Head Competition for Ketone Production

In Part 1 of this study (Cuenoud 2020), the pharmacokinetic differences (effects on blood levels) were compared for three ketogenic supplements in fifteen adults ages thirty-six to thirty-eight; eleven of the participants participated in each of the three treatments with at least a five-day washout period between treatments. The treatments were non-racemic D-betahydroxybutyrate (D-BHB) salts, racemic D+L-betahydroxybutyrate (D+L-BHB) salts, each with 12 grams of BHB combined with sodium, calcium, and magnesium, or 15 grams MCT oil (C8:0/C10:0 in 60:40 ratio) in a skim milk emulsion. Blood was drawn at 0, 15, 30, 45, 60, 120, and 240 minutes and analyzed for total ketones, total D-BHB + L-BHB, D-BHB, glucose, and insulin. Calculations were used, based on the measurements, to determine levels of L-BHB and acetoacetate.

- Blood ketones rapidly reached an average maximum of 1.2 mm/L with D-BHB, but just 0.62 mm/L for D+L-BHB and for MCT oil.

- The maximum D-BHB level was highest for D-BHB salts, then MCT oil, and lowest for D+L-BHB.

- Acetoacetate (AcAc) levels were highest for D-BHB, then D+L-BHB, and lowest for MCT oil.

- The ratio of acetoacetate to D-BHB was lowest for MCT oil (0.44) and highest for D+L-BHB salts (0.76), with D-BHB in between (0.63). MCT oil lowered the AcAc/D-BHB ratio from the baseline values while producing ketones.

- L-BHB levels increased with D+L-BHB salts (but not with D-BHB) and were still elevated at the end of four hours. This seems to indicate that L-BHB and D-BHB are utilized differently, metabolically speaking.

D-BHB salts appear to be the clear winner against equivalent amounts of D+L-BHB and MCT oil, for the potential to produce ATP. To enter the TCA cycle, glucose (through glycolysis), fatty acids, and ketones must first be converted to acetyl-CoA. D-betahydroxybutyrate converts first to the ketone acetoacetate then to acetyl-CoA. L-BHB does not convert directly to acetoacetate, and therefore may or may not contribute directly to production of ATP, but it could have other metabolic effects that are currently unknown. Of note, in another Cunnane study, ketone levels were measured after taking 20 grams of coconut oil, MCT oil alone, or in various combinations. While this small amount of coconut oil alone had little effect on total ketones, coconut oil had the highest ratio of acetoacetate to BHB (St-Pierre 2019) compared to MCT oil and any of the other combinations of oils.

The authors of the Cuenoud et al. study also state that conversion of BHB to acetoacetate requires that the cofactor nicotinamide adenine dinucleotide (NAD+) be reduced to NADH, and, therefore, a higher AcAc/D-BHB ratio might better preserve the mitochondrial NAD+/NADH ratio which has been associated with better health (Mattson 2018). This is discussed in further detail in chapter 10.

Cuenoud et al., Part 2: Ketones Also Provide Alternative Fuel for the Heart and Kidneys

In part 2 of their study (Cuenoud 2020), Cunnane and group measured ketone uptake by the brain and other organs from ketogenic supplements in a sixty-six-year-old healthy male. After fasting for six hours, the participant consumed two 12-gram servings of D-BHB salts 75 minutes and 30 minutes before imaging studies of the brain and whole-body (head to mid-thigh). The plasma ketone levels were between 0.9 and 1.2 mm/L during the first 30 minutes of scanning. There was marked increase in cerebral metabolic rate from acetoacetate as well as a marked acetoacetate uptake by the brain, heart, and kidneys, and other organs to a lesser degree. The heart normally uses glucose and fatty acids, and the kidney mainly uses fatty acids as fuel; this study confirms that these organs actively use ketones as well.

These results support the feasibility of using ketone PET imaging to evaluate organ uptake of exogenous ketones.

Other studies have demonstrated the potential for ketones to improve heart failure; help with recovery following a heart attack; improve cardiac status, cognition, and ability to overcome congestive heart failure; and improve development in children with severe multiple acyl-CoA dehydrogenase deficiency (Kadir 2020; Byrne 2020; Fischer 2019; Nielsen 2019; Van Hove 2003).

To learn more about the effects of exogenous ketone supplements on metabolic pathways related to aging and neurodegenerative diseases, please read the excellent review by Kovács, Brunner, and Ari (Kovács 2021).

How Many Ketone Salt Servings Are Safe?

The big limitation to how much ketone salts can be taken in a day are the salts themselves, and they may not be safe for everyone. Ketone salts products often have a high sodium content, which could increase blood pressure in people who are sensitive to sodium. Some people report water retention with puffy feet and hands when using ketone salts. People who take diuretics (water pills) and/or potassium supplements already have difficulty maintaining a normal balance of electrolyte and mineral levels, and taking ketone salts could upset the balance. For example, a serving of ketone salts could contain between 440 and 1600 mg of sodium. The Daily Recommended Intake of sodium for adults is 2,300 mg (about 1 teaspoon of table salt) and 1,500 mg for people with high blood pressure. Therefore, just one serving of higher-sodium ketone salts would not leave much room in the daily intake of sodium from other foods. Sodium in medications should also be factored into the total.

Some products have a high potassium content as an alternative to sodium, which could be a problem for people who take prescribed potassium or have another reason to limit potassium. To counter the issues with sodium and potassium, some companies balance them with calcium or magnesium BHB salts, which our bodies also require. Using such combinations could replace the need to take other mineral supplements.

A knowledgeable dietitian could help you factor the amounts of sodium, potassium, calcium, and magnesium into your diet. It is especially important to be mindful of the potential problems with ketone salts if you have a medical condition.

Also, the blood sugar and insulin levels tend to drop as ketone levels go up, and this is true when taking ketone salts. Blood sugar can drop rapidly, over an hour or less, and the change can be significant. Therefore, people who have high blood sugar or episodes of low blood sugar (hypoglycemia), and especially those taking insulin and/or oral diabetic medications, need to be aware that changes in blood sugar almost certainly will occur, and they should monitor blood sugar closely and work with their doctors to adjust medications, if indicated.

Ketone salts could be a problem for pregnant women, who already have a natural expansion in their plasma volume of 50 percent and tend to go into ketosis more easily than non-pregnant women. I do not recommend using ketone salts in pregnant and breastfeeding women, since the effects of acutely raising ketone levels on the developing fetus and newborn are not known.

Ketone salts could also be a problem for the elderly and for infants and children who generally need less sodium, potassium, and other minerals than young and middle-aged adults. As of 2021, ketone salts have not been studied in pregnant women, in the very elderly, or in young healthy infants and children.

More studies using ketone salts are beginning to emerge, and many others are in progress.

Ketone Salts Help Children with Rare Enzyme Deficiency

Johan Van Hove, MD, PhD, and associates treated three related children with a rare enzyme defect called multiple acyl-CoA dehydrogenase deficiency (MADD), using the sodium salt of betahydroxybutyrate. People with this defect are unable to use fat to produce energy after using up their stores of glucose. A two-year-old child, who was paralyzed and near death with a failing heart, was given the ketone salts and experienced nearly complete reversal, leading to improved cardiac status, and was walking and talking nineteen months after the treatment began. Similar improvements occurred in two other children treated with the ketone salts, beginning within days and continuing for months (Van Hove 2003). The relatively low blood levels of 0.3 mmol/L were in the same range in my husband Steve after he consumed coconut oil.

Start Ketone Salts Slowly and Increase as Tolerated

It is tempting to start with a whole serving of ketone salts in the hope of seeing maximum benefits right away, and this should be fine for healthy younger people. However, I advise that elderly people, infants, children, and people with medical conditions have their physician's approval and be closely monitored after weighing the risks and benefits. For an adult with Alzheimer's or Parkinson's, or for a child with epilepsy or autism, the benefits could outweigh the risks, so use of ketone salts is worth considering. For these special groups, I suggest starting with 1 or 2 level teaspoons once or twice per day, and, if there are no issues such as intestinal distress, consider increasing by the same amount every few days until arriving at ½ to 1 full serving once or twice per day. An alternative is to dilute a serving of ketone salts with water in a sports bottle, to take as smaller portions or sips throughout the day.

Since ketone salts can have a dehydrating effect, especially in the beginning, it is very important to get plenty of water and other clear liquids.

Ketones can suppress appetite, which is great if you need to lose weight. If you are too thin, you could add more calories to your diet with calorie-dense naturally ketogenic foods such as coconut oil, coconut milk, olive oil, butter, cheese, cream cheese, olive oil, butter, cream, avocado, and nuts.

Ketone Esters

Ketone esters are not completely new and were used decades ago in research, mainly outside of the United States. A 1961 article that was published in Russian on the synthesis of the sodium salt of betahydroxybutyrate from acetoacetate ester indicates that a ketone ester was already available at that time (Kondrashova 1961).

An ester is a molecule made by combining an acid with an alcohol. The ketones betahydroxybutyrate and acetoacetate are acids, which could be harmful to the stomach and esophagus if not properly buffered. The pure ketone acids alone are not good candidates to take orally. However, combining the ketone acid with an alcohol to make a ketone ester would essentially neutralize the harmful acid and makes it feasible to create an exogenous ketone supplement that is well tolerated when taken orally.

Biochemically speaking, the peak levels of ketones from ketone salts are dampened due to rate-limiting factors in the chemical pathways that affect how quickly they can be metabolized. By comparison, the sky is the limit for peak ketone levels with ketone esters (see side box on ketone ester versus ketone salts levels).

In 2010, two years after Steve's dramatic response to coconut oil, Dr. Richard Veech supplied us with the ketone ester he developed at the NIH, and Steve became the first person with Alzheimer's to take the ketone ester as a pilot study. One of my greatest honors was to co-author the publication of Steve's case report published in Alzheimer's and Dementia with Dr. Veech, Dr. Theodore VanItallie (see photo 4), and others (Newport, 2015). Sadly, Dr. VanItallie, who wrote

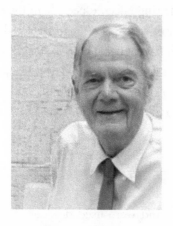

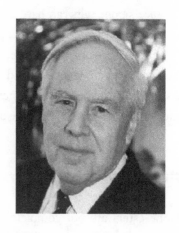

PHOTO 3. Richard L. Veech, MD, D.Phil.   PHOTO 4. Theodore B. VanItallie, MD

the foreword to my previous book, died just before his one-hundredth birthday in 2019, and Dr. Veech died a few months later in early 2020 at age eighty-four.

Dr. Veech received his medical degree at Harvard and his doctorate degree at Oxford University in the lab of the famous Hans Krebs. Dr. Veech spent his career at the National Institutes of Health near Washington, D.C., up until his passing. In the 1990s, he became laser-focused on the potential for ketones to serve as a therapeutic for Alzheimer's, Parkinson's, other dementias, multiple sclerosis, Huntington's, congestive heart failure, traumatic brain injury, and other conditions in which there is decreased glucose uptake into brain and nerve cells.

Dr. Veech met Kieran Clarke, PhD (photo 5), in 1993 when he gave a presentation at Oxford University and asked her to collaborate in studies of ketones and the heart. They learned that betahydroxybutyrate (BHB) allows the heart to pump more efficiently while using less oxygen than when it is fueled by an equivalent amount of glucose, and that BHB results in the production of nearly twice as much ATP as an equivalent amount of glucose (Sato 1995). In 2000, Veech and group reported that BHB protected survival of neurons and increased the size

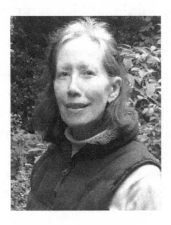

PHOTO 5. Kieran Clarke, PhD

of neurons and outgrowths of neurons when cell cultures were exposed to toxins that cause Alzheimer's and Parkinson's diseases (Kashiwaya 2000).

Veech and Clarke received a $10 million grant in 2003 from the Defense Advanced Research Projects Agency (DARPA) to develop a ketone drink that would rapidly increase ketone levels that otherwise would require many days of starvation to achieve. Veech and Clarke established a company called TDeltaS, Ltd., to administer the DARPA grants and license the patents coming out of the work, which now number twenty-five worldwide.

Dr. Veech and group tried various formulations of a betahydroxybutyrate ester and settled on (R)-3-hydroxybutyl (R)-3-hydroxybutyrate (R stands for "right," not "racemic"), which is a combination of D-BHB and D-1,3-butanediol, both in the non-racemic forms. The beauty of using 1,3-butanediol is that the molecule breaks apart to form more BHB in the liver after it is consumed. The rationale for this combination and its potential uses for Alzheimer's and other disorders is explained in a paper by Clarke and others (Soto-Mota 2020).

When the Veech ketone ester was given in food to an Alzheimer's mouse model versus a control group without ester, there was less beta amyloid plaque, fewer tangles, and less anxiety in the mice who received ketone ester (Kashiwaya 2013).

In a series of experiments in elite athletes, Clarke and collaborators reported a decrease in the breakdown of intramuscular glycogen and protein when ketone ester is taken before exercise, compared to taking carbohydrates alone. During a workout, D-BHB is anti-inflammatory and reduces exercise-induced oxidative stress that can damage cells. Post-workout, taking the ketone ester appears to expedite the resynthesis of glycogen by 60 percent and protein by double, allowing faster recovery (Cox 2016; Holdsworth 2017; Vandoorne 2017; Stubbs 2017; Clarke 2012).

Despite increasing awareness of the potential for ketones to help people with Alzheimer's, clinical studies beyond the pilot study in 2010 of my husband Steve have not yet come to fruition for Alzheimer's. However, on a positive note, the National Institute of Aging is conducting a twenty-eight-day randomized placebo-controlled trial of the ketone ester in one hundred fifty people with metabolic syndrome, which should be completed in the fall of 2023 (Avgerinos 2022). They will be taking twenty-five grams of betahydroxybutyrate three times daily. This is a big step in the right direction. The Veech ketone ester is expensive to produce, and the unusual bitter taste creates a challenge to find a suitable placebo. Dr. Veech's dream was to bring down the cost with mass-production to study the ketone ester for Alzheimer's, other neurodegenerative disorders, traumatic brain injury, radiation poisoning, and many other disorders. Even though we are awaiting study results, about 30 percent of people buying ketone esters use them for neurological and other medical disorders.

Veech's ketone ester is not yet recognized by the FDA for any clinical condition, pending studies, but is recognized by the FDA for use in healthy adults and for athletic performance. The BHB/BD ester was also found to be safe in twenty-eight-day toxicity studies of healthy adults (Soto-Mota 2019). There have been many anecdotal reports of people with Alzheimer's and other neurological disorders experiencing symptomatic improvement at lower doses (5 to 10 grams BHB) than used by athletes (usually 25 to 35 grams).

On a positive note, a study of the ketone ester reported improvement in blood-glucose control in people with type 2 diabetes (Soto-Mota 2021), a great step in the right direction. See the side box on this study for more details.

(R)-3-Hydroxybutyl (R)-3-Hydroxybutyrate Ketone Ester Improves Blood-Sugar Control in Type 2 Diabetes on a Typical Diet

Kieran Clarke, PhD, at Oxford University and group studied twenty-one people ages eighteen to seventy with type 2 diabetes using a continuous glucose monitor attached to the skin beginning one week before starting the (R)-3-hydroxybutyl (R)-3-hydroxybutyrate (BHB/ BD) ketone ester. Then, they drank 25 grams BHB/BD three times per day for four weeks, and recorded their mealtimes, sleep duration, physical activity, and any symptoms. They continued their usual medications, diet, and level of physical activity. Blood and urine were analyzed periodically for various metabolites. Mild nausea, mild headache, and mild intestinal upset were reported in <0.5 percent of doses of BHB/BD. Blood BHB levels averaged 3.1 to 3.8 mm/L. The HbA1C levels (which approximates the average blood sugar over about three months) dropped significantly from 7.7 to 7.2 percent on average. The average blood-sugar level dropped significantly from 140 ± 23 mg/dL to 133 ± 25 mg/dL (7.8 ± 1.4 mm/L to 7.4 ± 1.3 mm/L). There were no differences in blood pressure, fasting lipid profile, C-reactive protein (which screens for inflammation), and body composition. Taking BHB/ BH ester could allow type 2 diabetics to achieve better blood sugar control on their usual diet (Soto-Mota 2021). Combining BHB/BD with a low-carb diet could have an even greater impact.

A Ketone Ester Outperformed Racemic Ketone Salts BHB Levels but Lowered Blood pH More

In a Clarke and group study, when equivalent amounts of beta-hydroxybutyrate (BHB) were consumed as racemic salts versus (R)-3-hydroxybutyl (R)-3-hydroxybutyrate (BHB/BD) ketone ester, the peak ketone level was significantly higher with BHB/BD (2.8 versus 1 mmol/L on average). The BHB dose was roughly equivalent to 20 grams for someone who weighs 154 pounds or 70 kg. My concern is that the BHB/BD dose resulted in an average drop in blood pH from 7.41 to 7.31 and a drop in bicarbonate level from 23.6 to 17.0, reaching the lowest levels at about one hour after taking the drink, and with the values still not back to baseline two hours after taking the dose. The change in pH and bicarbonate could be metabolically significant and indicate that the acid load from the ester is not immediately compensated for by the body's ability to buffer it, possibly for two or more hours. Such a drop in pH did not occur with an equal amount of BHB ketone salts, remaining around 7.4, with bicarbonate no lower than 20 at any time in the study (shown in figure 3 of the report). The glucose level dropped about equally for both the ketone ester and the ketone salts from 5.7 mmol/L (102.6 mg/dL) to 4.8 mmol/L (86.4 mg/dL) one hour after the dose. Unexpectedly, the sodium and chloride levels increased more with the BHB-BD ester, which contained no sodium or potassium, than with the ketone salts; and the potassium level dropped about equally (Stubbs 2017).

Based on this information, I strongly recommend timing doses of BHB/BD at least 4 hours apart, since stacking doses too close together could potentially worsen acidosis.

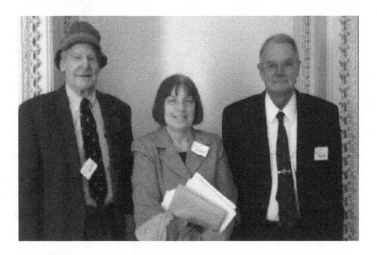

PHOTO 6. Dr. Mary Newport visits the U.S. Capitol Building in 2009 with Dr. Richard Veech (right), who invented the betahydroxybutyrate ketone ester, and Dr. George Cahill, Jr. (left), who discovered that ketones fuel the brain during starvation (Owen 1967).

How Much Ketone Ester?

How much ketone ester you might take depends on what you hope to accomplish. Competitive athletes generally take 25 to 35 grams for workouts to enhance their performance. When my husband Steve began taking the ester, what the best dose might be for someone with Alzheimer's was unknown. Dr. Veech suggested that Steve try various doses and that we aim for a peak BHB level of at least 4 mm/L or more. We found for Steve that a dose of 25 to 35 grams of the BHB/BD ketone ester rapidly raised ketone levels to the 5 to 7 mmol/L range (or higher) within thirty to sixty minutes, which is comparable to ketone levels that occur during prolonged fasting (see Steve's blood levels in figure 5.12).

For Steve, we settled on a dose that averaged 25 gm of ketone ester three times daily, which helped his symptoms tremendously. After a couple of years, it became obvious in his behavior and speech that when the BHB level was at its peak, he was much more alert; and when the level had come back down, he was less alert, and his language deteriorated. I thought a sustained-release form of the ester, even with a lower peak level, might provide more stability in his ability to function and interact. Hopefully, such a formulation will become available soon.

I am not advising people with a neurological disorder or other medical condition to take the BHB/BD or other ketone ester, pending the outcome of clinical trials. However, recognizing that people are tempted to try it, I suggest starting with a small dose, such as 2 or 3 gm BHB once or twice a day, and increase in small increments. Many people report better sleep, for example, with this tiny amount, and improvements in other symptoms with doses of 5 or 10 grams one or more times per day. Ketones as fuel will be available immediately, but effects on inflammation could take considerable time. Therefore, consistency, persistence, and patience are advised.

In early 2018, two companies launched the BHB/BD ester, marketing to athletes for performance enhancement with 25- to 32-gram serving sizes, though smaller amounts can easily be measured out. Two companies currently offer the BHB/BD ester—KetoneAid (https://ketoneaid.com) and TDeltaS (https://deltagketones.com). A third company, Juvenescence, offers a combination of the medium-chain triglyceride caproic acid (C6:0) in a ketone diester—Metabolic Switch Ketone Ester Fuel (https://juvlabs.com). Pruvit has a carbonated beverage called KetoUp that is free BHB with buffer added to reduce acidity. Many other variations on ketone ester, ketone salts, and "free" BHB products will soon appear on the market.

Issues with Consuming Ketone Esters

Taking ketone esters could be a blessing or a curse for someone who is diabetic and taking insulin or other medications. The blessing is that the ketone ester could help improve blood-glucose control. The curse is that the ketone ester, especially at higher amounts, can drop the blood-glucose level rapidly and substantially, leading to symptomatic hypoglycemia (low blood sugar) if the blood glucose

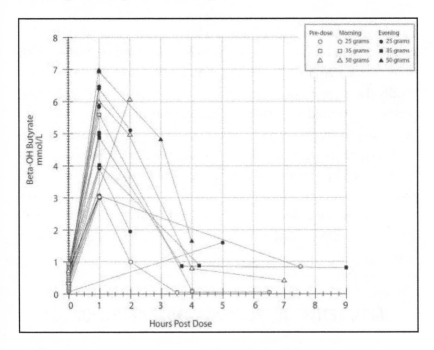

FIGURE 5.12. Steve Newport's betahydroxybutyrate levels with Precision Xtra at various doses of ketone ester.

is not monitored closely. The problem could be solved by wearing a continuous glucose monitor attached to the skin or checking blood-glucose levels frequently and by timing the dose of BHB/BD carefully in relation to dosages of insulin and other medications. I strongly urge diabetics to consult with their doctor before taking a ketone ester (or ketone salts).

MONITORING KETONE LEVELS

It is probably not necessary for healthy people who are transitioning to a low-carb ketogenic diet to measure ketone levels. However, this information could provide positive reinforcement. Ketosis is considered to be a level of 0.2 mmol/L or higher, and "mild nutritional ketosis" is reached at about 0.5 mmol/L and beyond (see figure 5.13). When transitioning from a higher carb to a low-carb ketogenic diet, it takes several days to see a significant increase in blood-ketone levels, which may rise for two or three weeks before leveling off. The ketone level usually fluctuates throughout the day, often lower in the morning and peaking in the mid-afternoon or later, and can vary considerably from person to person.

Using coconut oil and MCT oil routinely can help increase and sustain a baseline level of ketones. Exogenous ketone supplements can give you a jump-start on getting into ketosis. A typical serving of ketone salts could increase your baseline level from 1 mmol/L to 1.5 to 2.5 mmol/L temporarily, and 25 gm of ketone ester could double that level.

COULD KETONE SUPPLEMENTS CAUSE KETOACIDOSIS?

One concern doctors and diabetics often voice is whether ketogenic supplements can push a person into diabetic ketoacidosis. With diabetic ketoacidosis, the blood sugar is very high, and there is inadequate insulin on board to control the blood sugar. The body begins to break down fat rapidly to use as fuel, and extremely large amounts of ketones are produced in the process, making the blood dangerously acidic, since the body may not be able to compensate quickly enough to buffer the acids. The levels of ketones in diabetic ketoacidosis are many times higher (10 to 25 mmol/L) than the levels that can be reached by taking coconut oil, MCT oil, or ketone salts. Figure 5.14 shows the typical changes in BHB levels from the various ketogenic strategies.

On the other hand, taking large amounts of ketone ester stacked too close together could result in ketoacidosis (BHB 7.0 mm/L or higher), though not diabetic ketoacidosis. Ketone esters can increase ketone levels at least five times higher than ketone salts, depending on the dose. So, when taking ketone esters, closely monitoring the ketone level, especially in the beginning, is advised to determine the dose that works for you and to ensure that you are not getting into dangerous

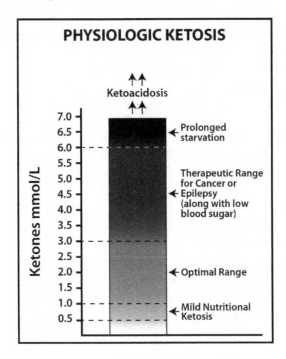

FIGURE 5.13. Physiologic ketosis represents a wide range of ketone levels. The optimal ketone level for individuals will depend on the goals they hope to achieve.

territory. Once you have established your ideal dose, you may not need to monitor your level as frequently.

Other reasons to monitor BHB levels more closely are when transitioning to a stricter ketogenic diet, when fasting, when trying a different ketone supplement or higher dose, or if you are ill, any of which could increase your BHB level.

> **KETOGENIC STRATEGY: KETONE LEVELS mmol/L:**
> Caffeine ➤ 0.2 to 0.3
> Coconut Oil ➤ 0.3 to 0.5
> Vigorous Exercise ➤ 0.3 to 0.5
> Overnight Fast ➤ 0.3 to 0.5
> MCT Oil ➤ 0.3 to 1.0
> Branched Chain Amino Acids ➤ 0.3 to 1.0
> Ketone Mineral Salts ➤ 0.5 to 1.0
> Classic Ketogenic Diet ➤ 2 to 6
> Starvation ➤ 2 to 7
> Ketone Esters (Oral or IV) ➤ 2 to 7 or higher
> Diabetic Ketoacidosis ➤ 10 to 25

FIGURE 5.14. Typical ketone levels obtained with ketogenic strategies, starvation, and diabetic ketoacidosis. Levels in diabetic ketoacidosis are many times higher than with ketogenic foods, exercise and overnight fasting, and ketone mineral salts.

Our Personal Experience with Exogenous Ketone Supplements

I have considerable personal experience with many different brands of ketone salts and ester products for myself and my husband Steve. Taking the Veech ketone ester had profound effects for Steve, reversing certain Alzheimer's symptoms during the first hours, days, and weeks, and sustaining his improvements for about twenty more months before he experienced serious setbacks again (Newport 2015). I have Alzheimer's on both sides of my family and began eating coconut oil when Steve did in 2008, and I have consistently used coconut oil, MCT oil, ketogenic diet, and ketone supplements, as they became available, as prevention strategies. Taking ketone salts every day helped me lose more than thirty pounds of fat over about four months in mid-2016. I travel extensively and like to try new foods wherever I go, which could easily put the fat back on. Using ketone salts and/or ester twice daily curbs my appetite and makes it much easier to maintain the weight loss. I sleep very well, never need a nap, have no aches or pains, and feel great at age sixty-nine. I take no prescribed medications, my blood pressure is normal at about 110/65, and my fasting blood sugar, insulin, and HbA1C levels are also normal.

METHODS OF MONITORING KETONES

Ketone levels can be measured in urine, in blood, or with a breath analyzer. Here are some of the differences.

Urine Ketone Test Strips

When blood levels of ketones become elevated, excess ketones filter out of the blood into the urine. Urine ketone test strips were originally developed for diabetics to help detect diabetic ketoacidosis if the blood sugar is elevated. Many companies sell urine test strips, which change color when ketone levels are elevated—usually the deeper the color, the higher the ketone level. The results do not measure your actual blood ketone level but can give you a rough idea of whether you are in ketosis and how deeply you are in ketosis.

A drawback is that urine test strips typically measure the ketone acetoacetate but not BHB, which is usually much more elevated than acetoacetate during ketosis. A decent level of BHB might not be reflected by a urine test strip. Also, if you drink a lot of fluid, ketones in the urine might be diluted and below the level detected by the urine test strip. Consider contacting the manufacturer directly if the package does not indicate which ketones the urine test strip tests for (see photo 7).

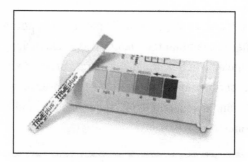

PHOTO 7. True Plus urine ketone strips. Most urine ketone strips measure acetoacetate and not betahydroxybutyrate.

Blood Ketone Monitoring

A blood ketone monitor using ketone test strips is a direct way to measure BHB levels. These monitors were developed for diabetics and come with a lancet holder and disposable lancets to prick your finger. The ketone test strips require only a small drop of blood and a matter of seconds to get results. The opposite of urine test strips, the ketone test strips do not detect the ketone acetoacetate but rather D-betahydroxybutyrate. The test strip does not contain the enzyme to detect the other form of BHB called L-betahydroxybutyrate. So, if you are taking a racemic mixture of D-BHB and L-BHB, you could have a higher level of total BHB than the test result indicates. Several different companies make blood ketone monitors, including Precision Xtra, NovaMax, and Keto Mojo, which are all available online. All three meters are capable of measuring ketones and glucose but require separate strips to do so. Currently, the Keto Mojo strips are the least expensive and their glucose test strip also measures hemoglobin and hematocrit.

It is possible to check glucose and ketone levels back-to-back with the same monitor if you are adept at swapping out the strips before the skin prick stops bleeding. I find it easier to set up a second monitor to test my blood sugar at the same time. These days, I mainly check my ketone and glucose levels to document how a new or different dose of an exogenous ketone supplement affects me. I also like to keep an eye on my fasting blood sugar every month or so. The fasting blood sugar tends to trend down (a good thing) when transitioning from a higher-carb to a low-carb ketogenic diet, and blood sugar may drop shortly after taking MCT oil, ketone salts, and ketone esters. Blood-glucose monitors are not very expensive, usually less than $40 with a starter set of glucose strips. At present, ketone test strips cost around $1 to $2 each, and glucose test strips cost much less (see photo 8).

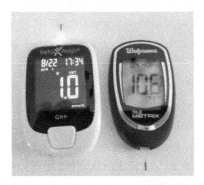

PHOTO 8. Monitoring blood ketone and glucose blood levels using two monitors set up to test blood glucose and betahydroxybutyrate from the same finger prick. Photo by Mary Newport.

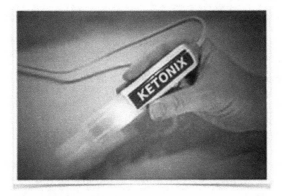

PHOTO 9. A ketone breath analyzer can be used repeatedly throughout the day to detect acetone and can be used to estimate blood ketone levels. Used with permission from Ketonix.

Ketone Breath Analyzer

Ketone breath analyzers measure the ketone called acetone. Acetone becomes elevated and is mostly exhaled when you are in ketosis, which accounts for the fruity breath some people experience. The breath analyzer gives a rough estimate of how deeply you are into ketosis. The monitor is pricy at $150 to $190 but is reusable, and you can monitor your level of ketosis as often as you like throughout the day. This could be helpful to detect ketosis while you are transitioning from a higher-carb to low-carb diet and to follow the trend in ketosis when trying various ketogenic strategies (see photo 9).

Direct Lab Ketone Testing

The most definitive way to measure ketone levels is through direct lab testing of blood. Both BHB and acetoacetate can be measured with these techniques. This kind of monitoring is most useful in ketone research where very precise levels are important. If you are having other lab work done, you could ask your doctor to include a ketone level if you want to go this route.

Ketone and glucose monitoring is strongly recommended for people on a strict ketogenic diet for epilepsy, cancer, or other serious medical condition, or when using moderate to high doses of ketone ester.

MONITORING OTHER PARAMETERS

Interest in the ketogenic diet and exogenous ketone supplements is growing rapidly as people experience the benefits for themselves and share this information with others. It helps to be aware of the possible pitfalls while transitioning to this lifestyle, which can often be avoided with careful monitoring and planning. It is important to consult with your doctor to help with monitoring if you are older or have medical conditions. What needs to be monitored depends on your age and health status and why you are adopting the ketogenic lifestyle.

Basic Monitoring

For everyone starting the ketogenic diet and/or taking exogenous ketones, it helps to keep a journal to record the date and baseline body measurements, particularly if you are trying to lose weight. If you are an athlete and already fit, these measurements may reflect changes in your body composition (less fat and more muscle). Some people report that their body shape changes despite no weight loss. Such measurements could tip you off to add calories if you are thin and worried about losing more weight.

Basic measurements could include:
- Weight
- Height
- Optional: Calculate BMI from height and weight (see Side Box below)
- Measurements around chest, waist, hips, and around the thickest parts of your upper and lower arms and legs
- According to NIH recommendations, a waist measurement greater than 35 inches (89 cm) for women and greater than 40 inches (101.5 cm) for men indicates a higher risk of heart disease and type 2 diabetes mellitus. Measure your waist just above the hip bones and after you breathe out.
- Measuring inches can provide encouragement when there is not much change on the scale. The same volume of muscle weighs more than fat, and you could be gaining muscle and losing fat.
- Blood pressure and heart rate/pulse. Most electronic blood pressure instruments measure blood pressure and pulse. You should consult with your physician if your blood pressure is too high (hypertension) or too low (hypotension). (Table 5.3 on Blood Pressure Status.)

- The NIH recently tightened blood pressure guidelines (see table 5.3).
- Normal pulse, after resting for at least ten minutes, is between 60 and 100; generally, a lower number indicates better cardiovascular fitness. People who are very fit may have a heart rate lower than 60, though this could be abnormal for someone with heart disease.
- Your pulse should be regular (pulsate evenly), and if it is irregular, you should consult with your physician right away.
- Optional: If you are very serious about changing your body composition and want to monitor this beyond calculating your BMI, you could request measurements of skin-fold thickness or consider having a more definitive test such as a DXA scan (dual energy x-ray absorptiometry) or plethysmography specifically for body composition, and repeat annually or after losing a large amount of weight to make sure you are not losing too much muscle mass.

BLOOD PRESSURE STATUS FOR ADULTS

BLOOD PRESSURE STATUS	SYSTOLIC (upper number)	DIASTOLIC (lower number)
Hypotension (low blood pressure)	Less than 90	Less than 60
Normal	Less than 120	Less than 80
Pre-Hypertension*	120 to 139	80 to 89
Hypertension* Stage 1	140 to 159	90 to 99
Hypertension* Stage 2	160 or higher	100 or higher

*Hypertension = High blood pressure
The above values are from https://www.nhlbi.nih.gov/health-topics/high-blood-pressure
For blood pressure values for children see tables at https://www.nhlbi.nih.gov/files/docs/guidelines/child_tbl.pdf]

TABLE 5.3. Blood-pressure status for adults from the National Institutes of Health.

Body Mass Index (BMI)

The BMI is a measure of body fat based on height and weight that applies to adults. The ranges are the same for men and women. The main limitations are that the BMI can overestimate body fat for athletes and others who are muscular and can underestimate body fat in people who have lost muscle, such as the elderly.

BMI Categories:
Underweight: Less than 18.5
Normal weight: 18.5 to 24.9
Overweight: 25 to 29.9
Obese: 30 or greater

The actual formula to calculate BMI is complicated. Instead, you can estimate your BMI with an online BMI calculator at: https://www.nhlbi.nih.gov/health/educational/lose_wt/BMI/bmicalc.htm.

Laboratory Monitoring

As you begin the ketogenic diet and/or an exogenous ketone supplement, during the first day to weeks, you could experience significant loss of water, electrolytes, and minerals leading to dehydration and electrolyte imbalances unless you take plenty of clear fluids and replace these nutrients. It is also likely that your fasting blood sugar and insulin levels will drop.

Also, ketone salts contain significant amounts of sodium and may contain varying amounts of potassium, calcium, and magnesium. This is an important consideration for children, the elderly, and people with medical conditions such as high blood pressure, edema (swelling), a history of abnormal levels of sodium, potassium, calcium, or magnesium, heart disease, diabetes, cancer, hormone abnormalities, kidney or liver disease, people who take blood thinners for any reason, or people who have any other chronic medical condition. It is crucial to involve your doctor before getting started with the ketogenic diet or exogenous ketones to avoid complications and to monitor blood levels of these electrolytes and minerals at baseline and periodically thereafter. Your doctor or a dietitian may be able to help you factor the minerals in ketone salts into your diet and adjust, for example, your potassium supplement to account for the amounts in ketone salts. People who are taking diuretics and/or potassium supplements and people who need to restrict their sodium intake might not be good candidates for taking ketone salts, but could do well with the ketogenic diet or a ketone ester with good support from their doctor and/or dietitian.

Screening Lab Work

Your doctor may wish to check blood levels before you embark on your ketogenic diet, or take exogenous ketone supplements and follow up with measurements of electrolytes, fasting blood glucose, and fasting insulin levels about six weeks later and periodically thereafter, depending on your age and health status (see figure 5.15 for a summary listing). Many of the blood tests listed here can be done as part of two tests called the Complete Blood Count (CBC) and the Complete Blood Panel (CMP) and could include:

- Electrolytes (sodium, potassium, chloride, bicarbonate)
- Minerals (calcium, phosphorus, magnesium)
- Tests for insulin resistance and diabetes
- Fasting blood glucose
- Fasting insulin
- HbA1C
- Calculation of HOMA-IR
- Lipid profile (Total, LDL, HDL, VLDL cholesterol, and triglycerides. LDL-P tests cholesterol particle size and may be a better indicator of heart-disease risk.)

- Kidney function (BUN, creatinine, and GFR)
- Liver function (ALT, AST, GGT)
- White blood count, hemoglobin, hematocrit, and platelet count
- Baseline studies for those with conditions such as thyroid disease or other hormone issues
- C-reactive protein. This is a test used to screen for inflammation and could be checked at baseline and followed if abnormal. Ketones are anti-inflammatory, and it would be interesting to see whether this test reflects your lifestyle changes over time.
- Omega-3 Index from DHA levels
- Vitamin panel

BLOOD WORK: SCREENING

Suggested blood work for nutritional screening and for peopole with cognitive/memory impairment:

Many of the blood tests listed here can be done as part of two tests called the Complete Blood Count (CBC) and Comprehensive Blood Panel (CMP).

- Electrolytes (sodium, potassium, chloride, bicarbonate)
- Minerals (calcium, phosphorus, magnesium)
- Tests for insulin resistance and diabetes:
  - Fasting blood glucose
  - Fasting insulin
  - HbA1C
  - Calculation of HOMA-IR
- Lipid profile (Total cholesterol, LDL-C, HDL-C, VLDL-C, triglycerides)
- LDL-P (LDL-cholesterol particle size)
- Kidney functions (BUN, creatinine, and GFR)
- Liver enzymes (ALT, AST, GGT)
- White blood count, hemoglobin, hematocrit, and platelet count
- Thyroid panel
- C-reactive protein to screen for inflammation
- Omega-3 Index from DHA level
- Vitamin panel
- ApoE phenotype
- Clotting studies (INR), for people taking certain blood thinners for any significant change in foods, vitamins, and other supplements.
- Evaluation for suspected infection, such as Lyme disease, candida, or other fungal infection.
- Further laboratory testing as indicated by abnormal screening results or unusual exposures, such as heavy metals in work environment.

FIGURE 5.15. Blood work to screen for status of electrolytes, minerals, and other health biomarkers.

- ApoE phenotype (to determine if you are a carrier of one or two ApoE4 genes, which carries a higher risk of Alzheimer's)
- Clotting studies for people who are on blood thinners: if your doctor allows you to try the ketogenic diet or exogenous ketones, it is important to check your clotting studies before you get started and within a week—or possibly sooner—after starting. Changes in diet can sometimes affect blood clotting for people taking warfarin or other medications.
- Evaluation for suspected infection, such as Lyme disease, candida, or other fungal infection
- Further laboratory testing as indicated by abnormal screening results or unusual exposures, such as heavy metals in work environment

BRING THESE GUIDELINES TO YOUR DOCTOR

Ketone salts and ketone esters are so new that most doctors don't know about them yet, much less about the potential of ketones to provide alternative fuel to the brain and other organs, reduce inflammation, and burn fat. I suggest that you bring this information to your doctor for guidance in what needs to be monitored. Your doctor may decide to pass this information on to other patients when they see how a ketogenic diet or exogenous ketones have improved your life.

CHAPTER SIX

OTHER SUPPLEMENTS
THAT MAKE SENSE

"Solve one problem, and you keep a hundred others away."

—Chinese Proverb

AVOID "SUPPLEMENTITIS": CHOOSE WISELY

When you or a loved one is dealing with a disease like Alzheimer's, it is very easy to develop a case of "supplementitis," and that was certainly the case for Steve and me. Steve could swallow a handful of supplements with one mouthful of water. We were ever hopeful that just the right supplement would come along to save him. I jumped on the bandwagon if a supplement seemed reasonable based on research, and would then have difficulty stopping it, even when there was no obvious effect. We were desperate for anything that could "freeze" his condition and stop the downward spiral.

Supplements are a multi-billion-dollar industry. We are bombarded constantly with TV commercials and print ads encouraging us to buy "memory" supplements, but the evidence is weak at best for most of them. Supplement companies can make a claim simply by adding a vitamin or other substance that has good evidence for cognitive support, such as vitamin B12.

Wouldn't it be great if we could just take a pill that would magically keep our brains from aging no matter what else we put in our mouths, and not have to do the hard work of eating a healthy diet? Supplements generally attempt to provide vitamins, minerals, and other micronutrients that our metabolism requires to assemble the building blocks from food into our cells, tissues, organs, and substances that allow cells to communicate.

For a brain supplement to be of value, it must be absorbed from the digestive tract, then must be able to cross the blood–brain barrier and arrive in a form the brain can use. The supplement should enhance the pathway in metabolism it is targeting and not cause harm by affecting unintended metabolic pathways. Many supplements are synthetic and have not been studied well enough to know how well they are absorbed, whether they cross the blood–brain barrier, and what form they take when they arrive in the brain, much less whether they are truly beneficial and not harmful. There are many unknowns in this regard, even with FDA-approved medications, and supplements receive much less scrutiny since they are considered food rather than drugs. This is of concern not only for adults but also for infants and children, and synthetic forms of vitamins and minerals are used to fortify foods for people of all ages.

BEWARE OF INTERACTIONS BETWEEN SUPPLEMENTS AND COMMON MEDICATIONS

Before taking a new supplement, it is important to know if it is compatible with any medications you are taking. Just because a supplement or medication is available over the counter does not make it safe for everyone. For example, ashwagandha has become popular as an anti-inflammatory supplement and for memory impairment, but the evidence is not strong. Ashwagandha can interfere with medications for high blood pressure, thyroid disease, diabetes, and immune suppression, and it can exaggerate the sedative effect of medications for sleep or anxiety. St. John's wort, a supplement used for depression, anxiety, poor appetite, and insomnia, has been banned from some countries due to reports of serious interactions with drugs taken for birth control, cardiac conditions, blood thinning (warfarin), suppression of the HIV virus, and many more. Heart complications have occurred during anesthesia in people taking St. John's wort for more than six months, and some research suggests that this supplement may worsen dementia in people with Alzheimer's.

A WHOLE-FOOD MEDITERRANEAN-STYLE DIET CAN PROVIDE MOST OF THE NUTRIENTS YOU NEED

It is best to get the naturally occurring forms of vitamins, minerals, and phytonutrients from whole, unfortified foods, since these natural forms will be recognized and processed normally by our metabolism. Eating a whole-food Mediterranean-style diet with its broad range of food groups, as detailed in chapter 4, is the easiest way to accomplish this goal without having to overthink it. Herbs and spices don't only add flavor; many contain antioxidants and other beneficial phytonutrients. Sea salt can provide many important trace elements that are removed when salt is refined, with the caveat that consuming some iodized salt is important for normal thyroid function.

Clearly, a keto diet and other ketogenic strategies can optimize utilization of the foods in the Mediterranean-style diet. Factory workers can load the assembly line with all the necessary parts and man the stations, but the finished product will not come out the other end if the power is not on. Cells require fuel to make ATP, the energy needed to manufacture thousands of proteins and other compounds to build cells and tissues and carry out many cell functions. When insulin-resistant cells don't take up glucose normally, ketones can provide the required fuel. Eating a healthy diet that provides a usable fuel to the body and brain creates a solid foundation for aging better. Supplements might not be necessary with healthy whole-food choices and should provide back-up insurance rather than acting as your basic strategy to keep your brain healthy. It is important to choose supplements that will help you achieve that goal.

Dozens of supplements are touted for memory and brain health. I have narrowed down the list to supplements that are often deficient in people with Alzheimer's and/or other neurological conditions and would be beneficial—but also not harmful. It can be difficult to reach the recommended daily allowances for a few vitamins and other nutrients that are critical to the brain, even with a healthy whole-food diet. Certain minerals like calcium, iron, copper, and zinc are required for brain health but can easily be obtained from foods. While taking a small amount is vital, taking too much of these minerals can be harmful, which will be discussed further in chapter 9 on things to avoid. In this chapter, you will find tables for each nutrient discussed, including the recommended daily allowances (when they exist), good food sources, and natural forms of supplements to look for when diet does not provide enough.

"Fact sheets" for consumers and health professionals, for vitamins and many other nutrients, are available on the NIH website (https://ods.od.nih.gov/), which is the source of information in this section where other publications are not cited.

Does a Popular Protein from Jellyfish Really Improve Memory?

Let's take a closer look at an actual study published on a protein from jellyfish by one of the leading memory-supplement companies (Lerner 2016). Prior to starting the study, the participants were given a self-reported cognitive test, called the AD8 (Galvin 2018), with "yes" or "no" questions asking whether cognition had changed over the past few years in eight areas. Zero or one question checked "yes" indicated normal cognition, and two or more "yes" answers indicated cognitive impairment. Participants took either the supplement or placebo for 90 days, and two-thirds of the 211 people received the supplement. Nine cognitive tests were administered at baseline and after 90 days. The results were not statistically significant for the supplement versus placebo for any of the nine tests. However, the results were reported as significant for subgroups receiving the supplement who had AD8 scores of 0 to 1 (cognitively normal) or 0 to 2 (normal to slightly impaired). If you look closely at the details, the 0 to 1 subgroup taking the supplement improved on four of nine tests, but the group taking the placebo also improved on four of nine tests, of which three were different tests. Similarly, for the 0 to 2 subgroup, the supplement and placebo groups each improved on five of the nine tests, though some were different tests. Through a miracle of statistical analysis, it would appear that there was statistically significant improvement for the supplement compared to placebo on all nine tests. The package says "improves memory" based on this study, and the article states that the supplement is intended for healthy non-demented individuals.

OMEGA-3 FATTY ACIDS—ALPHA-LINOLENIC ACID, DHA, AND EPA

There are two classes of polyunsaturated fatty acids (PUFAs), omega-6 and omega-3, that are essential for humans and all other mammals. We cannot make adequate amounts in our bodies, but they are critical to our overall health and brain health, including normal brain growth and development, visual acuity, and normal cognitive function from fetal life to old age. The good news is that we do not need very much of these essential fatty acids. The bad news is that many of us get far too much omega-6 fatty acids as linoleic acid (LA) and not enough of the right omega-3 fatty acids if we don't eat seafood.

The main plant source of omega-3 fatty acids is alpha-linolenic acid (ALA), which is found in natural plant oils and animal and dairy fat, but is especially rich in chia oil (64 percent of the oil) and flaxseed oil (55 percent of the oil). Flaxseed and chia oil are not great-tasting oils, but are easy to find in capsules. The main known function of ALA is to serve as a precursor for the very important omega-3 fatty acid called

DHA through a process called elongation (ALA is an 18-carbon chain and DHA has 22 carbons). EPA is another important omega-3 fatty acid that is created as an intermediate step in the pathway between ALA and DHA. The recommended daily allowance (RDA) for ALA is just 1.1 grams (1100 mg) for women and 1.6 grams (1600 mg) for men (IOM 2006). This amount was chosen to assure that an adequate amount of DHA is produced from ALA, but it is not so simple since the amount of DHA produced from ALA varies in individuals from 0.5 to 5 percent. This huge disparity is at least partly due to variants in genes that regulate the pathways to make DHA from ALA. See table 6.1 for ALA-rich foods and RDA.

Alpha-Linolenic Acid (ALA)
Recommended Daily Allowance (RDA) and Food Sources

RDA (Adults): Men: 1600 mg | Women: 1100 mg
Supplements: Inexpensive brands of flax oil and chia oil in capsule or liquid form can be found online and health food stores.

FOOD SOURCES	SERVING SIZE	ALA (mg)
English walnuts	1 oz	2570
Chia seeds	1 oz	2390
Flaxseed oil	1 tbsp	2420
Flax seeds	1 oz	2350
Canola oil	1 tbsp	1280
Soybean oil	1 tbsp	900
Black walnuts	1 oz	760
Olive oil	1 tbsp	107

Sources: IOM, 2006; NIH Dietary Supplement Fact Sheets- https://ods.od.nih.gov/factsheets/list-all/
USDA FoodData Central - https://fdc.nal.usda.gov/

TABLE 6.1. Alpha-Linolenic Acid (ALA): Recommended Daily Allowance (RDA) and Good Food Sources.

LA and ALA give rise to numerous longer-chain metabolites. LA gives rise to arachidonic acid (ARA), an omega-6 fatty acid that is critically important in the brain but is easily provided through diet. ALA gives rise to eicosapentanoic acid (EPA), which is further elongated to docosahexaenoic acid (DHA). Each of these longer-chain metabolites has important opposing functions in the brain and body. Getting the right balance of omega-6 to omega-3 fatty acids is important to keep certain aspects of metabolism in check, because excessive linoleic acid can promote inflammation and blood clotting and constrict blood vessels, resulting in increased risk of high blood pressure and its serious consequences. Omega-3 fatty acids have the opposite effects. There is much more detail on the problem of excessive linoleic acid in chapter 9.

The omega-3 docosahexaenoic acid (DHA) is rich in fish (some types more than others) and algae oil. There are small amounts of DHA in land animals, eggs, and dairy. DHA is the most abundant polyunsaturated fatty acid (PUFA) in the brain, where it is highly concentrated in cell membranes (40 percent of the PUFAs) and in the retina of the eye (60 percent of the PUFAs), which is an extension of the brain. DHA is anti-inflammatory, and supplementation with DHA reduces beta amyloid plaque and tau tangle pathologies in animal models of Alzheimer's.

The critical nature of DHA has come into greater focus in just the past two decades. In 2002, commercial infant-formula manufacturers began to add DHA to their products after supplementation studies in newborns revealed the importance of DHA to the development of normal visual acuity and stronger performance on IQ testing. Large population studies have shown that higher DHA levels and/or higher intake of fish in pregnant women are associated with lower rates of preterm birth and infant mortality. High fish intake has consistently outperformed simple supplementation with DHA, which has had inconsistent results, for example, in studies of delaying preterm birth (Almeida 2021; Hibbeln 2019). A manufacturer of fish oils once explained to me that fish oil contains more than two dozen different fatty acids—DHA just happens to be the most studied—and it is very possible that other fatty acids in fish have important functions in humans as well.

Certain enzymes are needed for ALA to give rise to DHA, and these enzymes are often deficient in people with Alzheimer's. People with Alzheimer's tend to have lower than average blood and brain levels of DHA, though it is not certain whether the low brain levels of DHA are a cause or consequence of Alzheimer's. Greater intake of fish in populations tends to correlate with lower rates of Alzheimer's disease. People who carry the ApoE4 gene are at greater risk than average for developing Alzheimer's and tend to oxidize DHA more rapidly than people without the ApoE4 gene, which alters the DHA. DHA also does not cross the blood–brain barrier as well in people who have the ApoE4 gene compared to those who do not (Norwitz 2021).

The most effective way to increase DHA in the blood and brain is to eat more fatty fish, fish roe (eggs), or other seafood, and next best is to take fish oil, algae oil, or krill oil. Algae oil is a good vegan source of DHA, since eating algae is how DHA makes it into fish and other seafood. Seafood, fish roe, and krill oil are rich in DHA that is bound to phospholipids and could be especially beneficial for people who are ApoE4, since DHA phospholipids appear to cross the blood–brain barrier more easily than free DHA (Patrick 2019). Taking a concentrated DHA supplement is also quite effective at increasing blood levels of DHA. DHA is bound to phospholipids in the cell membrane, especially phosphatidylcholine (which we will talk about in the next section). Fish oil comes in capsules, gummies, and liquid, sometimes flavored with lemon or orange, which could be helpful to people who cannot swallow capsules easily.

I eat fish (about half as salmon) and other seafood several times per week, and take both krill oil and a Norwegian fish oil concentrate that is rich in DHA, even though I do not carry the ApoE4 gene. There is little downside to taking more DHA than the recommended daily allowance of omega-3 fatty acids, unless the amount significantly upsets the balance of omega-6 to omega-3. No Upper Tolerable Limit (the limit above which adverse effects are more likely) has been established for omega-3 fatty acids.

Captain Joseph Hibbeln, former Chief of the NIH/NIAAA Section on Nutritional Neurosciences, and his associates have reported that benefits to cognitive development in infants occur with as little as 4 ounces of seafood per week intake by the pregnant mother, and benefits continue to increase up to 12 ounces of seafood per week; the same figures apply to growing children. It is reasonable to think that eating similar amounts of seafood could be equally beneficial to the aging brain. The review found no adverse effects at the highest level of fish intake, including consideration of mercury intake (Hibbeln 2019). Seafood contains other important nutrients like choline, iodine, vitamin B12, iron, vitamin D, zinc, and manganese.

The amount of DHA varies quite a lot between types of seafood. Salmon is one of the richest sources of DHA. Eating twelve ounces of salmon per week provides about 5 grams of DHA, which works out to about 700 mg of DHA per day (with additional EPA). Some types of seafood have just 10 to 50 percent of the amount of DHA in salmon (see table 6.2). A study of 485 adults >55 years old with age-related cognitive decline taking 900 mg DHA per day versus placebo for 24 weeks found benefit to learning and memory (Yurko-Mauro 2010).

HOW MUCH MARINE OMEGA-3 SHOULD I TAKE?

Surprisingly, there is no specific recommended daily allowance (RDA) for DHA or EPA. The best way to get enough DHA and EPA is to eat at least 12 ounces of fish and seafood per week, including at least one serving of fatty fish per week (Hibbeln 2019). Please see the discussion in chapter 4, along with a table showing fat, protein, and carbohydrate content of fish and seafood choices.

If you eat less than 12 ounces of fish and seafood per week or don't eat seafood at all, consider making up the difference with a supplement. EPA mostly converts to DHA in the body, so you can total EPA + DHA when figuring out how much to take. Many types of capsules, gummies, and liquid supplements are available, such as DHA concentrate, algae oil, fish oil, salmon oil, cod liver oil (which is also rich in

MARINE OMEGA-3 FATTY ACIDS DHA AND EPA

There is **no recommended daily allowance** for DHA and EPA.
Best Choice: Eat 12 ounces or more of seafood per week (Hibbeln, 2019).
For people who don't eat seafood, suggest:
• If no ApoE4 gene: **at least 500 mg/day DHA + EPA.**
• If ApoE4 gene (or unknown), or omega-3 index is low: **~700 mg/day DHA + EPA**
Optional: Take part of supplementation as krill oil.
Note: Some eggs, milk, and other foods are fortified with DHA.
Good Food Sources of DHA and EPA: Other foods may contain DHA and EPA

FOOD	SERVING SIZE	DHA (mg)	EPA (mg)
Cod liver oil	1 tbsp	1500	938
Salmon, Atlantic, farmed	3 oz	1240	590
Salmon, Atlantic, wild	3 oz	1220	350
Herring, Atlantic	3 oz	940	770
Sardines, drained	3 oz	740	450
Mackerel	3 oz	590	430
Salmon, pink	3 oz	630	280
Trout, rainbow, wild	3 oz	440	400
Sea bass	3 oz	470	180
Fish roe / caviar	1 oz	23	239
Tuna, canned	3 oz	170	20
Shrimp	3 oz	120	120

Sources: NIH Dietary Supplement Fact Sheets:https://ods.od.nih.gov/factsheets/list-all/
USDA FoodData Central - https://fdc.nal.usda.gov

TABLE 6.2. Marine sources of the omega-3 fatty acids DHA and EPA, suggested supplementation, and good food sources.

vitamins A and D), and krill oil. Some flaxseed and chia seed oil supplements also contain DHA from algae oil. See table 6.2 for good food sources and suggestions for supplementation with DHA and EPA.

Consider Checking Your Omega-3 Index

If you do not eat fish and/or take a fish oil or DHA/EPA supplement, you might ask your doctor to measure your Omega-3 Index with your next lab work.

Omega-3 Index = DHA + EPA levels in blood as a percent of erythro-cyte fatty acids. The omega-3 index in Japan, where seafood intake is high, averages 9 to 11 percent. In the U.S., where seafood intake is much lower, the average is 3 to 4 percent. Japan has one of the lowest rates of preterm birth and infant mortality and the highest average life expectancy in the world at eighty-one years for men and eighty-seven years for women (compared to seventy-seven years for men and eighty-one years for women in the United States).

CHOLINE AND PHOSPHATIDYLCHOLINE

Choline is essential to a healthy brain. We can make some choline in our bodies but not nearly as much as we need. The average American does not eat enough of the right kinds of foods to get an adequate supply of choline. U.S. women get only about half of the recommended requirement, and the need for choline is higher during pregnancy and lactation. Poor intake of choline is a big problem for their children, who may come up short during fetal life and early infancy, affecting the health and lifespan of those offspring.

In the brain, choline is found mainly as phosphatidylcholine in cell membranes, but also as free choline and some other choline metabolites (glycerophosphocholine, phosphocholine, sphingomyelin, and others). These are the same forms of choline found in human milk, and dietary intake influences the concentration of choline in human milk. Choline is also part of the important neurotransmitter acetylcholine, which is deficient in Alzheimer's disease, explaining many of the symptoms. Acetylcholine is important in memory, muscle control, and mood, and the enzyme that converts choline to acetylcholine is also deficient in the Alzheimer's brain. Increasing brain levels of acetylcholine is the mechanism for most of the approved Alzheimer's drugs. Choline's main metabolite is betaine, which is important in methylation, a process that occurs in every cell. Betaine affects the biological behavior of numerous enzymes, hormones, proteins, and vitamins. In addition to effects on the brain, depletion of choline through poor intake can lead to fatty liver and leakage of enzymes from the liver and muscles into the bloodstream, resulting in damage to those tissues (EFSA 2016; Wallace 2016).

The fetus has fifteen times the mother's blood levels of choline. Studies in humans show that better cognitive performance in children correlates with higher maternal choline intake during pregnancy and breastfeeding. In animal studies, the offspring of mice that were fed a low-choline diet had greatly reduced numbers of neural stem cells (which become mature brain cells) and smaller brains. Also, the normal layering of neurons in the brain was not complete, resulting in abnormalities in the structure and function of the brain (Wang 2016).

Could poor choline intake be a factor in autism? In a study of 863 children with autism and 123 healthy children, a diagnosis of autism, with or without regression in function, was 2.5 times more likely to occur in infants who received formula rather than exclusive breastfeeding for at least the first six months of life. Also noteworthy, receiving a formula without DHA and ARA (which was typical before 2002) increased the odds of autism with regression in function to thirteen times the rate of children who were exclusively breastfed (Schultz 2006).

DHA and choline are bound together in the plasma cell membrane, so another missing ingredient (of many) in infant formulas could be the right form of choline. The choline added to infant formulas is usually a synthetic form, such as choline bitartrate and/or choline chloride. These synthetic forms are not nearly so well-absorbed, reach much lower peak blood levels, and only stay in the bloodstream for about 30 minutes, compared to 6 to 12 hours for the naturally occurring forms found in foods like egg yolk or lecithin (Hirsch 1978; Smolders 2019). Synthetic forms of choline are also used in many supplements for all ages and to fortify foods.

Studies of Alzheimer's mouse models reported that lifelong supplementation with choline in the diet protected the brain from Alzheimer's, apparently by blocking plaque formation and activation of microglia (which occurs with inflammation). Similar changes in the brain occur with Parkinson's, other neurodegenerative diseases, and traumatic brain injury. In a mouse model of Down syndrome, choline

CHOLINE

Recommended Daily Allowance (RDA): Adults: Men: 550 mg, Women: 425 mg
Supplement suggestions: If you are unable to get enough choline from your food choices, make up the difference to meet the RDA.
• Concentrated phosphatidylcholine (PC) in liquid or capsule.
• Soy, egg yolk, or sunflower lecithin (usually 420 mg PC per 1200 mg capsule).

FOOD	SERVING SIZE	CHOLINE (mg)
Beef liver	3 oz	356
Egg, large	2	294
Salmon or beef, top round	3 oz	100-120
Fish roe	1 oz	
Soybeans, roasted	½ cup	
Chicken breast, lean ground beef, fish	3 oz	70-90
Wheat germ	1 oz	40-60
Kidney beans	½ cup	
Quinoa	1 cup	
Whole milk	1 cup	
Yogurt, plain or ricotta cheese	1 cup	
Brussel sprouts, broccoli, green beans, cauliflower, shitake mushrooms	½ cup	20-30
Cottage cheese	1 cup	
Whole grain rown rice	1 cup	
Peanuts/Sunflower seeds	¼ cup	
Tangerine, apple, carrots, kiwifruit	½ cup	≤10

Sources: NIH Dietary Supplement Fact Sheets: https://ods.od.nih.gov/factsheets/list-all/
SDA FoodData Central - https://fdc.nal.usda.gov

TABLE 6.3. Choline: Recommended Daily Allowance (RDA), Good Food Sources, and Supplements.

in the diet reduced cognitive deficits. Another animal study showed that offspring of mice who received low levels of choline had lifelong abnormalities on memory testing, whereas mice receiving adequate amounts of choline did not (Velasquez 2020). These studies support the idea that getting adequate choline in the diet is important to early brain growth and development and to how well the brain ages. Much more study of choline is warranted in humans.

The recommended daily allowance for choline is 550 mg/day for adult men and 425 mg/day for women (450 mg/day in pregnancy and 550 mg/day during lactation) (IOM 2006). Like DHA, it is possible to get enough choline in the diet if you know the right foods to eat (see table 6.3). Most choline-rich foods are from animal sources, so getting enough choline is a challenge for vegans, since usual serving sizes of the best plant sources barely supply 5 to 20 percent of the RDA.

Given the importance of choline, a supplement from a natural food source could provide good insurance. Soy lecithin, egg yolk lecithin, and sunflower lecithin are all rich in phosphatidylcholine and other brain phospholipids, and can be easily found in liquids and capsules. Depending on the brand, two capsules of lecithin could supply 400 mg of choline inexpensively. Back in 2008, I added soy lecithin to the coconut-and-MCT-oil mixture I gave my husband Steve to provide phosphatidylcholine and other important brain phospholipids. Fortunately, Steve liked choline-rich eggs very much and ate several every day. A few supplements are available that contain concentrated phosphatidylcholine extracted from lecithin, but they tend to be more expensive (see table 6.3).

MAGNESIUM

Magnesium is a critically important mineral for humans, but the U.S. population, on average, gets only about half the recommended daily allowance in the typical diet. Refinement and hybridization of grains and food processing have greatly reduced the magnesium content of the American diet overall, compared to a few decades ago. A serum magnesium level less than 1.7 mg/dl (0.75 mmol/L) is considered abnormally low, a condition called hypomagnesemia. When I was in practice in the newborn intensive care unit, it was common to see low magnesium levels in the new mothers as well as in their tiny babies. Magnesium is used intravenously in pregnant women to reduce out-of-control blood pressure, which can occur in preeclampsia, and to slow down contractions during premature labor.

Magnesium is required for more than 80 percent of metabolic functions, including more than 350 enzymatic processes. In many of these processes, magnesium must bind to ATP for the chemical reaction to occur. Magnesium is also required for enzymes involved in synthesizing DNA and RNA and maintenance of the structure and function of DNA and RNA. About 99 percent of magnesium is located within cells, mainly in bone but also in muscle, soft tissues, and other organs. Only about 1 percent of magnesium is in the blood and other body fluids outside of cells, mainly in the free-ionized form, but most magnesium in the body is attached to a variety of proteins and other compounds.

Magnesium plays a critical role in the brain and peripheral nervous system. Spinal-fluid levels of magnesium are higher than blood levels, indicating that magnesium is likely actively transported across the blood–brain barrier, but the mechanisms have not been fully worked out yet. Magnesium is required for the normal structure and function of synapses (the junctions between neurons) and is highly concentrated in mitochondria, playing a key role in many processes related to energy production and protein synthesis. Magnesium suppresses the production of damaging reactive oxygen species in various tissues, including the brain, and affects other pathways that keep inflammation in check.

Magnesium also promotes differentiation of neural stem cells into neurons. The spinal-fluid concentration of magnesium is lower in people with Parkinson's and Alzheimer's than in healthy people, but studies of blood-magnesium levels have been inconsistent. While animal studies have shown some benefit, studies of magnesium supplementation in people with Parkinson's and Alzheimer's have been disappointing (Yamanaka 2019; Kirkland 2018).

The body tries to hold on to magnesium, but excretion through the kidneys increases with age and in conditions like diabetes, leading to a greater risk of hypomagnesemia, which can affect nearly every organ. Early signs include weakness, poor appetite, fatigue, nausea, and vomiting and can progress to muscle cramping, numbness, tingling, and abnormal heart rhythms. Severe deficiency may cause seizures (Case 2021; Fiorentini 2021).

The body absorbs only about 30 to 40 percent of magnesium in foods, and this figure is not much better, at about 35 to 45 percent, for the common magnesium supplements. If you are low on magnesium, the digestive tract tends to absorb more but absorbs less than usual if your magnesium status is above normal. Taking calcium, high doses of zinc, or excess alcohol with magnesium, or having a gastrointestinal disorder with chronic diarrhea, can further interfere with magnesium absorption.

Of the dozen or so different types of magnesium supplements available, magnesium oxide is the least well absorbed and magnesium citrate one of the better choices. My personal favorites are magnesium glycinate and magnesium L-threonate. Several ketone salts products contain magnesium betahydroxybutyrate, another potential supplemental source that I take advantage of. Magnesium glycinate is simply magnesium bound to the amino acid glycine, which is also an inhibitory neurotransmitter mainly found in the spinal cord, brain stem, and retina. Magnesium glycinate is purported to have a relaxing effect conducive to sleep, but convincing evidence for this is scarce. Magnesium L-threonate is magnesium bound to L-threonate, a natural metabolite of vitamin C. In animal studies, magnesium L-threonate increased magnesium levels in the brain more than most other types of magnesium supplements. Studies of mouse models for diseases like Alzheimer's have reported that magnesium L-threonate had positive effects on cognition and increased the number of neural stem cells in the hippocampus, but human trial data is not yet available (Slutsky 2010).

Many magnesium supplements have a laxative effect, which can help prevent constipation for those eating a ketogenic diet. Some magnesium supplements are marketed specifically for constipation or for heartburn. Food and supplement labels are required to list the amount of elemental magnesium in the food, not the entire weight of the compound with magnesium.

If you do not mind eating two ounces of pumpkin seeds every day, with about 310 mg magnesium, you could easily meet the RDA from food, but few other food sources come close to this amount of magnesium in a typical serving. Two surprisingly good sources of magnesium are coconut milk and coconut water, which naturally provide other minerals like calcium, potassium, and sodium, as well as vitamins and other nutrients. Unrefined sea salt contains a significant amount of magnesium, but refined table salt does not.

When you total up the magnesium content you normally eat in a day, it is easy to see how difficult it is to meet the RDA, and you might not even come close. To prevent magnesium deficiency, consider using a supplement to make up the difference between what you get in your

MAGNESIUM

Supplements: Consider 50 to 120 mg/capsule to meet RDA if inadequate intake from diet.

Notes: Look closely at nutrient label for actual magnesium content per capsule or tablet. Factor magnesium taken laxative or antacid. High doses may cause diarrhea.

Best absorbed supplements: Magnesium as citrate, glycinate, and L-threonate (crosses blood brain barrier in animal studies).

Recommended daily allowance (RDA):

Adults ages 19-30:	Adults 31 and over:
Men: 400 mg Women: 310 mg	Men: 420 mg Women: 320 mg

GOOD FOOD SOURCES:	SERVING SIZE	MAGNESIUM (mg)
Pumpkin seeds, roasted	1 oz	155
Chia seeds	1 oz	100-110
Brazil nuts	½ cup	
Coconut milk	½ cup	
Almonds/Cashews	1 oz	60-80
Boiled soybeans/spinach	½ cup	
Quinoa	¼ cup	
Coconut water	1 cup	
Pecans, walnuts, peanuts, macadamias, sunflower seeds	1 oz	30-50
Black beans, kidney beans, chickpeas, whole grain brown rice	½ cup	
Whole grain oatmeal, unenriched	½ cup	
Plain whole fat yogurt	1 cup	
Cocoa powder	1 tsp	
Banana	1 medium	15-25 mg
Raisins	½ cup	
Avocado	½ cup, cubed	
Salmon, halibut, chicken, beef	3 oz	
Whole milk	1 cup	
Whole wheat bread	1 oz slice	
Most cheeses	1 oz	<12 mg
Apple/Carrot	1 oz	
Broccoli, cooked	½ cup	

Sources: NIH Dietary Supplement Fact Sheets: https://ods.od.nih.gov/factsheets/list-all/
USDA FoodData Central - https://fdc.nal.usda.gov/

TABLE 6.4. Magnesium: Recommended Daily Allowance (RDA), Good Food Sources, and Supplements.

diet on an average day and the RDA. Routinely taking very high doses of supplemental magnesium could interfere with absorption of calcium and other minerals and have unknown potentially negative effects. The front label of a supplement might show an amount of 2000 mg for the total compound, for example. The nutrient label on the back should list the amount of actual magnesium per serving. It may say something like "magnesium (as magnesium glycinate)." Also, be aware that a "serving" could be three or four capsules or tablets.

Magnesium supplements do not need to be expensive. While researching this section, I was able to find online magnesium glycinate for nine to twenty-one cents for 100 to 120 mg magnesium in capsule form. Magnesium L-threonate was about fifty cents for 100 mg. Magnesium supplements (including glycinate) come in tablet, capsule, powder, and liquid forms.

- Poorest absorption: Magnesium oxide
- Better absorption: Magnesium citrate, magnesium glycinate, magnesium L-threonate
- Known to cross blood–brain barrier (in animal studies): Magnesium L-threonate
- Ketones with magnesium: Ketone salts products contain magnesium if indicated on the nutrient label

Look in table 6.4 for recommended daily allowance and good food sources and suggestions for supplementation.

VITAMINS

Vitamins are essential nutrients found in food that are needed in small amounts in metabolism but cannot be made at all or in the full amount required by the organism (in this case, humans). Deficiency of a specific vitamin leads to a predictable set of disease symptoms. Twelve micronutrients meet the definition of a vitamin, though some also consider choline to be a vitamin. We have at least 20,000 genes that encode for at least 620,000 different proteins. There are more than 3,000 chemical classes with more than 1 million metabolites engaged in the intricate orchestration that is our metabolism. A tiny change in DNA could increase the amount of a metabolite that is present by as much as 10,000 times (Wishart 2019) (see figure 6.1). Given everything that could go wrong, it is amazing how often everything goes right in our metabolism. It is very likely that there are more essential nutrients yet to be identified.

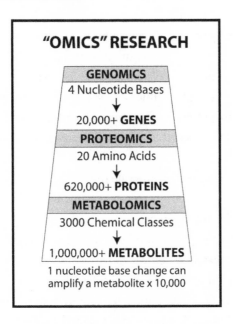

FIGURE 6.1. "Omics" research has revealed that more than 1,000,000 metabolites are at play in the human body (Wishart 2019). Vitamins are just a few of the metabolites that have been studied intensively. There is much more to learn. Graphic by Joanna Newport.

New fields of research, genomics, epigenomics, proteomics, metabolomics, lipidomics, and other "omics" are uncovering the effects of diet and dietary interventions on our genetic makeup and our metabolism. The information from such studies is accumulating at a rapid pace, but we are still very early in the process of fully understanding the differences between healthy and unhealthy patterns of metabolites and how these are affected by diet in various disease states.

I bring "omics" research up here because the essential vitamins we have known about for so long are just a tiny fraction of the million metabolites at play in the human body. Vitamins are essential organic nutrients needed for normal growth and health. You might think of vitamins as the nuts and bolts required to make the final product in an assembly line. "Omics" research is helping us to understand more about the effects of vitamins through studies of supplementation. Genomics research studies genetic differences between individuals and populations, as well as patterns of upregulation and downregulation of genes, for example, in a nutritional deficiency or in response to a dietary intervention. Likewise, proteomics and metabolomics research helps uncover changes in patterns of proteins and metabolites. There is little doubt that "omics" research will reveal many more essential vitamin-like substances.

If you eat a Mediterranean-style diet with a variety of whole foods from the full range of food groups, you should be able to get adequate amounts of the essential vitamins.

Remember when people used to eat liver on a regular basis, as well as other organ meats? When Steve was growing up, his family had a milk cow and a bull that they raised to stock their freezer with beef. I remember having beef-heart and beef-tongue soups as well as liver and onions at their house. The first time I signed up for Weight Watchers in 1972, the diet required a weekly serving of liver. These days, it is not easy to find liver in grocery stores in the United States. A 3-ounce serving of beef liver can easily provide the daily recommended intake of vitamin A and six of the eight B vitamins as well as CoQ10, iron, and other minerals. But excessive intake of vitamin A can be toxic, so eating liver every day would not be a good idea, for this and other reasons. There is concern that toxins may be stored in the livers of animals that are fed antibiotics, hormones, and pesticides. So I personally only eat liver and other organ meats from pasture-raised animals.

A complete discussion of the essential vitamins could fill its own book. I will discuss here the fat-soluble and water-soluble vitamins broadly, and then focus on a few vitamins that have been studied specifically for effects on brain atrophy, cognition, and Alzheimer's, and/or have important roles in energy metabolism. Whenever available, it is best to take vitamins in the naturally occurring forms found in food, because these may have better absorption and bioavailability than synthetic vitamins.

Another general consideration is whether there could be consequences for the average healthy person from taking mega-doses of vitamin C and certain B vitamins. Our metabolism is a complex and

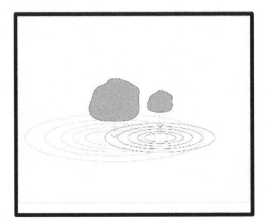

FIGURE 6.2. Our metabolism is a delicate balance, and too much of a good thing, even a vitamin, can have unintended consequences.

delicate balance, and a specific vitamin can impact many different metabolic pathways. If you drop a small rock into a glassy pond, a nice concentric pattern of ripples will radiate outward in all directions. If you drop a big rock into that radiating pattern, it will disrupt the pattern into chaos, sending the ripples off in many different directions (see figure 6.2). In other words, it is important to consider benefits versus risks. There is some evidence that mega-doses of, for example, vitamin C could be helpful for specific health conditions. But for general health, mega-doses of vitamins are probably neither necessary nor a great idea. Clinical trials using mega-doses to correct low blood levels of vitamins in Alzheimer's disease with the hope of improving cognition have been mostly disappointing.

THE FAT-SOLUBLE VITAMINS: A, D, E, AND K

Vitamins A, D, E, and K are the fat-soluble vitamins, meaning that they need fat to be well absorbed during digestion, and also that they are stored in our body fat and/or liver. Vitamin D3 is often found in a hard white pill, often with calcium carbonate, but can be taken in oil droplets or gel capsule with oil, which allow better absorption and higher blood levels. Many oil-based products are available with natural forms of vitamins A, D, E, and K alone or in various combinations. Table 6.5 shows the natural forms of the fat-soluble vitamins found in foods, the recommended daily allowances for adults, and good food sources.

Vitamin A (retinol) plays an important role in immune function, in maintaining vision, and for prevention of macular degeneration, and it appears to have an impact on neuroinflammation, mitochondrial dysfunction, and neurodegeneration. Many foods contain natural retinoids and carotenoids, which are metabolized in the body to the active forms of vitamin A. Theoretically, based on animal studies, supplementation with vitamin A could reduce neuroinflammation and Alzheimer's pathology, but human studies showing a benefit of vitamin A supplementation are lacking (Das 2019). Vitamin A levels can be measured but do not drop below normal until vitamin A is almost completely depleted. A normal plasma retinol level is at least 0.70 micromol/L (20 micrograms/dL).

Vitamin D (calciferol) is a hormone very important to bone health. It also regulates neurotransmitters and has anti-inflammatory, antioxidant, and neuroprotective properties. Low vitamin D levels have been associated with Alzheimer's and cognitive impairment, and vitamin D appears to play a role in reducing formation of beta amyloid plaques and tau tangles. Relatively small studies of vitamin D supplementation for prevention and treatment of Alzheimer's have had conflicting results (Sultan 2020). Vitamin D blood levels can be improved with supplementation. The best indicator of vitamin D status is serum 25-hydroxyvitamin D (25(OH)D), which is reported two different ways by labs:

- <30 nmol/L (<12 ng/mL) indicates deficiency with serious bone consequences (rickets in children or osteomalacia in adults).
- 30 to <50 nmol/L (12 to <20 ng/mL) is inadequate for bone and overall health.
- >50 nmol/L (>20 ng/mL) is adequate for bone and overall health.
- >125 nmol/L (>50 ng/mL) may indicate toxic level with risk of adverse effects.

FAT-SOLUBLE VITAMINS – A, D, E, K

VITAMIN	NATURAL FOOD FORMS	RDA MEN	RDA WOMEN	GOOD FOOD SOURCES
A	Retinoids, carotenoids	900 mcg RAE* (*RAE = retinoic acid equivalents)	700 mcg RAE* (*RAE = retinoic acid equivalents)	Liver, sweet potato, carrots, spinach, pumpkin, ricotta cheese, eggs, herring
D	Ergocalciferol, cholecalciferol	Age 19-70: 15 mcg (600 IU) Age >70: 20 mcg (800 IU)		Salmon, trout, mackerel, tuna, cod liver oil, (sun exposure)
E	Alpha and other tocopherols	15 mg as alpha-tocopherol		Wheat germ, safflower oil, sunflower seeds and oil, hazelnuts, almonds, walnuts, peanuts and peanut oil, corn oil, spinach
K	Phylloquinone, menaquinones	120 mcg	90 mcg	Natto, collards, turnip greens, spinach, kale, broccoli, pomegranate juice, soybeans and oil, edamame

Source: USDA FoodData Central - https://fdc.nal.usda.gov/

TABLE 6.5. The fat-soluble vitamins: recommended daily allowance (RDA), natural foods forms, and good food sources.

Vitamin E (alpha-tocopherol) is a potent antioxidant that stops the production of damaging reactive oxygen species when fat is oxidized (burned as fuel). Alpha-tocopherol is often used as an additive in food manufacturing to delay oxidation and spoilage of foods. Vitamin E also has an important role in supporting immune function and cell communication, as well as in lowering cholesterol. While low levels of vitamin E occur in people with Alzheimer's and cognitive impairment, intervention studies with vitamin E have been disappointing (Browne 2019). Vitamin E levels are not routinely measured, and there is not much information available on this.

Vitamin K (K1-phylloquinone, K2-menaquinone) is involved in blood clotting, bone formation, cell growth, cell division, and my-elination, and it may prevent brain cells from dying in response to the presence of beta amyloid plaques. Vitamin K can interfere with the effects of the common anticoagulant warfarin but is also used as a treatment when anticoagulation from warfarin is excessive. Low vitamin K levels have been associated with Alzheimer's and with cognitive impairment in some studies but not in others, and studies of vitamin K supplementation have not shown clear benefit in Alzheimer's (Alisi 2019). Vitamin K levels are not routinely measured except in people taking anticoagulants or with bleeding disorders. Vitamin K status can be checked in a roundabout way with prothrombin time, the time it takes for blood to clot, and the INR, which is a calculation using prothrombin time.

There are many excellent reasons to get adequate amounts of the fat-soluble vitamins for normal function of body and brain, but the evidence for a beneficial effect of taking supplements to prevent or treat Alzheimer's and other types of cognitive impairment is underwhelming.

THE WATER-SOLUBLE VITAMINS: B AND C

The B and C vitamins are water-soluble and are not stored for very long in the body, apart from vitamin B12. Therefore, regular intake of water-soluble vitamins is necessary. Like the fat-soluble vitamins, a well-balanced whole-food Mediterranean-style diet can supply the recommended daily allowances. It is hard to take too much of these vitamins, because the unused excess is mostly flushed out in the urine. Taking mega-doses does not necessarily equate to mega-blood levels. For example, an oral supplement of 1250 mg ascorbic acid (vitamin C) is sixteen times the recommended amount for women (75 mg), but it only doubles the blood level a person can achieve by eating vitamin C-rich foods.

Vitamin C (ascorbic acid) is a natural antioxidant in our metabolism and is also used for its antioxidant effects in processed foods. Vitamin C is important to the immune system; wound healing; the synthesis of collagen, myelin, many proteins, and several neurotransmitters; and maturation of brain cells. During digestion, vitamin C

VITAMIN C

NATURAL FOOD FORMS	RDA Men	RDA Women	GOOD FOOD SOURCES
L-ascorbic acid	90 mg	75 mg	Red peppers, orange or juice, grapefruit or juice, kiwi fruit, green peppers, broccoli, strawberries, Brussels sprouts, tomato or juice, melon, cabbage, cauliflower, lemon, or lime juice.

Source: USDA FoodData Central - https://fdc.nal.usda.gov/

TABLE 6.6. Vitamin C: Recommended Daily Allowance (RDA) and Good Food Sources.

improves absorption of a form of iron found in certain plants. Studies have not found a clear correlation between blood levels of vitamin C and cognitive performance. Increasing blood levels of vitamin C with supplementation does not appear to improve cognitive performance (Travica 2019). See table 6.6 on vitamin C for recommended daily allowances and good food sources. The plasma vitamin C level can be measured:

- >50 micromol/L indicates adequate level.
- <23 micromol/L indicates low level (called hypovitaminosis C).
- <11.4 micomol/L indicates deficiency with potential adverse consequences.

Originally, thirteen B vitamins were identified, named vitamin B1 through vitamin B13. However, five were eliminated because they were discovered to be neither vitamins nor essential, which explains the gaps in numbering (see table 6.7). The B vitamins as a group are required in hundreds of enzyme-catalyzed chemical reactions in all aspects of metabolism, and certain B vitamins are needed to activate other vitamins. Table 6.7 lists the natural forms of the vitamins that are found in foods and/or are biologically active in the body, the recommended daily allowances, and good food sources.

Vitamin B1 (thiamin or thiamine) plays such a critical role in energy metabolism, cell growth, development, and function that deficiency can be devastating to the heart and nervous system, which have a higher energy and oxygen consumption than most other organs. The active form of thiamin, called thiamin diphosphate (or thiamin pyrophosphate) is a coenzyme for two key enzymes in the biochemical pathways leading from glucose as fuel to the production of ATP. Thiamin diphosphate is required to convert glucose within the cell to ribose (a component of DNA, RNA, and ATP molecules). Thiamin diphosphate is also involved in amino acid and lipid metabolism, as well as in the synthesis of the neurotransmitters acetylcholine, GABA, and glutamate (Sambon 2021).

Thiamin deficiency is common. The early symptoms of thiamin deficiency include weight loss, lack of appetite, confusion, short-term memory loss, muscle weakness, and cardiac symptoms such as an enlarged heart. This can progress to either beriberi or Wernicke-Korsakoff syndrome. People with beriberi develop peripheral neuropathy (nerve pain and numbness), muscle wasting, and impairment of senses, motor functions, and reflexes, and they may go on to develop congestive heart failure with edema of the lower limbs. Supplementation can quickly cure beriberi. Wernicke-Korsakoff (WK) syndrome is more common than beriberi in the United States and can have an acute onset with life-threatening encephalopathy (widespread damage to brain function and structure). Mortality is 20 percent if untreated, and permanent brain damage occurs in 75 percent of those who survive, even if treated. WK begins with peripheral neuropathy and evolves to symptoms like severe short-term memory loss, disorientation, confabulation (confusion between reality and made-up memories), and psychosis. Additional symptoms identified in thirty-six hospitalized non-alcoholic veterans with thiamin deficiency included weakness and falling (75 percent), neuropsychiatric symptoms (72 percent), gastrointestinal dysfunction (53 percent), and loss of coordination (42 percent) (Mates 2020).

Thiamin deficiency may also play an important role in the progression of Alzheimer's disease. In the Alzheimer's brain, there are lower activity levels of thiamin-dependent enzymes in the pathway to production of ATP from glucose. Thiamin deficiency produces oxidative stress/mitochondrial dysfunction in neurons, death of neurons, loss of memory, plaque formation, and changes in glucose metabolism, all characteristic of Alzheimer's disease. Studies using animal models have shown improvement in these pathologies with benfotiamine, a synthetic thiamin supplement that converts to a natural biological form and will be discussed shortly (Sambon 2021).

Thiamin does not stay for very long in the body, and, therefore, a constant dietary supply is needed. Blood levels of thiamin are unreliable, and studies are not done routinely. The recommended daily allowance (RDA) for thiamin is 1.2 mg for men and 1.1 mg for women. It is not easy to get enough thiamin from food, since there is just 0.4 mg in some of the richest natural sources, such as a 3-ounce serving of pork or trout, or ½ cup of boiled black beans. Whole-grain brown rice and oatmeal have only 0.1 mg per ½ cup serving, and unfortified refined rice or flours have 1/10 of that amount. Refined white rice, wheat, and corn flour and foods made with them, like bread, pasta, crackers, cookies, and cereals, have been stripped of thiamin, riboflavin (vitamin B2), niacin (vitamin B3), and other nutrients (Allen 2006). Fortification of foods like refined flours and rice accounts for about half of dietary thiamin. Only added thiamin must be listed on food labels. Despite fortification, most people in the United States do not meet the recommended daily allowance.

Due to its critical role in glucose metabolism, the thiamin requirement is greater for people who eat a higher-carbohydrate diet and when there is a higher demand for energy, such as during physical labor, pregnancy, and lactation. Thiamin is important to infant cognitive and language development, as well as motor function. Blood levels of thiamin tend to be much lower in people with both type 1 and type 2 diabetes than in non-diabetics, so diabetics may need more than the recommended daily amount of thiamin. Because of problems with absorption, severe deficiency of thiamin can occur in chronic alcoholism and in people who have had gastric bypass surgery or have a gastrointestinal disorder. Thiamin can be lost from foods cooked in water, with leavening and baking. Amounts of thiamin greater than 2.5 mg in a meal are mostly unabsorbed. People with a high intake of raw fish can become deficient in thiamin due to the presence of an enzyme that inactivates the vitamin (Whitfield 2021; NIH 2021; Allen 2006).

Given the difficulty of getting adequate thiamin from food, and especially from a low-carb diet, thiamin supplementation is reasonable. Unfortunately, the natural forms of thiamin found in food (thiamin diphosphate or free thiamin) are not readily available as supplements. Most dry thiamin-fortified foods, like rice and flour, some infant formulas and baby foods, and many vitamin supplements, have thiamin in the form of synthetic thiamin mononitrate. Another synthetic form, thiamin hydrochloride, is used mainly in liquids since it is completely water-soluble. Absorption during digestion of these synthetic vitamins is slow and incomplete, and exposure to heat during cooking may degrade these compounds to some degree. While there is little doubt that the thiamin component of thiamin mononitrate has greatly reduced the prevalence of thiamin deficiency, I have a concern about the "mononitrate" component of the supplement. Most Americans eat processed foods containing thiamine mononitrate with nearly every meal and snack. I have been unable to find out how much, if any, of the mononitrate portion of the compound is absorbed during digestion. My concern is explained in more detail in chapter 9, on things to avoid in the section on nitrosamine compounds, which may cause brain insulin resistance, according to research by Dr. Suzanne de la Monte and group (De la Monte 2009; Tong 2009).

Synthetic thiamin hydrochloride is also present in some foods, infant formulas, and supplements, and it may be a better choice than thiamin mononitrate. Despite reliance on thiamin mononitrate and thiamin hydrochloride for fortification of refined grains and many other foods worldwide since the mid to late 1900s, there is surprisingly little information on digestion, absorption, and human safety testing for either of these supplements (PubChem 2021).

Another synthetic form of thiamin, called benfotiamine, which was developed in Japan in the mid-twentieth century, may provide a good option for thiamin supplementation, and it is readily available from several different companies in 100-to-300-mg capsules. Benfotiamine is absorbed more rapidly and completely and produces higher blood thiamin levels than thiamin mononitrate or thiamin hydrochloride. Benfotiamine, though synthetic, is converted to a fat-soluble metabolite, which is further converted to free thiamin, thiamin monophosphate, and the active form thiamin diphosphate. Benfotiamine could be used for fortification of foods and is probably a better choice, but it is not currently used this way.

Supplementation with benfotiamine has shown encouraging effects in studies for thiamin deficiency, type 1 and type 2 diabetes, diabetic kidney disease (nephropathy), diabetic polyneuropathy, diabetic retinopathy, Alzheimer's (see side box), blood-vessel damage in heavy smokers, and in alcoholism. Benfotiamine was also shown to rescue function in damaged heart-muscle cells and to have anti-inflammatory (decreased blood markers of inflammation) and antioxidant effects. Benfotiamine reduces blood levels of tissue-damaging advanced glycation end-products (AGEs), which increase when blood sugar is chronically elevated, as in diabetes (Sambon 2021). The dosages used in the various studies ranged from 250 mg to 1000 mg per day, and have not shown toxic or adverse effects in studies of use for up to eighteen months.

Benfotiamine Supplementation

If you decide to take benfotiamine as a supplement, I suggest:
- 100 mg per day for people who want to avoid deficiency
- 250 to 600 mg per day (with doctor's approval) for people who are prediabetic or diabetic, or have mild cognitive impairment, Alzheimer's, other neurological condition, or a disorder that may interfere with digestion and absorption of thiamin

Benfotiamine for Alzheimer's

Studies using standard thiamin supplementation for Alzheimer's have not reported improved cognition. However, in an uncontrolled pilot study, five people with mild to moderate Alzheimer's taking 300 mg per day of benfotiamine for eighteen months gained an average of 3.2 points of 30 points on the Mini-Mental Status Exam (MMSE), despite greater accumulation of beta amyloid plaque in the brain. One patient had a very significant increase in MMSE from 12 to 18 of 30 points (Pan 2016). In a larger study, seventy-five people with mild cognitive impairment or mild Alzheimer's were given either 300 mg of benfotiamine twice per day (n=34) or placebo (n=36) for twelve months. There were no adverse effects of taking benfotiamine, thiamin blood levels increased, and blood levels of harmful advanced glycation end-products (AGEs) decreased compared to controls. At twelve months, there was less decline on two sub-categories of the Alzheimer's Disease Assessment Scale-Cognitive, as well as on the Clinical Dementia Rating (Gibson 2020). While these results were not spectacular, a larger, longer study is justified.

Vitamin B2 (riboflavin) plays a major role in energy production, cellular function, growth, and development, and it may play a role in inhibiting inflammation. Information on a connection between riboflavin and Alzheimer's is lacking. The riboflavin requirement is easily achieved in food, and blood levels are not measured routinely.

Following absorption, Vitamin B3 (niacin), is converted in all body tissues to the coenzyme nicotinamide adenine dinucleotide (NAD, also written as NAD+), which is required by more than 400 enzymes to catalyze chemical reactions. NAD is converted to the coenzyme nicotinamide adenine dinucleotide phosphate (NADP) in all tissues except skeletal muscle. NAD is involved mainly in reactions that liberate energy as ATP from carbohydrates, fats, and proteins, but also in maintaining the integrity of our genes, controlling how genes are expressed, and communication between cells. NADP plays a role in maintaining antioxidant functions in cells and in reactions that build substances like fatty acids and cholesterol. High doses of niacin are absorbed, and some of the excess is stored in red blood cells. Blood levels of niacin are not considered to be reliable and are not considered routinely for general health assessment.

Declining blood levels of NAD are associated with many disorders of aging, such as cognitive decline, heart failure, and kidney failure. NAD levels can become greatly depleted in brain cells when there is an excessive level of the excitatory neurotransmitter glutamate. Increasing NAD levels is reported to have favorable effects in type 2 diabetes, metabolic syndrome, and non-alcoholic fatty liver disease, and it may even increase lifespan. So there is great interest in studying supplementation with various forms of niacin.

Supplementation with NAD precursors appears to increase levels more than taking NAD itself, leading to special interest in nicotinamide riboside, which naturally occurs in milk, and in a supplemental form that is generally recognized as safe (GRAS) by the FDA. Nicotinamide riboside (NR) is formed from niacinamide and ribose and does not cause flushing, which occurs with some niacin supplements. Ribose is a sugar that becomes a component of ATP, deoxyribonucleic acid (DNA), and ribonucleic acid (RNA), and all nucleotides, which are building blocks of DNA and RNA. NR supplementation increases NAD levels in multiple tissues, improves mitochondrial function (which increases ATP production), and appears to promote stem-cell regeneration, repair DNA, decrease brain inflammation, inhibit formation of beta amyloid plaques, and allow sirtuins (SIRT) to function. Sirtuins are protein metabolic sensors that help regulate cell health and homeostasis (Mehmel 2020).

NR was used in a small pilot study of people with mild cognitive impairment in which the dosage was increased to 1000 mg daily over six weeks and maintained for four more weeks. Improvements were seen using functional magnetic resonance imaging (MRI) and in day-to-day functionality, but not in cognitive testing, though this was a short-term study (Orr 2020).

In 2021, more than sixty clinical trials of NR using doses between 250 and 1000 mg (in four doses) daily have been completed or are recruiting for Alzheimer's, subjective cognitive impairment, mild cognitive impairment, Parkinson's disease, heart failure, kidney failure, metabolic syndrome, diabetes, and many other disorders involving energy metabolism or mitochondrial dysfunction. In toxicity studies, NR dosages up to 3000 mg were found to be safe (Conze 2016), though I would not recommend such a mega-dose pending high-dose studies. Given the safety profile and FDA GRAS status, it is reasonable to take an NR supplement.

Worth noting here, increasing blood ketone levels also boosts NAD levels (see side box).

Nicotinamide Riboside Supplementation. How Much?

Studies for a variety of disorders have used nicotinamide riboside at doses between 250 mg and 1000 mg per day. Here are my recommendations:

- For general brain health, 250 mg daily
- 250 to 300 mg two or three times per day, with doctor's approval, for someone with Alzheimer's, mild cognitive impairment, or other disorder mentioned in the discussion of Vitamin B3

Ketones Also Increase NAD Levels

Vitamin B3 (niacin) includes an active form called nicotinamide adenine dinucleotide (NAD, also written as NAD+), which serves as a coenzyme for many different biochemical reactions, including the production of ATP. A decline in NAD in the brain and an abnormally low NAD/NADH ratio occurs in age-related metabolic diseases and neurodegenerative disorders, like Alzheimer's. To generate ATP, glucose and ketones must be converted to acetyl CoA, which then enters the TCA (or Krebs) cycle, a series of chemical reactions leading eventually to production of ATP. Glycolysis (breakdown of glucose) requires conversion of four NAD molecules to NADH to produce acetyl CoA, whereas the ketone betahydroxybutyrate requires just one NAD molecule, and acetoacetate requires no NAD to produce acetyl CoA. Thus, ketones should, theoretically, help preserve availability of NAD in the brain. An animal study and a human study have confirmed this NAD-sparing effect:

- Healthy rats fed a ketogenic diet showed a regional increase of brain NAD/NADH ratio after just two days, which was sustained for three weeks (Elamin 2017).

You can read more on NAD and the other "great controlling nucleotide coenzymes" in a review by Veech, et al. (Veech 2019).

Vitamin B5 (pantothenic acid) is important to the synthesis of coenzyme A, which is essential to fatty-acid synthesis and degradation, production of ATP in the TCA cycle, and a great many other anabolic and catabolic processes, including ketone synthesis from fatty acids. B5 is also required for the synthesis of acyl carrier protein, which itself is needed for synthesis of fatty acids and innumerable metabolites. The recommended amount of B5 is easily met by eating many types of animal and plant foods. Some B5 is made in the intestine, and B5 is circulated on red blood cells throughout the body. Taking megadoses of pantethine has been touted to reduce LDL cholesterol, but this substance is not identical to the vitamin pantothenic acid, and long-term effects of taking megadoses of pantethine are unknown. Blood levels of pantothenic acid are not done routinely.

Vitamin B6 (pyridoxine) in its coenzyme forms is involved in more than 100 enzyme reactions mostly related to amino acid and protein metabolism but, also, carbohydrate and lipid metabolism, breakdown of glycogen (the storage form of glucose) to glucose, and production of glucose from certain amino acids (gluconeogenesis). B6 is also important to the production of neurotransmitters, immune function, formation of hemoglobin (which carries oxygen in red blood cells), and maintenance of normal levels of homocysteine. We will discuss more about homocysteine shortly. A pyridoxal 5′ phosphate (PLP) level >30 nmol/L is generally considered adequate, though the Institute of Medicine sets the level at >20 nmol/L.

Vitamin B7 (biotin) is required for five enzymes involved in the metabolism of fatty acids, glucose, and amino acids. B7 is also involved in cell communication and regulation of genes, and it impacts the structure and function of histones (spool-like structures that DNA wraps around). It is easy to get enough biotin in foods, though certain foods, like eggs, must be cooked for biotin to be activated. The normal level of biotin is set at 133 to 329 pmol/L in serum, though this may not be a reliable indicator of status. A normal 24-hour urine level is between 18 and 127 nmol.

Vitamin B9 (folic acid or folate) is vital to normal brain function and is found in a wide variety of foods (see table 6.7), mainly as tetrahydrofolate (THF). Tetrahydrofolate is converted after digestion in several steps to 5-methyl-tetrahydrofolate (MTHF), the main form of vitamin B9 found in plasma. About half of the folate in the body is stored in the liver. Folate acts as a coenzyme or helper molecule for other coenzymes in the production of DNA and RNA and in the metabolism of amino acids, such as homocysteine and methionine. Folate is required for methylation (see side box) in a specific chemical reaction that must occur during the formation of DNA for proper cell division to take place.

Gut bacteria in the large bowel also produce folic acid, which is absorbed, though it is unknown how—or even if—this form is used biologically. The fully oxidized form of B9 called "folic acid" is used for food fortification, and is absorbed during digestion, but it is unknown whether this form has any direct biological activity. Problems with methylation of folic acid due to genetic variations can cause unmetabolized levels of folic acid to build up in the blood. Abnormally high levels of unmetabolized folic acid combined with low vitamin B12 levels appear to double or triple the risk of cognitive impairment (Román 2019). Supplementation with 5-methyltetrahydrofolate (5-MTHR), the active form, rather than folic acid may be more effective and beneficial (Vidmar Golja 2020).

Pregnant women with low folic acid levels are more likely to have a child born with certain heart defects, cleft lip and cleft palate, or a neural tube defect, such as spina bifida. In spina bifida, the spine does not fuse normally, exposing the spinal cord, which leads to partial or total paralysis of the lower extremities, and the child often has increased fluid in the brain, called hydrocephalus. To help prevent these severe birth defects, since 1998 the United States has required fortification of breads, cereals, flours, corn meals, pastas, rice, and other grain products with 140 mcg of folic acid per 100 grams. Food-labeling advice is only required for added folic acid and not the natural content.

A serum folate level >3ng/mL is considered adequate but is sensitive to recent dietary intake. A better measure of longer-term status is erythrocyte folate, for which a level >140 ng/mL is considered adequate.

In the famous Nun Study of Aging and Alzheimer's Disease (see side box), a low folic acid level, attributed to low lifetime consumption of salad, was associated with a greater risk of cognitive decline and dementia and more severe brain atrophy. Higher folic acid levels strongly correlated with normal cognitive function in the nuns, even when there was a high concentration of beta amyloid plaque in the brain (Snowdon 2002).

Aging with Grace: The Nun Study of Aging and Alzheimer's Disease

David Snowdon and associates followed over many years a group of thirty nuns, who lived in the same convent, ate from the same kitchen, and shared a similar lifestyle and environment. Periodically, a battery of cognitive and language tests was administered, as well as lab draws to measure eighteen nutrients and other biomarkers. The nuns died between ages 78 and 101 and donated their brains. The nuns wrote autobiographies at the time they were admitted to the convent as young women. Analysis of their writings showed that the complexity of their word structure, vocabulary, and ideas, or lack thereof, correlated strongly with their risk for later dementia—less complexity correlated with greater likelihood of dementia.

Many of the deceased nuns had a high burden of beta amyloid plaque in their brains despite normal cognitive testing at their most recent assessment, which called into question the role of beta amyloid plaque as a cause of Alzheimer's disease. Low folic acid levels were the only micronutrient of eighteen that correlated with greater risk of dementia (Snowdon 2000). The study was memorialized in an intriguing book by David Snowdon entitled *Aging with Grace* (Snowdon 2002).

Vitamin B12 (cobalamins) is a group of compounds that contain cobalt, thus are called cobalamins. Like vitamin B9 (folic acid), B12 requires methylation to carry out many functions by serving as a methyl donor (see side box on methylation). B12 is required for conversion of homocysteine to methionine, which further converts to S-adenosylmethionine, a methyl donor for nearly 100 substrates, such as DNA, RNA, proteins, and lipids. B12 is also required in the metabolism of the short-chain fatty acid propionate, which is produced by bacteria in the gut from fiber as well as bacteria on the skin in oil glands.

The richest sources of vitamin B12 are liver, meats, fish, shellfish, and dairy products, and there is no B12 in most vegetables, so vegans are at a real disadvantage here. Use of certain drugs, like Metformin and specific antacids (proton pump inhibitors, Prilosec®, Prevacid®), as well as gastric bypass surgery, can decrease absorption of vitamin B12. Low vitamin B12 levels may increase the risk of dementia (study results are inconsistent). Numbness, burning, and tingling in the hands and feet are typical symptoms of deficiency. Vitamin B12 levels can be measured in blood, but high methyl malonic acid or homocysteine levels may be better indicators of vitamin B12 status:

- Serum or plasma vitamin B12 <200 to 250 pg/mL (148 to 185 pmol/L) indicates an inadequate level. The cutoffs for normal levels and units used to report vitamin B12 levels differ between labs.
- Experts suggest checking methyl malonic acid (MMA) level if serum or plasma vitamin B12 level is <150 pg/mL. An MMA level >0.271 micromol/L indicates vitamin B12 deficiency.
- Serum homocysteine level >15 micromol/L suggest vitamin B12 deficiency, but the results are also affected by folic acid status.

Studies have not clearly demonstrated that long-term B12 supplementation improves cognitive function (Román 2019). However, the two-year VITACOG study reported an average of 30 percent less brain atrophy and lower homocysteine levels, compared to those in the placebo group (n=113), in 110 people with mild cognitive impairment taking a combination of vitamin B12 (500 mcg cyanocobalamin), B9 (800 mcg folic acid), and B6 (20 mg pyridoxine). Those with the highest levels of homocysteine at baseline had the greatest reduction in brain atrophy (53 percent). The study reported no safety issues with this level of supplementation (Smith 2010). A follow-up study reported that this B-vitamin combination slowed cognitive decline, but only in people who also had a high blood omega-3 index (Oulhaj, 2016).

B-vitamin supplementation could be beneficial to brain health, particularly in people who don't obtain adequate amounts from their diet. There are many unanswered questions, such as the appropriate amount to achieve benefit, which could vary substantially from person to person. Roughly half the U.S. population has a gene variant that interferes with methylation, so natural methylated forms of B9 (5-methyltetrahydrofolate) and B12 (methylcobalamine) may improve the biological usefulness of these supplements.

See table 6.7 for a complete listing of the B vitamins, their natural food forms, the RDA, and some foods that are rich in each vitamin.

Common Gene Variants Undermine Methylation of B-Vitamins and Increase Homocysteine Levels

In a previous section, I mentioned the importance of choline in methylation of many different types of substances. Certain B-vitamins important to brain and nerve function (for example, B6, folic acid (B9), and B12) are also involved in methylation and remethylation. Methylation simply means transferring a methyl group, consisting of one carbon atom and three hydrogen atoms (CH3) from one substance to another. Many biochemical chain reactions require methylation.

Common variations in genes can lead to problems with methylation, which may lead to disease by affecting levels of vitamins B6, B9, and B12 and other important related substances. For example, a common variation in the MTHFR gene, which affects half the U.S. population, can lead to a high homocysteine level (>11 micromoles/L), which is associated with greater risk of heart attacks, psychiatric disorders, and double the risk of later-onset Alzheimer's disease. A high homocysteine level appears to increase leakiness of the blood–brain barrier, promote blood clotting and constriction of blood vessels, increase beta amyloid plaque and tau tangle formation, and interfere with production of several neurotransmitters. Disruption of DNA methylation has also been found in the brains of people who died with Alzheimer's disease.

Supplementation with the methylated forms of B12 and folic acid can greatly slow down the rate of brain atrophy (shrinkage) and cognitive decline in the elderly. Increasing levels with the right forms of these B-vitamins in food or as supplements can help reduce the blood level of homocysteine (Román 2019).

THE WATER-SOLUBLE B VITAMINS

VITAMIN	NATURAL FOOD FORMS	RDA Men	RDA Women	GOOD FOOD SOURCES
B1 Thiamin	Free thiamin, thiamin pyrophosphate or diphosphate	1.2 mg	1.1 mg	Whole grains, meat, fish and other seafood, black beans, other beans; small amounts in whole fat dairy. Heating reduces availability.
B2 Riboflavin	Flavin adenine dinucleotide, flavin mononucelotide, free riboflavin, riboflavin esters or glycosides	1.3 mg	1.1 mg	Eggs, liver and other organ meats, lean meats, seafood, poultry, almonds, yogurt, cheese, milk, mushrooms.
B3 Niacin	Nicotinic acid, nicotinamide, nicotinamide adenine dinucleotide (NAD), nicotinamide adenine dinucleotide phosphate (NADP); bioavailable derivatives: niacinamide, nicotinamide riboside	16 mg NE* (*Niacin Equivalents)		Beef liver, poultry, salmon, tuna, beef, pork, brown rice, peanuts, smaller amounts in other nuts, seeds, beans, vegetables, and potatoes. Some dietary tryptophan converts to niacin.
B5 Pantothenic acid	Pantothenic acid CoA, phosphop-antetheine, pantothenic acid, pantotheine; pantothenol (also called panthenol) is converted to pantothenic acid after consumption.	5 mg		Beef liver, shitake mushrooms, sunflower seeds, chicken, tuna, dairy, nuts, seeds, beans.
B6 Pyridoxine	Pyridoxine, pyridoxal, pyridoxamine, pyridoxal 5′ phosphate (PLP) and pyridoxamine 5′ phosphate (PMP)	Age 19-50 1.3 mg >50 yrs 1.7	Age 19-50 1.3 mg >50 years 1.5	Chickpeas, liver, tuna, salmon, poultry, beef, banana, dairy, nuts.
B7 Biotin	Biotin bound to proteins, free biotin	30 mcg		Beef liver, other organ meats, eggs (cooked), salmon, beef, pork, sunflower seeds, almonds, sweet potato, other nuts and seeds, spinach, broccoli, dairy.
B9 Folic acid, folate, folacin	Tetrahydrofolate (THF), or THF as polyglutamates; 5-methyl THF is main form found in bloodstream	400 mcg DFE (1 mcg DFE = 1 mcg food folate; differs for synthetic folates)		Beef liver, spinach, black-eyed peas, baker's yeast, asparagus, Brussels sprouts, romaine lettuce, avocado, eggs, beans, peas, nuts.
B12 Cobalamins	Methylcobalamin and 5-deoxyadenosylcobalamin; hydroxycobalamin and cyanocobalamin, become biologically active after they are converted to methylcobalamin or 5-deoxyadenosylcobalamin	2.4 mcg		Beef liver, clams, tuna, nutritional yeast, salmon, beef, dairy, eggs.

Source: USDA FoodData Central - https://fdc.nal.usda.gov/

TABLE 6.7. The Water-Soluble B-Vitamins: Recommended Daily Allowances (RDA) are for adults 19 and older except where indicated. The "good food sources" are listed in order of highest amounts per serving.

Supplementation with B-Vitamins: Some Things to Consider

While adequate amounts of some B-vitamins can easily be achieved by eating a variety of whole foods, getting enough thiamine, niacin, folic acid, and cobalamins can be a challenge. Taking a "B complex" vitamin could provide some insurance if the vitamins are in forms your body can use. Since most B-vitamins are not stored in the body and are water-soluble, excess amounts are mostly flushed out in the urine. Here are some considerations in choosing a vitamin B supplement:

- Vitamin B1 (thiamin): Look for thiamine hydrochloride instead of thiamin mononitrate in foods and other supplements. Consider supplementation with benfotiamine, especially if you are older or have memory or other cognitive impairment.
- Vitamin B3 (niacin): Consider nicotinamide riboside, especially if you are older or have memory or other cognitive issues.
- Vitamin B9 (folic acid): Look for the 5-methyl tetrahydrofolate (5-MTHF) form of folic acid, especially if you carry the MTHFR gene variant (about half the U.S. population) or do not know your status.
- Vitamin B12 (cobalamins): Look for the methylcobalamin form, especially if you carry the MTHFR gene variant (about half the U.S. population) or do not know your status.

THE MICROBIOME, FIBER, PROBIOTICS, AND PREBIOTICS

One of the longest nerves in the body, the vagus nerve, starts in the brain and travels throughout the entire gastrointestinal system from the mouth to the anus. The word "microbiome" has only been around for two decades and, for humans, refers to the community of microorganisms that live in and on the human body. About 95 percent of our microbiome lives in the gut (gastrointestinal tract), but the gut microbes sometimes find their way into the brain (see more on infection and

Alzheimer's in chapters 9 and 10). Overall, each individual lives with 10 to 100 trillion microbes consisting of thousands of different species of viruses, bacteria, and other types of organisms (Sochocka 2019). At this point, bacteria are the most studied microbes, since viruses are much more expensive and more difficult to study. The patterns of bacterial species in the gut vary considerably from population to population and are impacted significantly by diet.

Antibiotics save lives, but can also wipe out much of the normal microbe population in the gut and allow a potential disease-causing pathogen, such as Clostridium difficile or Candida albicans, to thrive. Infections can also alter the gut microbiome. Drinking chlorinated water prevents the spread of certain life-threatening pathogens, but could change the type of microbes we carry in the gut (Sasada 2015). Drinking spring water or using a filter or reverse osmosis to remove chlorine could be better alternatives. The big shift in the human diet over the past century has also affected the makeup of the gut microbiome.

The human microbiome project got its start in 2007, and the field of research exploring the "gut-brain axis" (interaction between the gut microbiome and the brain) for Alzheimer's and aging is in its infancy. Metagenomics (study of genetic material in a community of organisms or other environmental sample) and metabolomics studies are helping to identify microbiome patterns in different human populations and how these patterns change with dietary interventions. Research in animals and humans implicates alterations in the gut microbiome in neurodegenerative diseases like Alzheimer's, colorectal cancer, insulin resistance, metabolic syndrome, type 2 diabetes, obesity, allergies, inflammatory bowel disease, and heart failure (Giau 2018).

The gut and brain communicate by using inflammatory, immunological, hormonal, and neuronal signals. Certain harmful bacteria secrete substances that reduce the tightness between cells in the gut, allowing inflammatory substances to leak into the bloodstream. These inflammatory substances can then damage the blood–brain barrier, allowing inflammation to take hold in the brain. Neuroinflammation is associated with Alzheimer's, Parkinson's, autism, other dementias, and neurological disorders. Other tissues and organs can be affected by gut inflammation as well. A focus of gut microbiome research is to learn whether restoring a healthy microbiome could reduce dementia risk or improve cognitive performance in Alzheimer's and other cognitive disorders (Sochocka 2019).

Gut health, which requires a diversity of microbial species, could be maintained or restored by consuming fiber and fermented foods like kefir, yogurt, kimchi, kombucha tea, and fermented vegetables, or by taking probiotics with active cultures. Probiotic supplements sometimes come with a prebiotic to feed the bacteria. A fecal transplant from a healthy person is sometimes used to restore gut health, such as in someone whose microbiome has been depleted by prolonged treatment with broad-spectrum antibiotics. Parasitic infections can also upset the gut microbiome, and treating these infections could restore gut health.

Overgrowth of pathogens in the mouth that cause periodontal disease (tooth decay, gingivitis) increases the risk of Alzheimer's. Dental plaque, which leads to dental cavities, starts as bacterial biofilm and may pick up fungi and spirochetes and progress to gingivitis, or inflammation of the gums. Therefore, maintaining good oral health with brushing and flossing or water-flossing, good dental repair, and treating gingivitis are important. Oil pulling, a 4000-year-old Ayurvedic practice, is performed by swishing oil in the mouth and forcing the oil between the teeth for up to twenty minutes. Coconut oil is a particularly good choice for oil pulling, since lauric acid, which is half the fat in coconut oil, is known to be antimicrobial to oral pathogens like Streptococcus mutans and Candida albicans (Thaweboon 2011). Several studies of oil pulling using coconut oil have reported significant reductions in gingivitis and plaque, which leads to tooth decay (Peedikayil 2015).

Getting enough fiber helps the normal healthy bacteria in the gut to thrive. The whole-food Mediterranean-style diet provides fiber in vegetables, whole fruits, whole grains, beans, seeds, and nuts, and a fiber supplement might not be needed.

Fiber is indigestible, so it does not add calories to the diet or increase insulin levels, even though fiber is carbohydrate. There are two basic types of fibers, both of which are found in plants—insoluble and soluble fiber. Insoluble fiber does not dissolve in water but tends to promote secretion of mucus in the bowel, which helps bulk up the stool and keep bowel movements regular. Some examples of insoluble fiber are wheat bran, cellulose, and lignin. Soluble fiber dissolves in water and is fermented mainly in the colon, where it feeds bacteria, producing gases and biologically active byproducts, such as short-chain fatty acids, which have a beneficial impact on gut health. Short-chain fatty acids are converted to ketones and are absorbed and used as an energy source (Kimura 2011). For this reason, soluble fiber supplements are sometimes referred to as fermentable fiber or prebiotics. Some examples of soluble fiber include inulin (chicory root), oligosaccharides, resistant starches, beta glycans (from oats), and wheat dextrin. Psyllium is a combination of insoluble and soluble fiber, and is readily available as a supplement.

Chapter 4 offers more discussion on the importance of fiber; fiber is listed in the macronutrient tables for each food group that contains fiber. I recommend taking a fiber supplement to make up the difference between the amount of fiber in your food and the RDA. Fiber supplements come as tablets, capsules, powder, gummies, and forms that dissolve in water. Psyllium is a popular choice, since it contains both soluble and insoluble fiber and is usually well tolerated, but many more options are available. The daily recommended allowances (RDA) for fiber are (IOM 2006):

- For men ages 19 to 50:   38 grams
- For men ages 51 and over: 30 grams
- For women ages 19 to 50:   25 grams
- For women ages 51 and over: 21 grams

WHAT ABOUT COENZYME Q10?

Coenzyme Q10 (CoQ10) is a popular supplement, and is not a vitamin since it is normally made in the liver and in nearly all cells of the human body. Only a small amount of CoQ10 seems to come from foods, with organ meats providing the richest sources. CoQ10 operates within the mitochondria as an essential cofactor in the production of ATP, and is especially concentrated in tissues with high energy requirements, such as the brain, heart, kidneys, and muscles. CoQ10 is also a potent anti-oxidant that protects cells from damaging reactive oxygen species and facilitates breakdown of cellular waste products.

Levels of CoQ10 in the brain and retina tend to diminish with age and are even more diminished in the Alzheimer's brain. While researching CoQ10 as a possible supplement to consider, I learned that CoQ10 is synthesized and used mainly within mitochondria, and that the currently available supplements (ubiquinol and ubiquinone) do not appear to cross the blood–brain barrier or increase levels in the brain in animal studies, even with very high doses. In a human condition called "primary coenzyme Q10 deficiency," which results from gene mutations, supplementing with high doses of CoQ10 improves muscle and retinal symptoms but not neurological symptoms. Studies with currently available CoQ10 supplements for Alzheimer's and Parkinson's diseases have not shown benefit even at high doses. In some animal studies, very high concentrations of CoQ10 from supplementation showed harmful effects (Manzar 2020; Wear 2021).

Statins used to reduce LDL cholesterol are believed to interfere with production of CoQ10. LDL particles carry CoQ10 in the bloodstream and, along with LDL, blood levels of CoQ10 are reduced in statin users. However, studies are mixed on whether CoQ10 supplementation helps with muscle-related symptoms in people who take statins. It is possible that CoQ10 from supplements does not make it into mitochondria, where it does its job. For Alzheimer's disease and other neurodegenerative disorders with insulin resistance and mitochondrial dysfunction, in my opinion, the inadequate brain levels of CoQ10 could be related to insufficient fuel to drive the biochemical reactions that produce CoQ10 (and very many other important substances, like ATP).

Researchers are working on CoQ10 compounds that are more likely to make it into the brain, but studies showing benefit are lacking in humans at present. If these compounds prove to be the solution, there is potential to treat not only the disorders already mentioned, but also chronic diseases of the heart and kidneys, chronic obstructive pulmonary disease, and non-alcoholic fatty liver disease (Gutierrez-Mariscal 2020).

CHAPTER SEVEN

PUTTING YOUR PERSONAL PLAN TOGETHER TO FIGHT BRAIN AGING

"It takes three days to start a new habit or break an old habit."
—Unknown

Achieving healthy brain aging and prevention of Alzheimer's and other dementias may be possible with lifestyle changes. Diet is the most critical of these changes. If you choose to eat sugary drinks and a junk-food diet, which promote inflammation and insulin resistance, it is unlikely that taking exogenous ketones or other supplements will undo the negative effects. The Clearly Keto Whole-Food Mediterranean-style diet can provide the foundation for a lifestyle that will supply ketones as fuel to the brain, control blood sugar, help reverse insulin resistance, and reduce inflammation. Shifting your metabolism from burning glucose to burning fat as your primary fuel can get you on the road to healthier brain aging.

PUTTING YOUR PERSONALIZED PLAN INTO ACTION

You can pick and choose ketone-raising strategies that fit into your lifestyle to help you reach your goal of healthier brain aging (see figure 7.1). Here are some things to do and questions to answer as

KETOGENIC STRATEGY:	KETONE LEVELS mmol/L:
Caffeine ➤	0.2 to 0.3
Coconut Oil ➤	0.3 to 0.5
Vigorous Exercise ➤	0.3 to 0.5
Overnight Fast ➤	0.3 to 0.5
MCT Oil ➤	0.3 to 1.0
Branched Chain Amino Acids ➤	0.3 to 1.0
Ketone Mineral Salts ➤	0.5 to 1.0
Classic Ketogenic Diet ➤	2 to 6
Starvation ➤	2 to 7
Ketone Esters (Oral or IV) ➤	2 to 7 or higher
Diabetic Ketoacidosis ➤	10 to 25

FIGURE 7.1. Typical ketone levels obtained with ketogenic strategies, starvation, and diabetic ketoacidosis. Levels in diabetic ketoacidosis are many times higher than with ketogenic foods, exercise, overnight fasting, and ketone mineral salts.

you formulate your personal plan. The charts and tables mentioned here can be printed out from my website at https://coconutketones .com.

- Before putting your plan into action, consult with your doctor if you are elderly, have a medical condition, or are helping a child. Consultation with a dietitian experienced in the ketogenic diet is strongly recommended for people who require a strict version of the diet for epilepsy, cancer, or other medical condition.
- Consider whether to monitor ketone and/or glucose levels. Monitoring is particularly important for people with diabetes, for people taking high doses of ketone esters, and for people on a strict ketogenic diet for medical reasons.
- Write out your personal plan in a journal and jot down what you eat, keep track of carb grams, list recipes, document your progress in terms of weight and inches, and note changes to your plan as time goes on.
- Rid your home of sugary drinks and unhealthy foods to prepare for a healthier diet, and review the Clearly Keto Kickstart To-Do List in chapter 1, figure 2.

- Decide whether an overnight fast of at least ten hours or other type of fast will be part of your plan. During the fast, be sure to consume water or clear sugar-free liquids to avoid dehydration. Ketosis will be maintained or increase further if you drink coffee or tea with only added fat like coconut oil, MCT oil, butter, or cream.

- Are you able to do some exercise? What times of day work best into your routine? Morning exercise could kick-start your metabolism. What types of exercise will you engage in? Some combination of resistance and aerobic exercise geared to your comfort and age level, either together or at separate times, are ideal (see chapter 8).

- To plan your new diet, review the Clearly Keto Whole-Food Mediterranean-Style Diet Plan in chapter 4, figure 8.

- Use the Quick Reference Chart for Daily Planning (chapter 4, table 4.12) to calculate your protein requirement, choose your percent of fat, and determine how many grams of carbs you will eat per day.

- Consider whether coconut oil and/or MCT oil will be part of your plan. Remember to begin with small amounts of oil and increase slowly to avoid intestinal distress.

- Consider whether coffee or tea with caffeine and/or branched-chain amino acids will be part of your diet.

- Use the Quick Reference Chart for Meal Planning (chapter 4, table 13) to create two or three recipes for smaller meals and five to seven main meals to get you started.

- Refer to tables 1 through 9 in chapter 4 for each of the food groups to make planning easier. The nutrient breakdown for many other foods is available at the USDA FoodData website: https://fdc.nal.usda.gov.

- Consider buying a macronutrient counter such as *The Complete Book of Food Counts by Corrine T. Netzer* (see Resources).

- Refer to the Naturally Ketogenic Foods table (chapter 4, table 10) to plan some snacks.

- Decide whether exogenous ketone supplements will be part of your plan and where they will fit into your day (see chapter 5). Morning and mid-afternoon are good times to boost your ketone levels with these supplements, or you can sip smaller doses periodically throughout the day.

- Consider whether other supplements will be part of your plan. These might include choline, DHA/EPA, and vitamins and minerals that are not easy to get from diet alone (see chapters 6 and 9).

Take one step at a time as you build your personal plan. My own plan was years in the making, as I learned about the potential benefits of ketones and a ketogenic lifestyle. With such a plan, you will soon be on your way to healthier brain aging.

My Personal Routine with Diet, Fasting, Exercise, and Ketone Supplements

I have practiced overnight fasting for fourteen to sixteen hours for several years and, thanks to low-carb eating, I no longer wake up hungry during the night. To maintain physical strength, my morning wake-up routine includes 3 sets of 12 squats, 12 wall push-ups, and a 30-second wall plank which take no more than 8 minutes (see chapter 8 under Exercise). I build on the overnight fast by whisking coconut oil and MCT oil powders, a few drops of stevia, and cinnamon into coffee and have a serving of ketone salts or ketone ester mid-morning. When I get hungry, usually between noon and 1:30 p.m., I eat my largest meal, consisting of whole foods, including proteins, lots of vegetables, a very small portion of whole grains and sometimes legumes, with more fat grams than protein and carb grams combined. Fats always include virgin coconut oil and MCT oil and often butter, extra-virgin olive, or avocado oil. Around 3:00 or 4:00 p.m., I have a second serving of ketone salts or ester. During the rest of the day until 8:00 p.m. or so, I have two snacks: one snack consists of nuts and/or cheese, or my nut-and-seed granola with coconut milk, and the other snack consists of plain full-fat Greek yogurt or ricotta with grated unsweetened coconut, a few nuts, MCT/coconut oil mixture, and a few blueberries or strawberries (see Recipe section for these and other snack ideas). I never drink sugary beverages or keep sweets or other tempting high-carb snacks in my house.

Special foods and supplements: I eat at least 12 ounces of fish per week and get my vitamins and other important nutrients as much as possible from food. For added insurance, I also take fish oil (1 capsule with 500 mg DHA+EPA), krill oil (750 mg), vitamin D3 in oil (4000 IU), magnesium glycinate (400 mg), nicotinamide riboside (300 mg), benfotiamine (300 mg), and B-complex derived from foods.

Exercise: In addition to my morning functional exercise routine, I add a 20-minute workout using hand weights twice per week. I take a vigorous walk for thirty to forty-five minutes nearly every evening while I enjoy my music playlist, or I use an elliptical if the weather keeps me inside.

Rarely am I stomach-growling hungry, and I sleep and feel great!

PART **TWO**

Things to Do and
Things to Avoid
for Healthy Brain
Aging

CHAPTER EIGHT

LIFESTYLE CHOICES THAT CAN IMPACT HEALTHY AGING AND RISK OF DEMENTIA

"Sufficient sleep, exercise, healthy food, friendship, and peace of mind are necessities, not luxuries."

—Mark Halperin

BETTER LIFESTYLE CHOICES FOR HEALTHY BRAIN AGING

The impact of lifestyle choices on how well we age cannot be emphasized enough. If we are fortunate enough to reach age eighty-five, the odds of developing dementia are about 40 percent and increase with each birthday beyond that. Modifiable lifestyle choices appear to account for at least 30 percent of dementia cases worldwide, with diet at the top of the list. As discussed in part 1, the problem of inadequate brain energy is the earliest known abnormality in the progression of Alzheimer's disease. The brain can compensate for the decrease in energy for a while. However, as the energy-related and other abnormalities in the brain become too extensive, symptoms emerge and become apparent, first to the individual (Stage 2) and then to others (Stage 3 and beyond; see FAST score in chapter 8). There is a golden opportunity in the pre-clinical stage to fill in the growing gap in brain energy by eating a healthy diet and adopting strategies aimed at achieving nutritional ketosis. Healthy dietary choices can, for example, prevent, control, or reverse diabetes and its serious complications like blindness and kidney failure.

Many lifestyle choices beyond diet can also impact healthy aging. A personal choice to smoke could lead to chronic obstructive pulmonary disease (COPD) and possibly lung cancer. Consuming excessive alcohol could lead to fatal cirrhosis of the liver. Each of these conditions independently confers a higher risk of dementia, and the combination could lead to an early demise. How we choose to live can largely determine whether we will enjoy quality healthy aging or spend decades saddled with disability, dozens of medications, and hundreds of hours wasted in doctors' waiting rooms. It is never too late to make changes to try to prevent or delay dementia, but acting sooner will have greater impact since damage to the brain from poor choices is cumulative and tends to progress over time. We all know that a car will last longer and better if we stick with a regular preventive maintenance schedule. It makes sense to apply the same principle to our own brain and body to live longer and age better.

Prevention may be within your grasp, and you can take steps in that direction at any age . . . the sooner, the better!

LIFESTYLE RISK FACTORS BEYOND DIET

Let's take another look at the figure from chapter 4 to consider more closely the non-diet-related lifestyle risk factors (see figure 8.1). The data in this figure represent the number of lives that could have been saved if the risk factor had been eliminated. The Institute for Health Metrics and Evaluation (IHME) has determined that high blood pressure, at 10.44 million deaths annually, holds the greatest risk for preventable premature death. High dietary sodium intake, which can cause or worsen high blood pressure, accounts for another 3.2 million deaths, and reducing sodium could help. Smoking is the second-highest risk factor, accounting for 7.1 million deaths, with inhaling secondhand

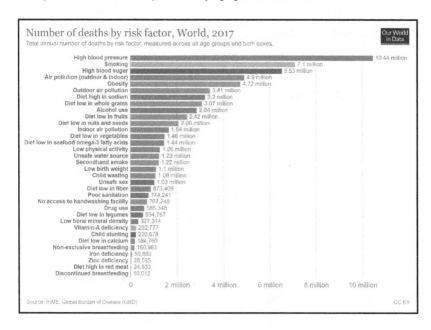

FIGURE 8.1. Numbers of Deaths by Risk Factors, World, 2017. Nearly 56 million people died in 2017. Source: Our World in Data: "Number of deaths by risk factor, World, 2017." From the Institute for Health Metrics and Evaluation. https://ourworldindata.org /grapher/number-of-deaths-by-risk-factor?country=~OWID_WRL from http://ghdx .healthdata.org/gbd-results-tool Open access permission.

smoke at 1.22 million deaths. Exposure to air pollution indoors or outdoors, lack of physical activity, alcohol consumption, drug use, and vitamin and mineral deficiencies are also important risk factors. This chapter will discuss these and other known risk factors for premature death, which are also risk factors for dementia.

Dementia is a massive growing problem worldwide, affecting both families and governments. Billions in research dollars have not led to a life-changing treatment, much less a cure, for Alzheimer's. In recent years, key organizations—including the National Institutes of Health, the Alzheimer's Association, and Alzheimer's Disease International— are supporting research to learn what modifiable lifestyle factors pose risks for developing dementia and whether intervening with better choices could prevent dementia. The focus has shifted to identifying people who are at risk before the disease becomes symptomatic (Stage 1 of Alzheimer's) and directing efforts toward treatment and prevention in this pre-clinical stage.

In 2017, the World-Wide FINGERS Network became the first global network of multidomain dementia-prevention trials, in which a combination of lifestyle interventions, such as diet, exercise, and cognitive training, are studied in individuals with repeated assessments for years. Miia Kivipelto, MD, PhD, is a Finnish neuroscientist who focuses on Alzheimer's and dementia and is a professor at the Karolinska Institute and at the University of Eastern Finland. She is one of the first researchers to conduct such a trial and has been the driving force behind this global effort. These and other studies present convincing evidence that prevention of dementia is possible (Marcos-Pardo 2020; Van den Brink 2019; Salas-Salvadó 2019; Qiu 2019; Rosenberg 2018; Rosenberg 2020; Yu 2020).

Based on the best evidence to date, recommendations by World-Wide FINGERS and other experts on lifestyle choices to prevent dementia and promote healthy brain aging include:

- Eat a healthy diet. Identify and control high blood sugar.
- Engage in physical activity.
- Consider intermittent fasting.
- Maximize your education, stay cognitively engaged, and challenge your brain.
- Stay socially engaged to avoid isolation.
- Get adequate sleep, but avoid medications to induce sleep.
- Do not smoke, and avoid second-hand smoke.
- Avoid excessive alcohol intake.
- Identify and control high blood pressure.
- Identify and treat sleep apnea.
- Identify and correct problems with hearing and vision.
- Take measures to reduce stress, anxiety, and depression through counseling and behavior modification as much as possible, rather than medications.

We will discuss each of these points in this chapter and then talk about some things to avoid in chapter 9.

EAT A HEALTHY DIET AND CONTROL BLOOD SUGAR

Of the more than 56 million deaths in 2017, the IHME attributes 28 million deaths to risk factors related to diet and nutrition, with high blood sugar third on the list at 6.53 million deaths and obesity fifth at 4.12 million deaths (figure 8.1). In part 1, we discussed the problems of insulin resistance, diabetes, obesity, and the brain-energy gap. A ketogenic whole-food Mediterranean diet could help overcome insulin resistance, put diabetes into remission, promote fat loss, and provide ketones to fill in the brain-energy gap.

ENGAGE IN PHYSICAL ACTIVITY

During the virtual 2021 Alzheimer's Association International Conference, a group of researchers, including Kivipelto, presented the results of their multi-domain interventional studies. During a panel discussion, they all agreed without hesitation that exercise is the next most important lifestyle choice after eating a healthy diet. Many studies have reported that regular physical activity may ward off cognitive impairment and Alzheimer's and may reduce symptoms of Parkinson's disease (Kim 2021; Ogino 2019; Rosenfeldt 2021; Schootemeijer 2020).

An eighty-nine-year-old family member had back surgery recently, and when he asked about physical therapy, the doctor said "Walk, walk, and walk." For people who have been couch potatoes, walking is the easiest way to get into the exercise habit. While our hunter-gatherer ancestors walked for hours every day searching for food, too many people today barely walk at all, much less engage in another form of exercise. The list of good reasons to change is long and supported by substantial scientific evidence. Just thirty to forty-five minutes of vigorous or sustained exercise increases ketone levels, and those levels can last up to nine hours, a phenomenon known as "post-exercise ketosis" that was first studied more than a hundred years ago. This is more likely to happen if a high-carbohydrate meal or snack is not eaten before the activity (Forssner 1909; Preti 1911; Courtice 1936; Passmore 1958; Rennie 1974; Koeslag 1979; Fery 1983).

Muscle Mass Shrinks with Age

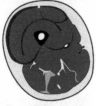 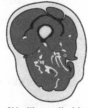 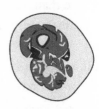

| Young Woman, Healthy
Age 24-26 | Older Woman, Healthy
Lifelong Exerciser, Age 74-76 | Older Woman, Healthy
Non-Lifelong Exerciser, Age 74-76 |

FIGURE 8.2. Exercise slows down loss of muscle mass with aging. This figure illustrates the difference in upper leg (top) muscle mass in young exercising women (ages twenty-four to twenty-six), lifelong exercising older women (ages seventy-four to seventy-six), and non-exercising healthy older women (ages seventy-four to seventy-six). Without exercise, muscle mass decreases, and fat invades and surrounds the muscle. Adapted from MRI images in Chambers 2020.

When you are walking, using a treadmill, bicycle, or elliptical, if possible, kick up your speed for 20 or 30 seconds every few minutes (called interval training) to enhance the benefits of aerobic exercise. Both insulin resistance and mitochondrial dysfunction are important features of Alzheimer's. Interval training has been shown to enhance the effect of exercise in overcoming insulin resistance and improving the function of mitochondria, where energy is made in our cells (Ruegsegger 2018). As discussed in chapter 5, walking at a moderate pace can nearly triple the uptake of energy as ketones in the brain (Castellano 2017).

Another issue of aging is the gradual loss of muscle and muscle strength leading, over time, to reduced functionality and endurance. Simple things that we previously took for granted, like getting up out of a chair, in or out of a car, and walking up steps may become more difficult. Figure 8.2 illustrates how muscle mass is lost with aging, especially in people who do not exercise routinely. Three muscle-sustaining tactics include eating enough protein (at least 0.5 grams per pound [1.1 gram per kg] of body weight), performing strength-training or resistance exercises several times per week, and using ketogenic strategies (fasting, ketogenic foods, ketogenic diet) to encourage more burning of fat as fuel.

Three Strength Exercises to Help Maintain Functionality

Strength exercises can help maintain functionality as you age, and do not require elaborate equipment or a lot of time. If you want to go further, you can add hand weights, gym machines, or resistance bands. A multitude of books, phone apps, and YouTube videos, many geared to seniors, can show you how to use weights or bands with exercise.

Simple exercises you can do at home in a few minutes can have surprising results over time. If you do just one exercise, choose "squats," since this exercise will help maintain leg strength and the ability to get up and down from a chair, walk, and negotiate steps with less fatigue and can contribute to a greater sense of physical security as you get older. You can also march or jog in place for a minute or so before and between sets of exercise to add an aerobic element to the exercise and warm up your muscles. Take your time! Slower rather than quick movement while doing strength exercises requires more muscle fibers and may be more effective.

Chair Squats: Taking the stairs instead of the elevator can help maintain leg strength, but if you live in a single-story home with just one step, like me, performing squats can be a good substitute (photo 1).

- If you are worried about balance, stand next to a kitchen counter with a chair positioned behind you.
- With your arms held straight out and feet about 12 inches (⅓ meter) apart, slowly bend at the knees and hips as if you are going to sit down; but just before you reach the chair, slowly stand back up again.

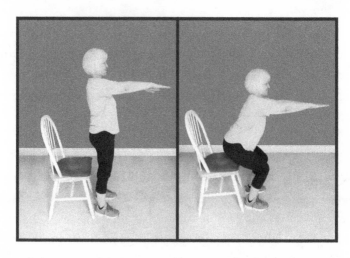

PHOTO 1. Chair squats in two positions.

- In the beginning, try to repeat these maneuvers at least five times, then slowly increase to sets of ten or more. As you get stronger, add a second or third set with a short rest between each set.

Wall Push-ups: Wall push-ups are a simple way to strengthen all the muscles in the arms, shoulders, and upper back (see photo 2).

- Stand about 18 inches (½ meter) away from a wall, facing it. If that distance is too challenging, move closer to the wall until your strength improves.
- Stretch your arms in front of you and flatten your hands against the wall.
- While leaving your feet in place, bend your arms until your face almost touches the wall, then slowly push back to the original position. Keep your back as straight as possible, which will also help strengthen the muscles in your back.
- In the beginning, try to repeat these maneuvers at least five times, then slowly increase to sets of ten, or more. As you get stronger, add a second or third set with a short rest in between each set.

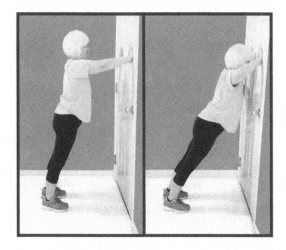

PHOTO 2. Wall push-ups in two positions.

- To further strengthen calf and ankle muscles, move your feet from the flat position to tiptoes as you move toward the wall during the push-up.
- As you get stronger, you might try switching from wall to floor push-ups.

Plank: This exercise is intended to strengthen your core, including your entire back, buttocks, and abdominal muscles. You can perform this exercise against the wall or from the floor as you get stronger (see photo 3).

- With arms bent at the elbows, place lower arms against the wall, and move feet about 18 inches from the wall and slightly apart.
- Alternatively, you can begin like a wall push-up, using your hands against the wall, and bend your arms until your face is a few inches from the wall.
- Tighten your back, buttocks, and abdominal muscles so that your body is straight, and hold that position for a minimum of 10 seconds. As you grow stronger, increase the time to 30 seconds or longer.
- Repeat the plank at least two or three times per exercise session.

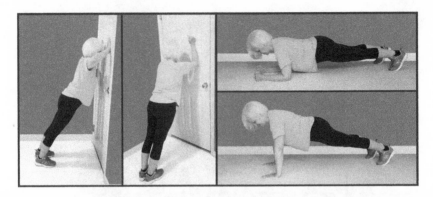

PHOTO 3. Wall or floor planks: four different positions to try.

Dementia-Friendly Exercises

The Mental Health Physiologists at the National Health Service of Greater Glasgow and Clyde, Scotland, kindly allowed me to include two charts of dementia-friendly seated and standing exercises to help maintain functionality (see figures 8.3 and 8.4). Cognitively healthy older people could benefit from these exercises as well.

INTERMITTENT FASTING CAN PROMOTE HEALTHY AGING

Intermittent fasting provides many health benefits, including higher ketone levels to help fill the brain-energy gap. Chapter 5 on other ketogenic strategies includes an extensive discussion of overnight fasting and other approaches to intermittent fasting.

MAXIMIZE YOUR EDUCATION, STAY COGNITIVELY ENGAGED, AND CHALLENGE YOUR BRAIN

According to the Alzheimer's Association Facts and Figures Report for 2020 (see https://alz.org), fewer years of formal education creates a higher risk of dementia due to lower socioeconomic status. People with

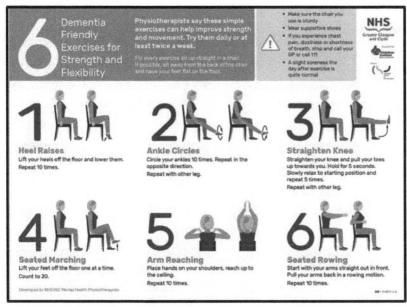

FIGURE 8.3. Dementia-friendly seated exercises. Used with permission from Mental Health Physiologists at National Health Service of Greater Glasgow and Clyde, Scotland at https://www.headsup.scot /media/264157/dementia-friendly-exercises-for-strength-and-flexibility-2020-12-a3-poster.pdf.

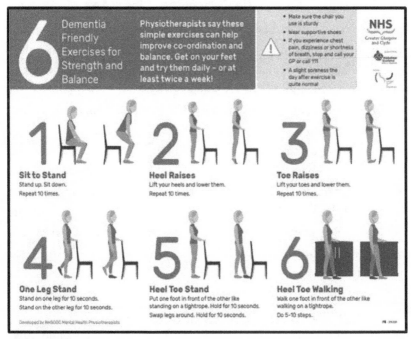

FIGURE 8.4. Dementia-friendly standing exercises. Used with permission from Mental Health Physiologists at National Health Service of Greater Glasgow and Clyde, Scotland at https://www.headsup.scot /media/264157/dementia-friendly-exercises-for-strength-and-flexibility-2020-12-a3-poster.pdf.

less education are more likely to smoke and develop medical conditions such as high blood pressure, obesity, diabetes, and heart disease, which are each risk factors for dementia. Having less money to live on often means a lower-quality diet, a tendency toward less physical activity, and the inability to afford treatment for medical conditions. While the risk of developing dementia is greater for people with lower levels of education, this can definitely happen to intelligent, highly educated people, including neurosurgeons, prime ministers, and presidents of the United States. Having more years of formal education is thought to build up "cognitive reserve," which may help protect against the development of cognitive impairment with aging. Cognitive reserve is the extent to which the brain can sustain damage without effects on intellectual capacity.

If you did not go to college, you are not doomed to develop dementia. Numerous studies suggest that stimulating your brain with mentally challenging activities may also help maintain cognitive reserve to protect the network connections in your brain (Ball 2002; Hall 2009; Sanjeev 2016; Staf 2018; Wilson 2002; Yates 2016). Many cognitive training programs have been developed for this purpose. Before purchasing such a program, ask whether clinical trials with good results have been performed, and request a preview of the program to determine if the program is challenging enough for you.

Learning something new is a great way to challenge your brain, and the possibilities are endless. Learn how to use a computer or tablet and how to get on the Internet if you do not know how. E-books and audiobooks can be stored on a tablet, computer, or smartphone. These versions save money and space on bookshelves, and many are available through free online or local libraries. Most newspapers now have online editions, saving many trees. Many news outlets have online streaming available to watch live or video clips of important and interesting stories. Harvard and other colleges offer free or low-cost online classes for topics ranging from the sciences to the arts. You can learn how to do almost anything, such as performing simple repairs, gardening, and art techniques, using free online options like YouTube, TikTok, and other social-media platforms.

If you play a musical instrument, learn new songs, and try to memorize them. If you like to sing, join a choral group. Learn new card games. Learn a new language. Research your family tree. Write an autobiography to pass down to your children and grandchildren. Take up a new hobby. Take a class. Work puzzles and mind games like Sudoku and crossword. Read, read, and read! Many of these activities have the added benefit of connecting you with other people, and the possibilities are endless.

STAY SOCIALLY ENGAGED TO AVOID ISOLATION

Staying socially engaged has never been more difficult than during the coronavirus pandemic that still affects how we go about our lives in early 2022. Social isolation can lead to loneliness, depression, and anxiety and, possibly, more rapid cognitive decline. Numerous studies suggest that becoming more socially engaged can change that. In one of the larger long-term studies (see side box), Dr. Bryan James and group at Rush Alzheimer's Disease Center in Chicago reported that people who are more socially active have much slower cognitive decline as they age (James 2011).

Frequent Social Interaction Slows Cognitive Decline

A group of 1138 people averaging age 79 and without dementia at baseline received a full battery of cognitive and psychological testing annually for up to 12 years. Participants were assigned a score based on how often they performed each category of the six activities listed below: once per year or less (1 point); several times per year (2 points); several times per month (3 points); several times per week (4 points); every day or almost every day (5 points):

- Go to restaurants, sporting events, or teletract [off-track betting], or play bingo.

- Go on day trips or overnight trips.

- Do unpaid community or volunteer work.

- Visit relatives' or friends' houses.

- Participate in groups, such as senior center, Knights of Columbus, Rosary Society, or something similar [like taking an adult education or art class].

- Attend church or religious services.

The points were totaled and divided by six to obtain a composite score. Higher scores indicated more activity. The highest possible score was 5.00. People at the 90th percentile averaged a score of 3.33, while the 10th percentile score was 1.83. People at the 90th percentile enjoyed a 70 percent slower cognitive rate of decline than people at the 10th percentile for all five cognitive domains tested. A 1-point increase in score correlated with a 47 percent decrease in the annual rate of cognitive decline. The authors showed that cognitive decline was not the cause of the infrequent social activity, but rather infrequent social activity resulted in faster cognitive decline (James 2011).

It is common for people to count down the days, minutes, and hours to retirement, only to find a big gap in their social life when they no longer have coworkers with whom to interact. The gap may be larger if a person lives alone and far away from children, grandchildren, and other family members, with infrequent phone calls and visits.

You can kill two birds with one stone—challenging your brain and staying socially connected—by learning to use a computer and the Internet if you do not already know how. One of my older family members resisted getting a computer for years because he did not want to be "one of the guys who sits on a computer all day," but now he loves it. The idea of using a computer or tablet may be intimidating. With just a little bit of help to get set up and learn a few basics like using a mouse, navigating a tablet, and getting on the Internet, a whole world of information and social connections by e-mail and on social media will open up. If you do not know how to type, apps can teach you step-by-step or you can hunt and peck, which will still get you there, albeit more slowly.

It is easy to sign up for a free account on websites like Zoom to have face-to-face video conversations, allowing people to celebrate birthdays and holidays with relatives and friends who are far away or practicing social distancing, to have work-related meetings, and even to hold international conferences with tens of thousands of people watching. In 2020, conferences and seminars of all types became virtual (online) for the first time. Many of these programs were free or much lower cost than their in-person events and open to everyone, such as Alzheimer's Disease International, which is geared to caregivers and people living with dementia, and the Alzheimer's Association International Conference, which focuses on the science but is also open to everyone who is interested. Many of the presentations in 2020 were live on Zoom or other platforms, and it was possible to ask questions and receive answers.

If you prefer to hold and read a printed book, spending time in a library or bookstore or joining a book club are great ways to challenge your brain and stay socially connected.

GET ADEQUATE SLEEP, BUT AVOID MEDICATIONS TO INDUCE SLEEP

Many people experience sleep disturbances as they age, for various reasons. Sleep problems are often exaggerated in people with mild cognitive impairment and dementia, including Alzheimer's. Poor sleep is a risk factor for developing dementia, and dementia can also lead to sleep disturbances. Likewise, poor sleep is common in people with obesity and diabetes and is also a consequence of these disorders, which are each independent risk factors for cognitive impairment and dementia (Van Cauter 2008). Even while sleeping, the brain requires a great deal of energy. Poor sleep is associated with dysfunction of glucose regulation with inadequate energy production in the brain.

In a review of studies encompassing 69,000 people, 15 percent of Alzheimer's cases were attributed to poor sleep, implying that Alzheimer's could be prevented if sleep duration and quality are improved. Obstructive sleep apnea was by far the greatest sleep-related risk for Alzheimer's and cognitive impairment. Excessive sleep (more than 8 hours) and shortened sleep (less than 7 hours) are both associated with Alzheimer's and cognitive impairment (Bubu 2017).

As people age, it may become more difficult to get to sleep and stay asleep as they experience more awake time during the night, resulting in less sleep overall. Sleep disturbances can lead to daytime sleepiness and frequent napping, which interfere with daytime activities and getting to sleep later that night—a vicious cycle. The circadian rhythm (our natural daytime/nighttime cycle) may weaken with age, leading to excessive sleepiness early in the evening, followed by waking early in the morning without the ability to get back to sleep (Borges 2019).

Since the 1970s, hundreds of studies of sleep duration, quality, and other sleep characteristics have been conducted in healthy people, in aging, and in many different conditions. Technological advances allow evaluation for sleep disorders, such as obstructive sleep apnea, which we will discuss in the next section. Polysomnography combines several technologies to evaluate various components of sleep, including measurement of the heart rate, breathing rate, chest movement, airflow through the nose, and percent of oxygen in the blood (oxygen saturation). Polysomnography can be performed overnight at home or in a sleep lab. At-home sleep studies can measure the important basic parameters. When performed in a sleep lab, a specially trained technician observes the study, which may include electroencephalogram (EEG) monitoring of brain waves and occasionally electromyogram (EMG) monitoring of muscle tone to determine the phase of sleep. Video observation is sometimes used to document seizures, restless legs, or other abnormal movements, and electrooculography (EOG) is sometimes used to study eye movement.

During seven to eight hours of normal sleep, there are four or five roughly ninety-minute cycles, during which we move between light sleep, deep sleep, and REM (rapid eye movement) sleep. During REM sleep, the eyelids move rapidly, vivid dreams occur, and muscle tone is low, which keeps us from acting out our dreams. Breathing, heart rate, temperature control, and blood pressure become irregular during REM sleep. Compared to other phases of sleep, REM sleep requires the same amount of energy as being awake, or more. The neurotransmitter acetylcholine is normally abundant during REM sleep but is deficient in Alzheimer's. As the night goes on, periods of REM sleep tend to get longer and take up more of the sleep cycle. Repeated disruptions of deep sleep and REM sleep, or deprivation of either phase, have consequences that can affect cognition and quality of life. Getting six hours of sleep or less for just two weeks has the cumulative effect of losing two full nights' sleep and can lead to decreased alertness, slower problem-solving, a slower reaction time, and inappropriate reactions. Sleep deprivation affects the very short-term memory (called working memory) that we need to accomplish a simple activity. These problems worsen as the average duration of sleep decreases. Inadequate sleep is not good for the heart, either. Sleep deprivation for just one night can raise hormone levels that increase heart rate and blood pressure (Bah 2019).

As we age, sleep may become less efficient at carrying out special functions the brain can only accomplish during sleep. Deep sleep appears to be the opportunity for the brain to recover from the day's activities and is also called the "slow-wave" phase, based on what the EEG pattern looks like. The brain's requirement for energy decreases during deep sleep, and certain components of food are converted to complex proteins, facilitating repair of muscle and other tissues. During deep sleep, growth hormone and certain appetite-related hormones are secreted, and the brain removes toxins that have accrued while awake through river-like channels called glymphatics, which empty into the spinal fluid. Without adequate deep sleep, toxins, such as beta amyloid and tau, can accumulate in the brain to form the characteristic plaques and tangles of Alzheimer's (Xie 2013; Boespflug 2018).

Dreaming occurs during REM sleep. Motor learning and conversion of short-term memories to long-term memories are thought to occur during REM sleep, and some types of memory formation occur in deep sleep as well. Establishment of synapses (connections between brain cells) and removal of defective synapses occur during REM sleep. Cell division is also active during REM sleep (Peever 2017).

An abnormal REM sleep pattern may be an early symptom of Lewy body dementia, Parkinson's disease, progressive supranuclear palsy, corticobasal degeneration, and multiple system atrophy. Inadequate REM sleep can result in increased anxiety, irritability, poor concentration, increased appetite, hallucinations, and aggressive behavior. In Alzheimer's, the changes in the brain affecting sleep can become so pronounced that the phase of sleep may be difficult to determine, even using polysomnography.

People with Alzheimer's tend to wake up more often and stay awake for longer periods than people without the disease. Normal circadian rhythm, which controls when we are awake or asleep, can also be disrupted. Circadian rhythm is complex, and one factor involves the balance of the hormones cortisol and melatonin, which cycle over twenty-four hours. In Alzheimer's, Parkinson's, and some other neurological disorders, the cycle of melatonin release, regulation of heart rate and blood pressure, and temperature control may be disrupted. Unlike most people, people with Alzheimer's may experience increased urine production at night compared to the daytime (Fifel 2021).

It is common for people with Alzheimer's to be up and about for hours during the night, then sleep throughout much of the daytime, which is quite difficult for the people living with them. Caregivers tend to lose hours of sleep as a result. I knew a doctor who told caregivers to "make" the sleepy person with dementia stay awake and walking in the daytime to encourage sleeping at night, but this practice is exhausting and time-consuming for caregivers, who already have enough on their plates. A sleepy person is also at greater risk of falling. At the point that Steve began having long periods of nighttime awakening, I hired paid caregivers to spend the night with him. This allowed me to get enough sleep to continue working and take calls from the hospital without disturbing Steve. This was a very sad moment for our marriage, since we needed to set up a separate room for Steve with a caregiver close by to keep him safe.

Deficiency of acetylcholine in Alzheimer's partly explains the sleep disturbances. Many drugs can interfere with REM sleep, including antidepressants, stimulants, and, ironically, certain "sleep aids," by blocking the production of acetylcholine, which is needed for quality REM sleep. This effect on REM sleep explains why people feel foggy and lethargic the day after taking these medications. The sleep aids at issue include diphenhydramine (Benadryl®), doxylamine (found alone or in Nyquil® and other cold remedies), and other antihistamines.

Sleep medications like zolpidem (Ambien®), eszopiclone (Lunesta®), and zaleplon (Sonata®) are good at inducing sleep but can interfere with REM and other sleep parameters. Many instances of sleepwalking, sleep-eating, and even sleep-driving with accidents have been reported in people taking these drugs, leading to an FDA box warning to alert people to these possible side effects. The benzodiazepine class of drugs, such as alprazolam (Xanax®), temazepam (Restoril®), lorazepam (Ativan®), and valium, are typically used for anxiety but are sometimes prescribed for sleep. These drugs were intended for short-term use, three days at most, but are sometimes prescribed for years. Benzodiazepines can cause increased drowsiness, confusion, loss of several hours of memory preceding the medication, and a rebound effect of worsening insomnia (Bah 2019). Some other drugs used to treat depression and seizures are under study for sleep but also carry a long list of potential side effects.

It is common for doctors to prescribe medications for urinary problems, which often interfere with sleep. However, some medications intended to control the bladder and improve urine flow, like tamsulosin (Flomax®) and oxybutynin (Ditropan®), also work by blocking acetylcholine. Anticholinergic medications may have side effects like dryness of the mouth, blurred vision, drowsiness, constipation, trouble urinating, confusion, and hallucinations. Most of the approved Alzheimer's medications work to increase availability of acetylcholine in the brain, so it does not make sense to take medications with the opposite effect. Chapter 9 includes more information on anticholinergic medications.

The need to urinate frequently or loss of bladder control (incontinence) is a common cause of sleep disruption in later years. It is not unusual for women and men to get up multiple times during the night to urinate, and many find it difficult to get back to sleep. Some people cannot get to sleep out of fear that they will soil the bed. Placing a disposable or washable underpad on the bed and wearing disposable underwear with an extra pad inserted, if necessary, could provide less worry and more sleep. Several brands of disposable underwear pull up and fit well under clothing without being obvious. External catheters for men and for women could provide relief for people with frequent nighttime incontinence. Most people know that urinals are available for men, but many do not know that urinals designed for women are also available. Urinals could work for someone who can stand but cannot easily walk to use the toilet. One genius caregiver used a good old-fashioned flexible ice bag for her bedbound husband to urinate in.

When I first began making home visits with elderly patients, I was quite surprised that many women over age eighty, and most over ninety, reported a problem with leakage of urine, often quite significant. The uterus and bladder tend to droop as people age and create the sensation of having to urinate frequently. For men, enlargement of the prostate can block the flow of urine, so the urine builds up in the bladder, and the bladder may not empty well, creating a constant annoying sensation of having to urinate. For either sex, when the bladder does not completely empty, there is risk of urinary-tract (bladder or kidney) infection. Surgery may be needed to correct an enlarged prostate or a fallen uterus if there is no good alternative. A visit to a urologist could determine if there is a treatable problem.

In people with Alzheimer's and other dementias, loss of bladder and bowel control are an unfortunate part of the progression of the disease in the later stages. The need to urinate or have a bowel movement can be a great source of anxiety and agitation, and the person with dementia cannot always voice the need to use the toilet. Poor cleanup after a bowel movement often precedes incontinence and is a setup for urinary-tract infections. Inflammation from infection can cause anxiety and confusion in someone who normally seems to be cognitively intact, and these symptoms will usually subside as the infection responds to treatment. A sudden increase in anxiety and confusion in an older person or someone with dementia should prompt a check for urinary-tract infection.

Another common problem affecting sleep is gastroesophageal reflux disorder (GERD), also called "heartburn" or indigestion. It normally takes about 2½ to 3 hours for the stomach to digest and empty out after eating. If food, alcoholic beverages, or soft drinks are consumed too close to bedtime, undigested material and stomach acid can come up (reflux) into the esophagus (tube connecting the back of the throat and the stomach). Breathing may stop when this occurs, interrupting sleep; and, even worse, this material can be inhaled into the lungs, which can cause choking in the short-term and inflammation and damage to the lungs and esophagus. Coughing during the night may be a sign of reflux. Most people can figure out which foods give them heartburn, and these should be avoided.

An adjustable bed that allows the head of the bed to be raised is a good investment for people with GERD, and it may be covered by Medicare or other insurance. Alternatively, sleeping on a wedge-type pillow or stacked pillows could take advantage of gravity to hold food down in the stomach while sleeping. If simple measures do not fix the problem, a visit to a gastroenterologist (GI doctor) is in order, to ensure that nothing more serious is going on, such as an ulcer or esophageal cancer, and to advise on other potential treatments. Various medications can treat GERD, but, like most medications, these can be a double-edged sword, so risks versus benefits should be considered. Avoiding foods that provoke stomach acid, allowing at least a three-hour gap between eating and bedtime, and elevation of the head of the bed are the key first steps to controlling GERD.

An over-the-counter sleep medication worth a try is melatonin, a hormone that normally increases during sleep, but we tend to produce less as we get older. Unfortunately, studies of melatonin for Alzheimer's have conflicting results. It is possible to get melatonin in a short-acting form to induce sleep and in an extended-release form to help keep a person asleep. A wide range of doses is available (1 to 20 mg), but more is not necessarily better. Some sleep experts recommend avoiding high doses of melatonin due to potential adverse effects (headache, dizziness, nausea, daytime drowsiness, low blood pressure, depression). They advise starting with the lowest dose available, such as 1 mg, then increasing gradually, watching for improved sleep and side effects. Melatonin is available as pills, gummies, and liquid.

Many people report sleeping better after adopting a healthier low-carb diet, when using an intermittent fasting/time-restricted eating approach, and also after adding MCT oil, coconut oil, ketone salts, or ketone esters to their regimen. Some people report more frequent, more vivid, and more memorable dreams. There are few studies on the effects of ketogenic strategies on sleep.

Gill and group (Gill 2015) studied forty-seven overweight men and women with erratic eating schedules, documenting their eating patterns and activity levels for three weeks with a smartphone application and an actigraphy wristband. Actigraphy detects movement and surrounding light and can record time in bed, sleep, and daytime activities. These erratic eaters were found to suffer from metabolic "jet lag," which affects circadian rhythm and sets a person up for chronic illnesses like diabetes and metabolic syndrome. Then, eight people in a subgroup were instructed to fast overnight and eat within a ten- to eleven-hour window in the daytime for sixteen weeks, but were not told how much or what to eat. They continued to wear the "actigraphy" bracelet. They ate fewer calories, lost an average of fourteen pounds (6.37 kg), and reported longer duration of sleep and feeling more energetic. These benefits continued for at least a year.

Brain cells need energy to sleep and accomplish tasks like growth and repair that only occur during sleep, and the age-related brain-energy gap could impair these processes. A person with brain insulin resistance can have plenty of glucose available, but affected cells in the brain are starving because glucose cannot enter the cell. This could also explain why some people wake up hungry and feel the need to eat during the night. Eating a high-carb snack in the evening before sleep is conducive to nighttime eating; a high-carb meal or snack with simple sugars sends insulin levels up, and hunger returns when the insulin level goes back down. Improved sleep with ketogenic strategies could simply be the result of providing ketones to fuel the activities of sleep-related brain cells. Hopefully, more studies will be forthcoming on specific ketogenic strategies and their effect on sleep.

Here are some non-drug strategies that could help improve the duration and quality of your sleep, as well as your overall quality of life:

- Maintain a regular time for going to bed and waking up in the morning. Allow adequate time to get between seven and eight hours of sleep.
- Limit liquids to sips for at least two to three hours before bedtime, to eliminate or reduce nighttime trips to the bathroom.
- Empty your bladder before bedtime, and see a urologist if you have not been evaluated and treated for problems with bladder control or frequent urination.
- A room that is either too cold or too warm can interfere with sleep. Find a room temperature that is conducive to sleep for you. If you are sharing your bed, partners may need to find some combination of room temperature, nighttime clothing, and bed covers that is comfortable for both.
- Avoid overstimulating activities before bedtime. Keep the bedroom environment quiet and dark. Too much ambient light, too much blue-light screentime (smart TVs, smart phones, tablets, and computers) or sound from a television or radio can interfere with sleep. Blackout shades could cut down on bothersome window light.
- To avoid falls when getting up to use the bathroom, consider inexpensive plug-in motion-detector night-lights to illuminate the pathway and the bathroom.
- Avoid looking at the clock if you have trouble getting to sleep, because this tends to increase anxiety about sleep.
- Limit napping, and avoid spending unnecessary time in bed in the daytime.

- Establish consistent mealtimes, and avoid eating for at least three hours before going to bed. If you experience heartburn, choking, or coughing during the night, see a gastroenterologist for evaluation and treatment.
- Take a walk or engage in other physical activities, which may encourage a good night's sleep.
- Avoid stimulants such as alcohol and chocolate in the late evening and drinks with caffeine after noon. Caffeine is a long-acting stimulant for some people and may make it difficult to "shut off" the brain at bedtime. Chocolate, while healthy for other reasons, may contain theobromine, a compound similar in effect to caffeine. Some medications and drugs are stimulants as well. Check with your doctor or pharmacist if you suspect that a medication is interfering with your sleep.
- If your brain is overstimulated, thinking about the day's events, or worrying about family matters, and if caffeine is not the issue, try venting about the day's events with a spouse or friend, but not too close to bedtime.
- If you are lying awake, worried about the next day's events or about an idea that pops into your head, writing down your thoughts could help your brain to calm down.
- Concentrate on relaxing your facial muscles, which can help take your mind off other thoughts.
- If you still have trouble getting to sleep and staying asleep, if you snore, or if you routinely feel like you have not gotten enough sleep, talk to your doctor about having a sleep study to evaluate for the possibility of sleep apnea, which carries a high risk of dementia if not recognized and treated.

Trazodone could be an option for severe persistent insomnia. Trazodone was developed originally as an antidepressant in the 1980s and was FDA-approved for this use in 1981. Since then, trazodone has been used more often to treat insomnia, since it has a sedating effect and is only mildly effective for depression. Trazodone works by increasing duration of sleep and, specifically, slow-wave sleep, which may help reduce accumulation of beta amyloid plaques that are associated with Alzheimer's. Trazodone does not have anti-cholinergic effects like most other sleep aids and many antidepressants. By two weeks after starting trazodone, most people do not report daytime drowsiness or a negative effect on cognition. In a four-week study, there were fewer episodes of wakening and longer duration of sleep for people with Alzheimer's (Camargos 2014). Another study reported that twenty-five older people who were not taking trazodone declined 2.6 times more on cognitive testing over four years than twenty-five matched people who took trazodone (La 2019).

A Cochrane review of sleep medications reported that there was no evidence that melatonin or ramelteon (Rozeram) helped with sleep in people with Alzheimer's, and there have been no trials of benzodiazepines for sleep in Alzheimer's. However, the authors concluded that the evidence for trazodone warrants larger studies (McLeery 2016).

IDENTIFY AND TREAT SLEEP APNEA

Untreated sleep apnea is a risk factor for mild cognitive impairment, Alzheimer's, and vascular dementia (Bah 2019; Kuo 2021). Sleep apnea can also increase blood pressure or cause chest pain or pressure (angina) in people with coronary artery disease, atrial fibrillation, or congestive heart failure, and it can even trigger seizures. Not long after my husband Steve began having seizures in 2013, we observed that he stopped breathing while he was sleeping for up to thirty seconds. A home sleep study revealed that Steve had periods of central sleep apnea, almost certainly tied to progression of Alzheimer's and Lewy body disease. Steve was treated with continuous positive airway pressure (CPAP), explained shortly, which effectively reduced the number of apneic episodes and may have prevented seizures.

Normally, an adult at rest breathes about twelve to sixteen times per minute, or about every four to five seconds. A decrease in blood oxygen and a build-up of carbon dioxide between breaths triggers the next breath by way of sensors, called chemoreceptors, in the brain's respiratory center. "Apnea" means cessation of breathing and can occur in two ways, called central apnea and obstructive apnea. "Central apnea" occurs when the respiratory center fails to give the signal to breathe for ten seconds or longer. There is no chest movement or struggling with central apnea, and the oxygen concentration in the blood can drop rapidly. In "obstructive apnea," the person attempts to breathe but the airflow is blocked, and this type of apnea typically occurs only during sleep. The chest moves with attempts to breathe, but air does not successfully move into the lungs. Snoring is a tip-off, and the person may appear to struggle or gasp. Age-related weakening of the muscles and other tissues in the throat area leads to collapse of the airway while trying to inhale. The tongue may fall and block the airway when sleeping on one's back, and build-up of fat in the tissues around the throat can also block airflow. Obstructive apnea can occur in older people of all sizes, but is more common in people who are overweight.

"Hypopnea" is a reduction of airflow of at least 30 percent from normal. Breathing is shallow and/or slow, and the person may appear pale, gray, or blue if the episode is prolonged due to a drop in oxygen concentration in the blood.

People with sleep apnea tend to wake up frequently and experience daytime sleepiness and lack of energy, along with headaches, irritability, and sometimes depression. Chronic sleep deprivation from apnea can negatively impact memory and the ability to pay attention and to organize and carry out tasks; therefore, the person may appear to have symptoms of dementia. Treating sleep apnea could significantly improve these symptoms.

A polysomnogram (discussed in the previous section on sleep) to evaluate for sleep apnea can be conducted in a sleep lab or at home. For the more basic home sleep study, equipment and supplies are sent by mail, and the study is typically conducted for two nights of sleep. The company typically provides good instructions and a link to a video demonstrating how to set up the device, which consists of nasal prongs to measure airflow through the nose, an oxygen and pulse sensor attached to the finger, and a band placed around the chest to record chest movement/rate of breathing. The equipment with the recorded studies is mailed back and read by a physician certified in sleep medicine and/ or pulmonology, who makes recommendations for appropriate treatment, if indicated.

The most effective treatment for sleep apnea is continuous positive airway pressure (CPAP), in which a bedside instrument is used to increase the pressure of air flowing into the lungs through tubing connected to a mask. The mask fits over the nose and mouth for mouth breathers, or is applied to the nose for non-mouth breathers. Alternatively, nasal prongs that fit into the nostrils may be used in place of a mask. A doctor prescribes the amount of pressure, based on results of the sleep study. The higher pressure helps keep the airway open and stimulates deeper breathing. For people with central apnea, the instrument can be set up to send out a puff of air to trigger breathing. For people with severe disease, bilevel positive airway pressure (BIPAP) may be ordered, which has different pressures set for inspiration and expiration. These devices are so smart that they can continuously record airflow with breathing and document the duration and frequency of apneic and hypopneic episodes. A smartphone application allows the patient to see their overnight results, and the information is also provided to the patient's physician.

Moderate to severe central apnea can also be treated with an implanted device similar to a pacemaker that stimulates the phrenic nerve that controls the diaphragm, the large muscle separating the chest and abdominal cavities, that expands and contracts with breathing. Another effective type of implanted device for obstructive sleep apnea stimulates the hypoglossal nerve and causes the tongue to move away from the airway with each breath (Strollo 2014).

Central apnea is quite common in premature newborns, due to immature brain development. Caffeine is an effective treatment for infants, but caffeine too late in the day may interfere with sleep in an adult. I could not find any medication that is effective to treat sleep apnea in an older person. On the other hand, medications that significantly depress breathing and worsen or cause sleep apnea are not good choices as sleep remedies, including barbiturates (phenobarbital, Seconal®) and narcotic painkillers (tramadol, codeine, hydromorphone, oxycodone, oxycontin, morphine, and others).

Consider the possibility of sleep apnea and have a discussion with your physician if you snore, feel excessively tired and lack energy in the daytime, wake up frequently, have headaches when you wake up in the morning, feel irritable or depressed, or have symptoms of cognitive impairment, such as poor memory or "brain fog." Sleep apnea can cause neurodegenerative changes in the brain, and treatment with CPAP could slow down the rate of cognitive decline (Kuo 2021).

DO NOT SMOKE AND AVOID SECOND-HAND SMOKE

We have known for more than fifty years that smoking tobacco causes lung cancer. Heart disease is the leading cause of death in the United States and in the world overall, and smoking is a leading risk factor for heart disease. Nearly half a million deaths annually in the United States can be attributed to smoking. Chronic obstructive pulmonary disease (COPD) is a severely disabling condition, most often caused by tobacco smoking, that may lead to a dependence on oxygen which severely limits a person's freedom. COPD can also occur with chronic exposure to secondhand smoke, air pollution, and unhealthy air in the work environment.

Death from COPD seemed especially tragic to me as a hospice doctor when it was the result of a bad, completely avoidable choice the person had made, years earlier, to smoke. It is common for people with COPD to continue smoking despite constant shortness of breath and angina (chest pain). One of my hospice patients with COPD and lung cancer, a lady in her forties, also had severe chronic back pain. During one of my visits, she sat next to an open window, smoking, started to cough violently, then sobbed uncontrollably due to a sudden increase in her severe chronic back pain. It was heartbreaking to witness this level of addiction. I acknowledged that she had been advised to quit repeatedly throughout her life but, as gently as possible, pointed out that smoking the cigarette directly triggered the episode of severe back pain. I suggested that using an electronic vaping device, at least some of the time, could reduce her coughing fits and back pain, recognizing that smoking cessation was unlikely for her.

An estimated 2 billion people use tobacco products globally, and there are more than 44 million tobacco users in the United States alone. Smoking is responsible for an average ten-year reduction in life expectancy in the U.S. (Durazzo 2014). The Institute for Health Metrics and Evaluation (IHME) estimated for 2019 that smoking tobacco accounted for 7.69 million of the more than 56 million deaths globally and was second only to high blood pressure as a risk factor for premature death. Smoking was also responsible for the equivalent of 200 million years of living with disability (GBD 2020).

Tobacco smoking is a major risk factor for cognitive impairment and dementia (Zhong 2015) and appears to be responsible for 4.7 million cases of Alzheimer's disease worldwide (Durazzo 2014). Smoking causes shrinkage of the entire brain—as well as the hippocampus and nearby structures, where memories form. Smoking increases levels of tissue-damaging reactive oxygen and nitrogen species—thereby causing neuroinflammation, which accelerates the formation of the beta amyloid plaques and neurofibrillary tangles seen in Alzheimer's.

Animal studies have demonstrated that exposure to tobacco smoke at levels equivalent to human smoking and exposure to secondhand smoke both promote formation of tangles. Other studies have demonstrated that nicotine, separate from the other components of tobacco smoke, directly leads to formation of tangles (Durazzo 2014). Smoking can further increase the risk of vascular dementia by promoting hardening of arteries in the brain (called cerebrovascular disease) and increasing the risk of stroke.

Passive smoking—exposure of nonsmokers to secondhand smoke—is a known risk factor for several diseases. Nonsmoking spouses of smokers have a 30 percent greater risk of lung cancer (Fontham 1994). Infants of mothers who smoke and infants exposed to smoke in the home have at least double the risk of sudden infant death syndrome (SIDS) (Anderson 2019; Anderson 1997). Studies also suggest that passive exposure to smoke in nonsmokers is a risk factor for more rapid cognitive decline and for dementia (Stirland 2018; He 2020).

Disability and premature death from tobacco smoking are almost entirely preventable. People often begin smoking cigarettes in their preteens or teens out of curiosity and pressure from peers, then find it difficult to quit because the nicotine in tobacco is so addictive. Many other substances in tobacco directly inflict damage to the delicate airways and air sacs in the lungs. Smoking can damage the heart muscle and blood vessels in the heart, leading to atherosclerosis (hardening of the arteries) and a heart attack. Nicotine raises blood pressure, and high blood pressure is the strongest risk factor for heart attack, cardiac death, and stroke. Smoking produces carbon monoxide in the blood, which reduces the amount of oxygen carried to the heart, the brain, and all other tissues and organs. Low oxygen levels constrict the arteries that feed and provide oxygen to our brain and body. Smoking delays wound healing, lowers resistance to infections, and increases the severity of gum infection. Smoking also increases acute and chronic inflammation. Cancer in the oral cavity, throat, and neck are much more common in smokers (Aghaloo 2019; CDC 2021). Smokers often appear older than their chronological age due to premature aging of the skin, a tip-off that internal organs are aging more quickly as well.

Smoking Cessation Can Slow Down Cognitive Decline

Zhong and group reviewed and analyzed results of 37 studies of tobacco smoking and dementia from all causes, including more than 960,000 individuals followed for two to forty years. There were 14,935 cases of dementia from all causes, of which 5,816 were diagnosed with Alzheimer's and 1,406 with vascular dementia. Compared to people who had never smoked, current smokers showed 1.30 times the risk of developing all-cause dementia, 1.40 times the risk of Alzheimer's, and 1.38 times the risk of vascular dementia. The risk for all-cause dementia increased by 34 percent for each twenty cigarettes smoked per day. Former smokers showed no increased risk of all-cause dementia, Alzheimer's, or vascular dementia compared to the non-smokers (Zhong 2015).

Choi and group studied data for 46,140 men aged sixty years and older collected over a 7-year period. The men were divided into 4 groups—continual smokers, short-term quitters (smoked less than 4 years), long-term quitters (smoked 4 years or longer), and never-smokers. Dementia was eventually diagnosed in 1,644 people. As the total amount of tobacco exposure decreased from continual smokers to short-term quitters, long-term quitters, and never-smokers, the risk of developing dementia from all causes significantly decreased. The risk of developing Alzheimer's and vascular dementia was much less for non-smokers and long-term quitters (Choi 2018).

These two large studies certainly make the case for smoking cessation and, better yet, never smoking at all.

The take-home message is to stop smoking, no matter what age you are. Your brain will benefit, and so will every other organ in your body. Smoking-cessation programs using several different strategies are widely available. One controversy is whether use of electronic cigarettes (e-cigarette) substitutes one set of problems for another. Guidelines for testing the effects of e-cigarettes are in progress (Aghaloo 2019). It is important to stay away from generic vaping products to avoid unknown contaminants that may seriously damage the lungs. One smoking-cessation method involves gradual reduction of nicotine, using an e-cigarette. A good friend and a close family member who were both long-term heavy smokers successfully quit smoking and then slowly weaned off the e-cigarette. It is not easy to quit smoking, but it is possible.

AVOID EXCESSIVE ALCOHOL INTAKE

Disorders related to excessive alcohol consumption account for about 6 percent of deaths globally and about 5 percent of the "global burden of disease" (death and loss of human health related to disease). The

World Health Organization rates alcohol misuse among the top five risk factors for disease, disability, and death. People who are alcohol-dependent have symptoms of withdrawal if they stop drinking and are three to four times more likely to develop Alzheimer's than those who are not alcohol-dependent. The risk is especially high for alcohol-dependent people in the sixty-five to seventy-nine age group (Zilkens 2014). The risk is greater for women consuming smaller amounts of alcohol than men.

It is common for people with alcohol consumption to also smoke, and the combination may bring about the onset of Alzheimer's four to six years sooner than in people who engage in neither habit. A study reported that, when three risk factors were present in individuals—smoking, alcohol misuse, and the ApoE4 gene—a diagnosis of Alzheimer's occurred on average ten years sooner than in people who had none of these risk factors (Harwood 2010).

In a large review of studies that included more than 131,000 people, moderate alcohol consumption increased risk of Alzheimer's by about 20 percent. Drinking enough alcohol to lose consciousness just once in twelve months more than doubled the risk of Alzheimer's and quadrupled the risk for vascular dementia (Kivimäki 2020).

Why Is Excessive Alcohol Intake So Bad for the Brain?

Alcohol increases inflammation in the brain, promotes shrinking of the brain (atrophy) with loss of neurons, and can damage the brain due to episodes of hypoglycemia (low blood sugar). Alcohol can cause depression and seizures. Excessive alcohol consumption can indirectly increase the risk of dementia by causing liver and kidney damage, coronary artery disease, diabetes, high blood pressure, abnormal heart rhythms, and stroke (Kivimäki 2020). Alcohol consumption increases risk of falls and other accidents that may result in traumatic brain injury, another important risk factor for Alzheimer's.

Malnutrition with nutrient deficiencies is common in people with alcoholism and can have a serious impact on brain health. For example,

B-vitamin thiamin is required in the production of the energy molecule ATP, and deficiency of thiamin from alcohol misuse can reduce ATP production and can also damage the blood–brain barrier. Thiamin is often deficient in people with Alzheimer's. Studies of Alzheimer's mouse models show worsening of plaque formation when the mice are deficient in thiamin (Venkataraman 2017). Heavy alcohol consumption also has a toxic effect on neurons that make dopamine, which are already greatly depleted in people with Parkinson's disease (Peng 2020).

Eliminating or reducing alcohol consumption could increase lifespan, improve quality of life, and reduce the risk of Alzheimer's and other dementias. It is possible to reverse some of the damage to the brain and improve cognition if alcohol use is discontinued (Venkataraman 2017).

While some studies suggest that small amounts of alcohol intake may be protective of the brain, excessive intake is clearly harmful. Further, a small amount for one person could be too much for another. For some of us, consuming just one serving of an alcoholic beverage is enough to temporarily upset the balance of neurotransmitters in the brain, which explains the "buzz" and effects on coordination, alertness, and behavior.

How Much Alcohol Intake Is Too Much?

The National Institutes of Health/National Institute on Alcohol Abuse and Alcoholism (NIH/NIAAA) recommends intake of no more than one serving daily for women and men over age sixty-five, and no more than two servings for younger men, with a serving defined as 12 ounces of beer, 5 ounces of wine, or 1.5 ounces of distilled spirits. Intake of alcohol is not recommended for people who have experienced alcohol dependency, people taking certain prescription and over-the-counter medications, and those with "certain medical conditions." In addition, the NIH-NIAAA recommends avoiding alcohol consumption when driving or operating machinery, and when planning to "participate in activities that require skill, coordination, and alertness." It makes sense

for people with mild cognitive impairment, Alzheimer's, or other dementia to consider discontinuing most, and maybe all, alcohol intake.

Here are some things to consider related to alcohol and reducing
your risk of cognitive impairment, Alzheimer's, vascular, and other dementias:

- Do not use the Mediterranean diet as a reason to start drinking
  alcohol. You can get phenolic compounds like resveratrol from eating grapes.
- If you do not drink now, do not start!
- If you have a history of alcohol dependency, avoid alcohol use.
- Consider strictly limiting or eliminating alcohol intake if you have
  memory or other cognitive impairment.
- If you are more sensitive than others to the effects of alcohol but
  still want to imbibe, figure out what serving size achieves that goal
  without negatively affecting your coordination, alertness, and behavior.
- If you have no history of alcohol dependency, limit alcohol intake
  to no more than one serving per day for women and men over age
  sixty-five, and no more than two servings for younger men (1 serving = 12 ounces of beer, 5 ounces of wine, or 1.5 ounces of distilled
  spirits).
- Check with a pharmacist or the package insert for all prescription
  and over-the-counter medications you take, to determine if they
  are compatible with alcohol consumption.
- If you think you may have a problem with excessive alcohol intake,
  check out the NIH/NIAAA website (www.niaaa.nih.gov).

Ketogenic Diet Helps Alcohol-Withdrawal Symptoms

People with alcohol-use disorder (alcoholism) have impairments in
several areas of cognition, and their brains, when sober, tend to use

more acetoacetate and less glucose as fuel. One study admitted thirty-three people for alcohol detoxification to a hospital of the NIH/ National Institute of Alcohol Abuse and Alcoholism. Participants were assigned to either a ketogenic diet (KD) or a standard American diet (SAD) for three weeks. The KD group saw a 39 percent drop in use of benzodiazepines for withdrawal symptoms, compared to an increase in use of 187 percent in the SAD group. The KD group experienced lower alcohol-withdrawal scores and reduced alcohol craving. Magnetic resonance spectrometry brain imaging showed higher levels of the ketones acetone and acetoacetate (betahydroxybutyrate could not be measured accurately) and reduced brain markers of inflammation only in the KD group (Wiers 2021).

IDENTIFY AND CONTROL HIGH BLOOD PRESSURE

High blood pressure, also called hypertension, is the leading risk factor globally for premature death and disability and is responsible for 10.44 million deaths per year, mainly due to strokes and heart diseases, such as heart attacks from coronary artery disease, heart failure, and atrial fibrillation. In 2017, a half million deaths in the United States were attributed to high blood pressure as either the cause or a major contributing factor. Clinical trials report that treatment of high blood pressure reduces the risk of stroke by 35 to 40 percent, risk of heart attack (myocardial infarction) by 15 to 25 percent, and of heart failure by up to 64 percent (SPRINT 2015).

High blood pressure is common: a survey from the National Center for Health Statistics (NCHS) reported a new diagnosis of high blood pressure in 27 percent of adults within the last year (NCHS 2019). High blood pressure is a diagnosis for 75 percent of people aged sixty-five and above and can usually be controlled through lifestyle changes and medications (SPRINT MIND 2019).

Blood pressure is the pressure exerted by blood against the walls of blood vessels as the blood is pumped from the heart through the arteries coursing through the body. When blood pressure is measured, two numbers are generated, usually written as 120/80, for example. The first number is the systolic blood pressure, which is the maximum pressure during a heartbeat, and the second number is the diastolic blood pressure, which is the lowest pressure that occurs when the heart is resting briefly between two heartbeats. Blood pressure normally fluctuates throughout the day in tune with the twenty-four-hour circadian rhythm and can change with position (lying down, sitting, standing) and level of activity (sleeping, awake but resting, walking, running). Nervousness, stress, and pain can produce an increase in blood pressure. Anxiety during your doctor visit can increase your blood pressure, sometimes called "white-coat syndrome" (Whelton 2017).

An optimal blood pressure reading is less than 120 systolic and less than 80 diastolic. While older treatment guidelines were more liberal, allowing systolic blood pressure up to 140, the most recent guidelines for best health are to aim for less than 120 systolic and less than 80 diastolic blood pressures (Whelton 2018); higher levels in middle-aged people carry a greater risk of dementia later in life (Meng 2014). The Systolic Blood Pressure Intervention Trial (SPRINT) Research Group study of more than 9,300 people reported that targeting a systolic blood pressure less than 120 compared to less than 140 significantly reduced stroke, heart attack, heart failure, and death from other serious cardiac events (SPRINT 2015). This held true in a follow-up study of more than 2,600 people ages seventy-five or older (Williamson 2016). In an analysis of 96,000 people in fourteen studies, lowering blood pressure reduced the risk of dementia and mild cognitive impairment (Hughes 2020). Other studies concluded that it is especially important for people who have the ApoE4 gene to control high blood pressure to prevent Alzheimer's and other dementias (Rajan 2018; Ding 2020; Ouk 2021).

Please see table 8.1 for normal and worrisome values for blood pressure in adults.

BLOOD PRESSURE STATUS FOR ADULTS

BLOOD PRESSURE STATUS	SYSTOLIC (upper number)	DIASTOLIC (lower number)
Hypotension (low blood pressure)	Less than 90	Less than 60
Normal	Less than 120	Less than 80
Pre-Hypertension*	120 to 139	80 to 89
Hypertension* Stage 1	140 to 159	90 to 99
Hypertension* Stage 2	160 or higher	100 or higher

*Hypertension = High blood pressure
The above values are from https://www.nhlbi.nih.gov/health-topics/high-blood-pressure
For blood pressure values for children see tables at https://www.nhlbi.nih.gov/files/docs/guidelines/child_tbl.pdf]

TABLE 8.1. Blood pressure status for adults from the National Institutes of Health. Source: https://www.nih.gov.

High blood pressure refers to a consistent increase above normal blood-pressure levels. Chronic high blood pressure can damage the arteries leading to the brain, heart, kidneys, eyes, and extremities. The effects of chronic high blood pressure and abnormal fluctuations in blood pressure can result in cognitive impairment and vascular dementia, and can contribute to the abnormalities in Alzheimer's and other types of dementia. In hypertension, small blood-vessel disease may lead to microscopic bleeding, damage to brain tissue, and death of small areas of brain tissue (Ma 2020). Chronic high blood pressure can also cause inflammation in the walls of the blood vessels and buildup of calcium and plaques (atherosclerosis or hardening of the arteries) which can narrow the opening and reduce blood flow to the brain or other organs. The walls of the blood vessels can become thicker, making them less elastic in response to blood-pressure fluctuations, causing further damage. A history of stroke is also a risk factor for vascular dementia and Alzheimer's. Biochemical dysfunction and inflammation with the release of inflammatory substances are consequences of stroke and are major factors affecting the brains of people with Alzheimer's and other dementias (Vijayan 2016).

Stroke is second only to heart disease among the leading causes of death worldwide and is a common consequence of poorly controlled high blood pressure. Each year, nearly 800,000 Americans suffer from a stroke. A stroke can happen at any age, beginning with the fetus in the womb, but is much more common in people over age fifty-five.

A stroke occurs when blood flow to part of the brain is interrupted by a blockage in a blood vessel. A clot can lodge in a blood vessel, blocking the flow of blood (ischemic stroke), for example; or, less often, a hemorrhage occurs in the brain (hemorrhagic stroke), such as from an aneurysm, a weak, dilated area in a blood vessel. Large to very small blood vessels can be involved, and the location and size of the area affected in the brain dictates the symptoms. Symptoms tend to come on suddenly and can include limpness of the arm and/or leg on one side of the body, numbness of an extremity, general weakness, facial drooping, slurred speech, intense headache, blurred vision in one or both eyes, loss of balance and coordination, dizziness, confusion, difficulty expressing a thought, or a sudden change in behavior. With a "mini-stroke," also called a "transient ischemic attack" (TIA), symptoms may appear suddenly but typically disappear after an interval ranging from minutes to less than twenty-four hours. It is possible to recover from a larger stroke with intensive physical therapy, but permanent disability is common.

A history of TIA predicts a much greater risk for a larger stroke and, therefore, immediate evaluation and treatment could prevent serious disability or death. People with a history of TIA have four times the risk of developing dementia compared to people who have not had a TIA (Tariq 2018). Medications called "clot dissolvers" can possibly reduce damage and death from a stroke or heart attack caused by a clot, when given as soon as possible after symptoms appear. Therefore, an immediate call for emergency services is in order.

Most strokes are preventable through modifying lifestyle factors, especially by controlling blood pressure, but also by controlling diabetes, treating atrial fibrillation, and discontinuing tobacco smoking. Fifty percent of strokes are related to high blood pressure, and uncontrolled high blood pressure increases risk of a stroke by four to six times (Vijayan 2016). Controlling blood sugar can help control blood pressure and is especially important for people with metabolic syndrome, pre-diabetes, or diabetes. People who have diabetes who have a stroke are much more likely to suffer disability or death than those who do not have it. It is common for people to have mixed dementia with the typical abnormalities found in Alzheimer's and in vascular dementia.

At least 90 percent of high blood pressure cases are due to genetics and lifestyle choices, including excess salt, caffeine, alcohol, or licorice intake, eating a "Western"-style high-carbohydrate diet, smoking, and lack of exercise. High blood pressure is also common in people who have insulin resistance, metabolic syndrome, prediabetes, and diabetes. Obesity and sleep apnea are risks for high blood pressure. Blood pressure also tends to increase as we age, due to atherosclerosis and chronic low-grade inflammation. Recreational drugs like methamphetamines and cocaine can increase blood pressure. Likewise, high blood pressure can be an adverse effect of specific prescription and over-the-counter medications, like birth-control pills, certain antidepressants, antipsychotics, steroids, anti-inflammatory medications, and decongestants such as pseudoephedrine, and herbs such as St. John's wort and Ma Huang, which contains ephedra. People with high blood pressure should consider alternatives to these medications.

Hypertension is often a result of hormone abnormalities, with 5 to 10 percent of cases secondary to hyperthyroidism, low levels of aldosterone and renin, hyperparathyroidism, or Cushing's disease, or another hormone abnormality. Hypertension can also occur when there is narrowing of the aorta or arteries to the kidneys, or a pheochromocytoma or paraganglioma tumor. These possibilities should be considered in the evaluation of high blood pressure, and blood tests can screen for many of these causes.

As mentioned, an optimal blood-pressure reading is less than 120 systolic and less than 80 diastolic. The highest blood-pressure levels tend to occur in the morning and evening, and the lowest levels occur during the night. People with high blood pressure typically do not experience obvious symptoms, even when the blood-pressure level is very elevated. Some people report morning headaches, vertigo, light-headedness, or tinnitus (buzzing or ringing in the ears) when blood pressure is high.

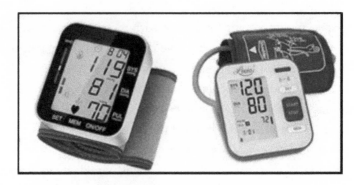

PHOTO 4. Blood-pressure cuffs for wrist (left) and arm (right).

Since most people do not have symptoms, high blood pressure is usually picked up through screening in a physician's office or clinic. A single blood-pressure reading measures just one point in time and may or may not reveal whether a person has high blood pressure. Unfortunately, the average healthy person may visit their doctor just once a year, or perhaps much less often, and has few opportunities for blood-pressure checks. Thus, many people are not aware that they have high blood pressure. It may be worthwhile to invest $30 or so in an electronic device to check your blood pressure periodically at home. There are devices that wrap around the wrist, and others that use the standard cuff found in a doctor's office (see photo 4). Pushing a button starts the device, and the pulse and blood-pressure readings appear in about 30 seconds. For the cuff-style blood-pressure monitors, it is important to use the correct size to get an accurate measurement. If you have a very large or very small arm, a pharmacist may be able to help determine your size. The bottom of the cuff is positioned just above the bend in the elbow.

For the most accurate blood-pressure reading, avoid caffeine, smoking, or exercise for at least thirty minutes beforehand, rest quietly for at least five minutes, and take the measurement while sitting straight up with both feet flat on the floor. Take two measurements a few minutes apart, because you may have slightly different results due to the normal fluctuations in blood pressure.

I suggest measuring your blood pressure at various times of the day while at rest. Then write the readings down in a journal, which you can take to your next doctor visit. If your blood-pressure readings are consistently or often greater than 120/80, a discussion with your doctor is in order. Current guidelines for diagnosis require two or three abnormal blood-pressure measurements taken at two or three different office visits. If there is concern, the doctor may prescribe an outpatient twenty-four-hour blood-pressure study. It is imperative to seek medical attention immediately for readings greater than 180 systolic or 120 diastolic, since a stroke or heart attack may be imminent and treatment could save your life.

The underlying cause of hypertension will dictate the course of treatment. For example, treatment may be different for high blood pressure due to hormonal or blood-vessel abnormalities, compared to high blood pressure due to lifestyle factors. When other treatable conditions are eliminated, lifestyle changes are the first line of treatment for mild to moderately high blood pressure. Smoking cessation, avoiding excessive alcohol intake, eating a healthier diet, reducing sodium intake, and engaging in aerobic and/or resistance exercise at least four days per week are a good place to start. Changing each of these factors individually can lower blood pressure, but combining them can have additive effects.

For blood-pressure levels above 130 systolic or 80 diastolic that do not respond to lifestyle changes, medication may be indicated. The type of medication prescribed will depend on the cause. Many people require two or more medications that act through different mechanisms to control their blood pressure, and these medications need to be compatible with each other, which the doctor or pharmacist can determine. It is important to be aware of common side effects and report these to your physician. For example, some medications to treat high blood pressure can, ironically, cause abnormally low blood pressure, light-headedness, or fainting, in which case the doctor should be contacted immediately since a reduction in dosage or discontinuation may be warranted to prevent injury from a fall.

In 2018, a task force organized by the American College of Cardiology and American Heart Association published a comprehensive set of Clinical Practice Guidelines for physicians on prevention, evaluation, and management of high blood pressure. This provides an invaluable detailed analysis of the evidence to guide physicians on care of people with high blood pressure, but may also be of interest to the public (Whelton 2018).

EAT A HEALTHY DIET AND LIMIT SODIUM INTAKE TO CONTROL BLOOD PRESSURE

A loss of just 5 to 10 percent of body weight can bring blood pressure into the normal range for some people. Many different types of diets can help with weight loss, including a whole-food Mediterranean-style diet, since it also tends to reduce blood sugar, curb cravings and feelings of hunger, and provide vitamins, minerals, and many other nutrients in their natural forms. Adding the component of nutritional ketosis, as discussed in chapter 4, has many benefits for healthy aging, including blood-pressure reduction and weight loss.

The Mediterranean and DASH (Dietary Approaches to Stop Hypertension) diets can help reduce and control blood pressure (Ozemek 2020). Both diets emphasize eating fruits and vegetables, whole grains, fish, poultry, legumes (beans), seeds, and nuts, and limiting red meat. A true Mediterranean-style diet places more emphasis than DASH on eating healthy fats, including moderate amounts of full-fat dairy products. The DASH diet discourages fat, including full-fat dairy, and limits daily sodium intake to 2,300 mg for most people, and to as little as 1,500 mg for people who still need better blood-pressure control. Several studies reported that reducing sodium intake to 1,500 mg daily was equivalent to taking one blood-pressure medication, whereas consuming more than 5,700 mg of sodium daily wiped out the effect of blood-pressure medication (Ozemek 2020). Fruits and vegetables are rich in fiber, potassium, calcium, and magnesium, each of which can help control blood pressure (Whelton 2018). It is possible to merge the best features of the DASH, Mediterranean, and low-carb diets.

POTASSIUM-RICH FOODS

FRUITS: Apricots, avocados, bananas, dates, melons, oranges, orange juice, prunes, prune juice, tomatoes, and tomato juice.

VEGETABLES: Broccoli, Brussels sprouts, potatoes, spinach, sweet potatoes, tomatoes.

PROTEINS: Beans, fish (cod, halibut, rockfish, salmon, trout, tuna), lentils, nuts and seeds, meat, milk, poultry, yogurt.

OTHER: Coconut water, whole grain brown and wild rice.

FIGURE 8.5. Potassium-rich foods.

Sodium is the most abundant mineral in our body fluids and is an essential nutrient that we must get from food. Mechanisms involving our kidneys and hormones, called the renin-angiotensin system, keep sodium and water in balance in the body. Water retention with puffiness in hands and feet can occur from eating too much salt and can increase blood pressure. Many people are sensitive to excess sodium, and people with type 2 diabetes tend to retain sodium due to high insulin levels, which could partly explain their greater likelihood of high blood pressure (Brands 2012).

As in standard table salt, sodium can be bound to chloride but is also a component of other molecules important to metabolism and brain function. Chloride and potassium are also abundant and essential minerals. Low-sodium salts often substitute potassium chloride for some of the sodium chloride. Potassium supplementation can help reduce blood pressure. Many foods are naturally high in potassium (see figure 8.5). For people with certain conditions, such as chronic kidney disease, excess potassium could be detrimental. Therefore, use of a potassium supplement and the dosage should be guided by your physician.

So, how much sodium should we eat every day? The average American consumes 3,400 mg of sodium per day, which may be too high for someone with high blood pressure (Ozemek 2020). A large twenty-one-country epidemiological study reported that communities with very high intake of sodium, over 5,000 mg per day on average, had significantly higher rates of stroke and cardiovascular disease (Mente 2018). Higher intake of potassium was associated with lower rates of these diseases. If you have high blood pressure, your doctor will almost certainly recommend limiting sodium intake.

On the other hand, trying to eliminate sodium from the diet could be detrimental because sodium is essential to many bodily functions. Based on the best evidence, the Institute of Medicine (IOM) Dietary Reference Intakes (2006) recommends a minimum of 1,500 mg per day for adults through age fifty as "adequate intake" and an upper limit of 2,300 mg for adults of all ages (Institute of Medicine, 2006). People who take certain diuretics or sweat a lot in their jobs or in athletics will lose more sodium in urine or sweat than average. When glucose appears in urine due to high blood glucose, sodium is pulled into the urine as well. Your doctor or dietitian could help determine if you need more than the recommended sodium intake.

Most sodium in the diet (77 percent) is added to food during processing. Just 12 percent comes from the natural sodium content of food, 6 percent is added while eating, and 5 percent is added while cooking (IOM, 2006). The standard food-industry practice of adding too much sugar and salt to otherwise bland processed foods encourages us to come back for more. Therefore, an easy way to reduce sodium intake is to stop eating so much processed food! Manufacturers must disclose sodium content on nutrition labels, which can help you decide which products to avoid. The amount of sodium in table salt is generally about 40 percent of the total weight—about 600 mg in a quarter teaspoon. So, take it easy with the saltshaker and avoid adding more than needed while cooking.

The main source of vital iodine in the typical American diet is iodized salt. The U.S. government requires fortification of salt with iodine to prevent iodine deficiency, the leading preventable cause of intellectual and developmental disabilities. Iodine is a crucial nutrient for cognitive development in infants and cognitive health in adults. Iodine deficiency also causes goiters and hypothyroidism. The NIH recommendation for iodine is 150 micrograms (0.15 mg) daily, the amount in about ½ teaspoon of table salt in the United States. However, salt used to make processed foods is almost never iodized. Some of the richest natural sources of iodine are nori seaweed, cod, oysters, Greek yogurt, milk, and eggs.

The NIH website has an excellent guide on "Tips to Reduce Salt and Sodium" based on the DASH Eating Plan (NIH on Sodium), including examples of significant differences in sodium content between several fresh and more processed foods. This guide suggests that you:

- Choose fresh, frozen, or no- or low-sodium canned vegetables, and add your own seasoning.
- Choose fresh or frozen poultry, fish, and meats instead of processed meats, such as those that are marinated, canned, smoked, brined, or cured. Ham is particularly high in sodium. Many meats and poultry, deli meats, bacons, and some cheeses contain a high content of salt, and some also contain sodium nitrites (discussed in chapter 9). Chain restaurants, delis, and grocery-store meat counters should be able to provide nutrition information for their products.
- Limit the amount of salt added to food during cooking and from a saltshaker.
- Look for the sodium content on the label. Skip or limit processed foods with higher amounts of sodium such as frozen meals and pizza, canned soups and broth, salad dressings, soy sauce, instant or flavored cereals, rice, pasta, and packaged mixes.
- Rinsing canned foods such as tuna and beans will remove much of the salt.
- Choose unsalted nuts and seeds.
- Add herbs and spices, lemon, lime, or vinegar in place of salt to enhance flavors.

MEDITATION, YOGA, MUSIC, AND SLOW BREATHING FOR BLOOD-PRESSURE CONTROL

Yoga, breathing techniques, and meditation have been used for thousands of years to enhance health and promote a sense of well-being. Behavioral techniques reported in studies that help reduce blood pressure include slow or paced breathing, guided breathing, yoga, listening to music, transcendental meditation, and "mindfulness" meditation. These practices can be done easily at home, have no downside, and could help control or reduce elevated blood pressure due to stress or anxiety. Numerous free phone apps are available for these behavioral techniques.

The normal rate of breathing is between twelve and twenty breaths per minute. Slow or paced breathing is generally set at six or eight breaths per minute for five to ten minutes or longer. This technique reduces blood pressure and pulse through an effect on specialized pressure-sensing neurons (called baroreceptors) located in the arch of the aorta as it leaves the heart and in the carotid arteries, which circulate blood to the brain. Blood vessels dilate in response to slow breathing, which allows the heart rate and blood pressure to drop. This effect occurs in people with high and normal blood pressure.

Guided breathing uses music or some other method to direct the pace of breathing. The effect of reducing heart rate and blood pressure may occur after a single session, and the daily practice of guided breathing can reduce blood pressure long-term (Li 2018). In a study of 87 people, listening to relaxing music had a slightly more positive effect on blood pressure than slow deep breathing guided by a musical pattern under the same conditions. After eight weeks, the systolic blood pressure was ten points lower in the music group versus eight points in the guided-breathing group, and both groups had a five-point drop in diastolic blood pressure (Kow 2018).

Meditation is used to promote inner awareness, and some forms use a mantra—repetition of a sound, word, or phrase—to accomplish that. Eight studies of transcendental meditation reported an average reduction of four points in systolic and two points in diastolic blood pressure (Ooi 2017). Another review of nine studies found no effect of transcendental meditation on blood pressure (Gathright 2019). A study of a breathing meditation program and lifestyle training in people with stage 1 hypertension (>130 systolic) reported a twelve-point drop on average in systolic pressure over one year, with 92 percent under 130 systolic. By contrast, 50 percent of the "lifestyle only" control group dropped below 130 systolic, averaging a reduction of just 1.5 points (Chandler 2020).

Fu and co-authors analyzed 120 studies of non-drug interventions to reduce blood pressure and found that the DASH low-sodium diet had the greatest effect overall, with good evidence for a beneficial effect of aerobic exercise. There was also enough evidence to support interventions like meditation, yoga, tai chi, and qi gong (Fu 2020).

Mindfulness-Based Stress Reduction is taught in a workshop or series of classes over several weeks. This program focuses on techniques to increase mind and body awareness to reduce stress, anxiety, depression, pain, and the related physiological effects, such as high blood pressure, and to experience more joy, serenity, and non-judgmental awareness in daily life. Meditation is part of this program. More than 1,000 reports and at least 100 randomized controlled trials have been published on this program, including many that studied effects on blood pressure. The Mindfulness-Based Blood Pressure Reduction (MB-BP) program teaches techniques to enhance self-regulation through attention control, self-awareness, and emotion regulation along with the DASH diet, salt reduction, weight loss, increased physical activity, avoidance of alcohol, and adherence to prescribed medication. In one study, forty-three people attended at least seven of ten MB-BP classes. Results showed that systolic blood pressure was down by about 6 points on average for the whole group and was down by 15 points in people with stage 2 hypertension (>140 systolic) after one year (Loucks 2019).

Since high blood pressure is the leading risk for death and puts us at risk for dementia and poor brain aging, it behooves each of us to check our blood pressure regularly, do everything in our power to prevent high blood pressure, and control high blood pressure if we already have this problem.

Identify, Prevent, and Control High Blood Pressure

There are many different steps you can take to control blood pressure. Here is a summary:
- Check your blood pressure periodically. If it's greater than 120 systolic or 80 diastolic, see your doctor for evaluation and possible treatment.

- If you snore, are overweight, or feel like you are not sleeping well, request an evaluation for sleep apnea.
- Avoid processed foods and eat a whole-food diet with a variety of vegetables, fruits, nuts, seeds, legumes, fish, poultry, and dairy.
- Control blood sugar by eating a low-carb, higher-healthy-fat Mediterranean-style, DASH, or combination diet.
- Keep sodium intake between 1,500 and 2,300 mg per day. Aim closer to 1,500 mg if you have high blood pressure.
- Eat some foods every day that are rich in potassium, unless your doctor advises otherwise due to a specific medical condition.
- Engage in aerobic and/or resistance exercise at least four times per week for at least thirty minutes, if possible.
- If you are overweight, work to lose at least 5 to 10 percent of your body weight.
- Avoid excessive alcohol intake.
- Stop smoking.
- If you have high blood pressure, if any of your medications list high blood pressure as a possible side effect, ask your doctor for an alternative, if available.
- If you take medication for high blood pressure, report blood pressure readings under 100 systolic, light-headedness, or fainting to your doctor.
- Work to reduce stress, anxiety, and depression; doing so can lower blood pressure and improve your overall quality of life.

REDUCE STRESS, ANXIETY, AND DEPRESSION THROUGH COUNSELING AND BEHAVIOR MODIFICATION

It is easy for someone who is not living your life to tell you to relax and not get so stressed out. How are you supposed to do that? Juggling a job and family responsibilities are stressful when everyone is healthy, but few jobs are more stressful than caring for a spouse, parent, or child with Alzheimer's, autism, or other serious disability, or someone at the end of life. Caregiving can be all-consuming, leaving little time to take care of one's own personal and healthcare needs. Most of us will become a caregiver for our spouse or parents at some point in our lives, and that job could last for years. I was caregiver for my husband Steve for fifteen years after he began to show the signs that evolved into Alzheimer's disease.

Stress can negatively impact health and quality of life. Chronic stress carries a higher risk of high blood pressure, coronary artery disease, increased inflammation, impaired immune function, slower wound healing, and higher levels of stress hormones (Alzheimer's Association 2020). Chronically high cortisol levels, for example, can increase blood pressure and blood sugar, reduce glucose uptake into the hippocampus where memories are formed, and interfere with sleep. All of these are risk factors for dementia.

Depression and anxiety are common, and they often occur together. About 5 percent of adults report regularly having feelings of depression, and 11 percent report worry, nervousness, or anxiety (NCHS 2019). Depression occurs in about 32 percent of people with dementia as part of broader neuropsychiatric symptoms, and an additional 16 percent have a diagnosis of major depression. Common symptoms of depression in dementia include poor appetite, low energy, irritability, social isolation, and sadness (Watt 2021). Among family caregivers of people with dementia, 30 to 40 percent report depression and high levels of emotional and physical stress in the people they care for (Alzheimer's Association 2020). So, if you are a caregiver for a loved one with dementia and are overly stressed and depressed, you are not alone.

Depression was one of my husband Steve's earliest symptoms of Alzheimer's, and his doctor thought this caused his memory problems at age fifty-one. However, it was more likely the opposite, since Steve was well aware that he was losing his accounting skills and other cognitive abilities. Steve began counseling in 2001 (at fifty-one), which continued through 2013 when he became homebound. As his caregiver and a working physician, I constantly experienced an undercurrent of stress, anxiety, and depression. I began counseling in 2007 when Steve was spiraling downward, and continued for one year after he passed away in 2016. With your counselor, you can speak your mind confidentially without judgment. A counselor can help you see your options more clearly to make important decisions.

Some Non-Drug Interventions Work as Well as, or Better Than, Drugs to Treat Depression in People with Dementia

A systemic review and meta-analysis of more than 25,000 people in 213 trials compared non-drug therapies to usual care for treatment of depression in people with dementia (Watt 2021). The highest-ranked non-drug therapies that were significantly more effective than usual care in reducing symptoms of depression included:

- Cognitive stimulation combined with exercise and social interaction
- Cognitive stimulation combined with cholinesterase inhibitor (the typical drugs for dementia)
- Cognitive therapy alone
- Massage, acupressure, or touch therapy
- A combination of psychotherapy, reminiscence therapy, and environmental modification
- Some other therapies that showed some benefit in relieving symptoms of depression included:
  - Exercise alone
  - Occupational therapy
  - Animal Therapy

CAREGIVING: A SPECIAL KIND OF STRESS WITH SPECIAL NEEDS

Caregiving is a job that one may acquire gradually and by default. A parent, child, or spouse affected by dementia or other progressive neurological condition will require more assistance as time goes on. As many as 40 percent of family caregivers of people with dementia report having no paid assistance. The healthcare system in the United States is not designed to proactively identify people with dementia and follow through with the kind of education and support caregivers need to keep their loved ones at home. Resources for caregivers are mostly local and few and far between. Family caregivers must often reinvent the wheel, learning as they go about how the disease progresses and how to take care of someone with that disease. Caregivers tend to learn from other caregivers about what to expect and how to deal with problems, but many have no one at all to guide them, much less help them. It seems that most primary care and neurology physician practices are not equipped to provide this type of education, guidance, and support. Insurance companies and Medicare are even less likely to reimburse physicians for the staff they would need to coordinate and implement these types of services. Governments around the world are undertaking these types of initiatives to keep people at home for the duration of their lives whenever possible. Hopefully, such an initiative will happen in the United States as soon as possible.

These are the steps I believe would greatly improve the experience of the person with dementia and their caregiver(s):

* When the patient or their caregiver senses a problem with memory or other cognitive function, the primary care physician or qualified staff member carries out a standardized screening test, such as the Montreal Cognitive Assessment (MoCA) and Mini-Mental Status Exam (MMSE), which are not difficult to administer or score. Currently, many doctors rely on a question or two, such as "Who is the president?" or "What year is it?" In my job doing in-home health-risk assessments for people in the Medicare or Medicaid

programs, the standard cognitive screening consists of having the person remember three words and a clock-drawing test. That is not enough!

- If the MMSE or MoCA screening test score is abnormal, the primary care doctor should then refer the patient to a neurologist or Alzheimer's/dementia center for a comprehensive evaluation and treatment.

- If testing indicates mild cognitive impairment or dementia, a nurse case manager and/or social worker would be assigned to coordinate care and educate the patient and family about the disease, how it progresses, what problems to anticipate, and how to manage these problems proactively. For example, a new caregiver may not know that wandering from home is common, can begin without notice, and can have tragic consequences. In my area, a fifty-seven-year-old woman with early-onset dementia wandered from home for the first time and crossed a busy road with an unfortunate fatal consequence.

- The case manager or social worker would provide information on local caregiving groups, online forums, and organizations or individuals who can provide respite care. Periodic respite care would be covered by Medicare, Medicaid, or private insurance.

- When in-person office visits become difficult, a physician or nurse practitioner and visiting nurse would perform home visits. Telemedicine visits would be another option.

- When the patient becomes bedbound or otherwise difficult to bathe due to physical or behavioral issues, in-home services utilizing nursing assistants would be provided daily to assist the caregiver. They would be covered by Medicare or other insurance. Currently, such services are limited and may be funded by insurance for just a few hours per week, if at all, leaving the caregiver to fend for themselves during the other hours. This type of care is well beyond the financial means of most families. The lack of reasonable assistance with in-home care is a major factor leading to placement in assisted-living or nursing homes when the exhausted caregiver can no longer cope with the deteriorating situation. Incontinence of bowels is often the deciding factor. Sadly, assisted living is only available to those who can afford it. Most states require the patient and their spouse to virtually deplete their assets before the government will pay for assisted living through the Medicaid program, potentially leaving little or nothing for the surviving spouse, who could end up in a similar situation. In addition, many facilities do not accept Medicaid, openings are few, and waiting lists are long.

• The case manager and/or social worker should discuss hospice care and help the caregiver determine optimal timing. Most people receive hospice care at home, and many people with end-of-life conditions are eligible long before anyone suggests it. People with dementia are usually eligible for hospice care when unable to walk without assistance (see FAST side box). At that point, the person is often incontinent most of the time and speaks few if any intelligible words. This last stage of dementia may continue for months to years, and hospice care can remain in place so long as the person continues to decline. Recertification occurs after the first six months and every three months thereafter. Hospice provides aides to assist with bathing and bed changes, and home visits by nurses, doctors, and social workers to provide counseling along with provision of medications, incontinence supplies, and equipment like adjustable beds and oxygen concentrators.

FAST—Functional Assessment Staging of Alzheimer's Disease

The FAST score is used to determine eligibility for hospice care through Medicare. Generally, people with dementia are eligible at Stage 7C or sooner, if they have had significant recent weight loss or have another life-limiting medical condition (Reisberg 1988). This score also provides a sense of how Alzheimer's and some other dementias usually progress over time.

STAGE 1. No difficulties, either subjectively or objectively.

STAGE 2. Complains of forgetting location of objects. Subjective word-finding difficulties.

STAGE 3. Decreased job function evident to coworkers. Difficulty in traveling to new locations. Decreased organizational capacity.

STAGE 4. Decreased ability to perform complex tasks (e.g., planning dinner for guests, paying bills).

STAGE 5. Requires assistance in choosing proper clothing to wear for day, season, and occasion.

STAGE 6A. Difficulty putting clothing on properly without assistance.

STAGE 6B. Unable to bathe properly (e.g., difficulty adjusting bath-water temperature) occasionally or more frequently over the past weeks.

STAGE 6C. Inability to handle mechanics of toileting (e.g., forgets to flush the toilet, does not wipe properly or properly dispose of toilet tissue) occasionally or more frequently over the past weeks.

STAGE 6D. Urinary incontinence, occasional or more frequent.

STAGE 6E. Fecal incontinence, occasional or more frequently over the past week.

STAGE 7A. Ability to speak limited to approximately a half dozen different words or fewer during an average day, or during an intensive interview.

STAGE 7B. Speech ability limited to the use of a single intelligible word in an average day.

STAGE 7C. Ambulatory ability lost (cannot walk without personal assistance).

STAGE 7D. Ability to sit up without assistance lost (e.g., the individual will fall over if there are no lateral rests [arms] on the chair).

STAGE 7E. Loss of the ability to smile.

Home Hospice Care—Our Experience and a New Career Path for Me

After Steve spent two weeks in the hospital in 2012, I needed help due to his erratic sleeping pattern and incontinence. I hired caregivers, since I was working and was often called emergently to the hospital. After Steve had his first prolonged seizure, complicated by a head injury and lack of oxygen, he became completely dependent. I made the difficult decision to stop working at that point. Paying several full-time caregivers is an expensive proposition, and we were fortunate to have saved for decades for retirement. Nearly a year after his first seizure, Steve stopped eating and drinking and was accepted into hospice care. As an anticonvulsant medication wore off, he began to eat and drink again, and Steve lived another eighteen months.

After depleting Steve's retirement account and dipping heavily into my own, I had little choice but to go back to work. I was so impressed with the hospice aides, nurses, the physician, and a social worker that I became a hospice doctor, which was more compatible with Steve's condition than emergency newborn care. After thirty years of caring for newborns, providing hospice care was an unexpected and rewarding practice at the other end of the spectrum. About three years later, after Steve had passed away, I transitioned to performing home health risk assessments for Medicare and Medicaid patients with a very flexible schedule that allowed me to travel internationally to speak about ketones and Alzheimer's disease. I gained valuable experience in caring for people with dementias and other neurological conditions, as well as many end-stage and chronic conditions. This work pulled me up out of my isolated view of living with dementia and gave me a greater appreciation for the suffering that people and their families go through in nearly every neighborhood every day. I thought I might learn about the true meaning of life by doing hospice work, but must report that I did not!

CONSIDER NON-DRUG OPTIONS FOR ANXIETY
AND DEPRESSION, WHENEVER POSSIBLE

There are clearly situations for which antidepressant or antipsychotic medication is indicated and can save lives, such as severe depression with suicidal thinking or dangerous, aggressive behavior. On the other hand, medication is too often the first resort and an "easy out" for treating anxiety and behavioral symptoms. Non-drug behavior modification options could be just as effective without the risk of serious side effects. For example, benzodiazepines like Xanax® (alprazolam) used to treat anxiety are intended for short-term relief but are often prescribed for years; prolonged use can lead to disturbing side effects, and withdrawal effects can be prolonged and severe. Xanax is a short-acting drug that can have a rebound effect of increased anxiety when the dose wears off. Counseling and education in stress reduction techniques could be a better alternative for chronic anxiety.

The power of music for relief of stress, anxiety, and mild depression is very real. Listening to anything by the Beatles or Beethoven lifts my mood. For my husband Steve, Willie Nelson, Neil Diamond, and Barry Manilow were his favorites long before the dementia set in, and playing their music would distract and calm him when he became anxious in the later stages of Alzheimer's. A wonderful documentary called Alive Inside (available on YouTube.com) shows how listening to familiar music can transform a non-communicative person into someone who sings and experiences joy once again.

Antipsychotic drugs (Haldol®, Zyprexa®, Abilify®, and Seroquel®, for example) are too often prescribed for anxiety, agitation, and/or insomnia for elderly people and people with dementia, despite FDA "Black Box Warnings" specifically stating that these drugs are "not approved for dementia-related psychosis" due to "increased mortality risk" and may also cause "increased suicidality risk in children, adolescents and young adults with major depression or other psychiatric disorders." Side effects of concern include tardive dyskinesia (abnormal movements) and akathisia (the inability to sit still). Antipsychotic drugs are particularly dangerous for people with Parkinson's disease and Lewy body dementia, who can suffer severe, acute worsening of parkinsonism including severe tremors, muscle rigidity, and neuroleptic malignant syndrome, which carries a 20 percent mortality if not recognized and treated.

Antipsychotic Drugs Can Be Dangerous for People with Diagnosed or Undiagnosed Parkinson's and Lewy Body Dementia

My husband Steve developed symptoms of neuroleptic malignant syndrome (massive sweating, fever, muscle rigidity, increased confusion) after he was given just a few doses of Haldol for confusion during a hospital stay. I soon suspected that Steve not only had Alzheimer's disease, but likely had Lewy body dementia as well, which was confirmed by autopsy of his donated brain after he passed away.

During my three years as a hospice physician, two female patients with dementia came to hospice under my care because they had stopped eating and drinking and had become bedbound. On exam, I noticed muscle rigidity and tremors, and each patient was receiving Seroquel, an antipsychotic. This medication was clearly contraindicated for one of the women who'd had Parkinson's disease for years. The other woman likely had unrecognized Lewy body dementia. A few days after stopping the medication, both women began eating and drinking again and, after a few weeks, were walking, enjoying activities, and doing so much better that they were able to be discharged from hospice care.

Antipsychotics are not FDA-approved for people with dementia. Yet no other medications are available to effectively address the behavioral problems (agitation, anxiety, aggression, depression, hallucinations, schizophrenia-like symptoms) that occur in many people as they decline. Thus, doctors often prescribe these medications off-label. Unfortunately, due to the lack of suitable behavior-controlling drugs, antipsychotics (including the highly toxic Haldol) are often overused as first-line drugs to treat people with dementia when behavioral issues appear in hospitals, nursing homes, and assisted living facilities. Many prescribing physicians, often not psychiatrists or neurologists, and nurses who administer medications confuse the serious adverse effects of antipsychotic medications with progression of dementia symptoms. An estimated 50 to 75 percent of nursing-home residents are given antipsychotic medications, but less than 5 percent of these medications are prescribed by mental health–care providers who are most familiar with them (Saltz 2004).

When there is no reasonable alternative (such as when a person is a danger to themselves or others), the smallest possible dose of an antipsychotic or anti-anxiety drug should be used to reduce the extreme behavior to a tolerable level. This practice could decrease the likelihood of serious adverse effects. For some people, a quarter or half of the smallest available dose may be effective. Even with small doses, these drugs can slowly accumulate in the brain, and a formerly active person can become overly sedated, almost immobile, and may drool, which warrants a dosage reduction. Certain behaviors, such as severe agitation and violent behavior, may be temporary phases during the progression of dementia. It is reasonable for families to ask for periodic reevaluation of their loved one every few months to determine if the medication can be reduced or discontinued.

Antipsychotics should be prescribed by providers who are highly trained in the use of these medications. The American Geriatrics Society recommends that antipsychotic drugs be reserved for people in whom all other non-drug options have been exhausted.

Behavior-modification techniques to reduce anxiety and agitation in people with dementia could be effective alternatives to drugs. Common situations can provoke anxiety and agitation, sometimes extreme, in people with dementia, such as bathing, going to bed, and the inability to communicate the need to urinate or have a bowel movement.

False beliefs also provoke anxiety for patients and caregivers, such as "this is not my home" or "they are stealing from me" or "you are not who you say you are." A person who is reasonably cooperative and rational in the daytime may become much more confused and anxious in the evening, sometimes called "sundowning" or "sundowner's syndrome." A wonderful educational series of videos on how to deal with these issues using a comforting positive behavioral approach is available from Teepa Snow, a highly experienced professional dementia caregiver (https://teepasnow.com). Educational and emotional support from others who have experienced these problems can be invaluable.

SUPPORT GROUPS CAN BE A SOURCE OF HELP AND EMOTIONAL SUPPORT

People with dementia and their caregivers often become isolated and lonely. Both caregivers and people with dementia can find immense help and emotional support by connecting with others who are in the same boat through online forums, social-media groups, and local support groups. By necessity, the COVID-19 pandemic opened a world of online group support. Local chapters of the Alzheimer's Association, Catholic Charities, and many other religious and non-religious organizations offer educational programs, support groups, individual and group counseling, and case management for people with dementia and their caregivers. Some organizations provide day care or other respite care services for several hours per week to several days in a row to give caregivers a break (see Resources for suggestions).

IDENTIFY AND CORRECT PROBLEMS WITH HEARING AND VISION

Hearing and vision impairment are common in people with dementia and, especially when uncorrected, can add considerably to the burden on the affected person and their caregivers, since considerably more supervision and assistance is needed to carry out everyday activities. Screening and treating people with dementia for hearing and vision impairments can improve quality of life and sensory functional ability to the degree that people with dementia may require less assistance from caregivers (Leroi 2020).

Screening periodically for hearing loss is important as we get older. Most people gradually lose hearing ability with age, clearly some much more than others. This loss of hearing can be frustrating to the impaired person and the people they live with. A hearing-impaired person may seem confused even when they are not. Hearing loss can lead to less interaction with others and social isolation. If you frequently need people to repeat themselves, you might have a correctable hearing problem. Hearing-aid technology has improved remarkably in recent years, and effective lower cost options are on the market. Correcting a hearing problem can enhance your own life and help your family and friends maintain their sanity!

Vision problems are also common as we age, and it is important to have regular eye exams to detect and treat correctable problems. Vision impairment increases the risk of serious falls and can affect independence, such as the ability to drive and run errands, engage socially, and move around the house.

Nearly everyone will develop presbyopia—problems seeing up close due to loss of elasticity in the lens of the eye—beginning around age forty, which is easily corrected with reading glasses. Glaucoma is a common condition with no obvious symptoms that can lead to blindness if not treated. Glaucoma can be easily detected by checking the pressures in the eyes, and prescription eye drops can return the pressure to normal, though occasionally surgery is required. Cataracts are common as the lenses of the eyes become cloudy or develop defects that interfere with normal vision. Replacing our natural lenses with artificial lenses is a brief surgical procedure that opens a world of color and sharper focus. Macular degeneration is a condition that results in deterioration of the retina of the eye, creating holes in vision that gradually enlarge. Some forms of macular degeneration are treatable, and treatment is more successful if detected early with a dilated eye exam.

About 40 percent of people with diabetes develop diabetic retinopathy, which can lead to blindness but is also treatable if detected early. Good blood sugar control through a consistent low-carb diet could prevent diabetic retinopathy and other diabetes complications.

The lifestyle risk factors discussed in this chapter are tightly interconnected with each other. Each choice you make provides an extra layer of protection for your brain and body as you age. In the next chapter, we will talk about some specific things to avoid that could add a few more layers of protection to enhance healthier brain aging and avoid dementia.

CHAPTER NINE

AVOID THESE THINGS TO PREVENT DEMENTIA AND ENJOY HEALTHIER BRAIN AGING

"We are not given a good life or a bad life. We are given life, and it's up to you to make it good or bad."

—Unknown

IN SEARCH OF A LONGER HEALTHSPAN

Throughout history, humans could only expect to live into their thirties on average, mainly due to deadly infections like smallpox and cholera, and this did not change until relatively recently. One hundred and twenty years ago, the average lifespan in the United States was just forty-one years, and infections took an extraordinary toll on infants and children. Mortality related to childbirth was high, and nearly one in four infants died during the first year of life. Only three of five children made it to age twenty.

Important public-health initiatives over the past two and a half centuries dramatically extended lifespans, beginning with variolation in Asia, a practice which protected people from smallpox by exposing them to the less dangerous cowpox. The true smallpox vaccine was developed in the late 1700s by Edward Jenner and completely eradicated the very deadly smallpox infection globally about 180 years later. Older Americans like me have a scar on our upper arm from the smallpox vaccine we received as children. Younger Americans no longer require this vaccine.

As population density increased in cities, and drinking milk became more prevalent, lethal infections from contaminated milk became more common, especially in children. Around 1865, when the newly invented microscope revealed that microbes likely caused infections, Louis Pasteur developed a sterilization technique, called pasteurization, initially for wine and later milk. The practice of pasteurization finally took hold in the United States about fifty years later and tremendously reduced milk-related fatal infections from tuberculosis, diphtheria, typhoid, listeria, and scarlet fever. Chlorination of drinking water gained steam beginning around 1912 in several large cities in the United States, reducing waterborne infections, such as typhoid fever, tenfold. By 1935, mainly thanks to these measures, infant mortality had been cut in half in the United States, and the average expected lifespan had increased from forty-one to more than fifty years.

Since 1914, vaccines have been introduced for pertussis (whooping cough), tuberculosis, diphtheria, polio, tetanus, rabies, measles, rubella, mumps, chicken pox, Hemophilus influenza (a bacteria), malaria, dengue fever, meningococcal meningitis, pneumococcal pneumonia, shingles, and many more. The flu kills tens of thousands of people in the United States alone every year, and the flu vaccine is revamped every year to try to match the expected epidemic strains. More recently, the COVID-19 vaccines have saved countless lives and may also need to be revamped periodically, as mutant forms of the SARS CoV-2 virus spread.

In 1930, Alexander Fleming noticed that penicillin killed bacteria in a discarded petri dish, and Howard Florey and Ernst Boris Chain further explored this phenomenon. The Merck company began to mass-produce penicillin in the early 1940s, saving countless soldiers during World War II and millions more people since. Numerous other types of antibiotics as well as antifungal, anti-parasitic, and some antiviral medications have followed. Many other advances in pharmaceutical and surgical treatments, prenatal and obstetrical care, newborn, pediatric, and adult intensive care have contributed to the average lifespan we enjoy in the United States today, now seventy-seven years for men and eighty-one years for women. For an interesting, in-depth read on the subject, I highly recommend the New York Times article "How Humanity Gave Itself an Extra Life," by Steven Johnson (Johnson 2021).

Though we have doubled our lifespan in the past century, we now live long enough to develop chronic conditions and related complications and are much more likely to develop dementia. Age is the biggest risk factor for Alzheimer's. At age eighty-five, the odds of dementia are about forty percent and increase for every year we live thereafter.

Along with extraordinary advances in public health, medical, and surgical care, the global population has exploded from about 1.8 billion people in 1920 to 7.8 billion in 2020. Mass production of food has been necessary to feed so many people, but the quality of our food has deteriorated in the process, since the costs are so enormous. The process of hydrogenation decreased the cost of production and extended the shelf life of fats and oils and foods containing them, but at the cost of introducing damaging trans fats into our diet. The practice of heating oils to high temperatures for deep frying and reusing them produces numerous toxic lipids. Since 1970, high-fructose corn syrup has become ubiquitous in beverages and processed foods but is highly inflammatory and may set the stage for diabetes, fatty liver, and many other disorders. Synthetic chemicals, used to preserve, color, and flavor foods, could have biological consequences as well.

Along with welcome technological advances in transportation have come serious pollution of air and soil. Avoidable practices, like tobacco smoking and head-butting contact sports, have led many people down an unhealthy path, affecting quality of life as we age.

Changing just one major lifestyle choice can impact aging of the brain, heart, and nearly every other organ in the body. In the previous chapter, we discussed making positive changes in major lifestyle factors to improve aging and prevent cognitive decline. In this chapter, we will discuss some things to avoid, many diet-related, to further enhance healthy aging.

- Avoid excessive sugar, fructose, and especially high-fructose corn syrup.
- Avoid foods made with trans fats and reused oils and reduce linoleic acid in the diet.
- Avoid nitrosamine compounds, processed meats, and other overly processed foods.
- Avoid taking anticholinergic prescriptions and over-the-counter medications.
- Avoid infections, like COVID-19, and get vaccinated.
- Avoid activities with significant risk of head injury.
- Reduce exposure to air pollution, if possible.
- Avoid excessive intake of iron and other metals.

AVOID EXCESSIVE SUGAR, FRUCTOSE, AND ESPECIALLY HIGH-FRUCTOSE CORN SYRUP

Accelerated brain aging and greater risk of premature death are just two important reasons that eating too much sugar is bad for your health. The average consumption of sugar in the United States has increased from just over six pounds per person in 1822 to well over one hundred pounds per year (Guyenet 2012) (see figure 9.1).

Table sugar is roughly half glucose and half fructose, and fructose is by far the sweetest of all sugars, the impetus for creating high-fructose corn syrup (HFCS). Surprisingly, more than 90 percent of fructose is converted to triglycerides in its first pass through the liver. Unlike glucose, fructose does not stimulate insulin secretion and is not stored as glycogen. However, excess fructose consumption promotes insulin resistance in the liver. Blood fructose levels are typically about 1 percent of glucose levels. However, when blood glucose is elevated, fructose levels can become very high and provoke formation of damaging advanced glycation end-products (AGEs) within certain cell types like the lens of the eye, in the kidneys, and in the nerves outside of the brain (Gugliucci 2019). Damage to these tissues can lead to cataracts, kidney failure, and peripheral neuropathy, all common complications of diabetes.

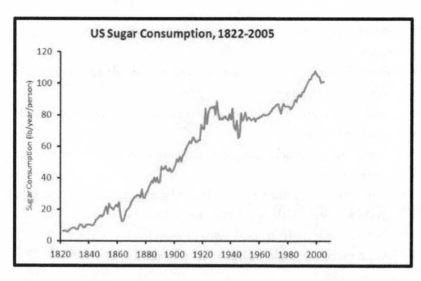

FIGURE 9.1. U.S. sugar consumption, 1822 to 2006. From Guyenet, "By 2606 the US diet will be 100 percent sugar." S. Whole Health Source: Nutrition and Health Science www.wholehealthsource.blogspot.com February 18, 2012. Previously published with permission from Stephan Guyenet.

High-fructose corn syrup (HFCS) was first marketed in the early 1970s by companies in the United States and Japan. Corn syrup is normally made from cornstarch. An enzyme is used to convert some of the glucose in corn syrup to fructose, yielding HFCSs that contain 44 or 55 percent fructose by weight. HFCS is easier and cheaper to make than granulated sugar and is used extensively in processed foods and sweetened beverages. Consumption of HFCS in the United States has increased from zero to sixty pounds per person annually since 1965 and appears to be the driving force in the huge increase in total sugar consumption since the early 1970s (see figure 9.2). Some other foods naturally high in fructose include agave nectar, honey, molasses, maple syrup, fruit, and fruit juices and, therefore, are not good substitutes for table sugar, especially in larger amounts.

Here are some compelling reasons not to eat so much sugar (and especially fructose).

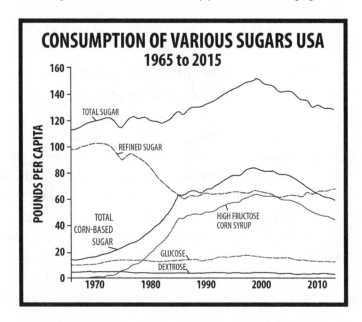

FIGURE 9.2. Annual consumption of sugar types in the United States from 1965 to 2015. Starting at "0" on the y-axis from bottom to top, the lines indicate: high-fructose corn syrup (HFCS), dextrose, glucose, total corn-based sugars, refined sugar, total sugar. HFCS increased from 0 lb. per capita in 1966 to more than 80 lb. per capita in 1980 and most recently at about 60 lb. per capita in 2015. Source: Data from USDA food consumptions databases. Adapted from figure at https://commons. wikimedia.org/wiki/File:US_Sweetener_consumption,_1966_to_2013.svg Permission/Attribution: Royote, CC BY-SA 4.0 <https://creativecommons. org/licenses/by-sa/4.0>, via Wikimedia Commons.

High Sugar Consumption Is Associated with Higher Risk of Diabetes

Increased sugar consumption in a population is associated with greater risk of diabetes (Basu 2013). Insulin resistance associated with type 2 diabetes and metabolic syndrome can be overcome with a low-carb diet (Feinman 2015). Therefore, a high-sugar diet likely causes or contributes to insulin resistance.

High Sugar Intake Is Associated with Accelerated Brain Aging

Chronic high blood sugar, insulin resistance, and diabetes are all associated with greater risk and earlier onset of cognitive decline. Sugar-sweetened beverages are associated with accelerated aging of the brain in terms of shrinkage and decline in delayed-memory recall (see side box on Pase study). A higher fasting blood-glucose level is associated with greater risk of dementia. In one study, people who did not have diabetes with blood sugars averaging just 115 mg/dl over the preceding five years were 1.18 times more likely to have dementia than those with blood glucose of 100 mg/dl. People with diabetes with an average blood glucose of 190 over the preceding five years were 1.4 times more likely to develop dementia than diabetics with an average blood glucose of 160 mg/dl (Crane 2013). There is much more on sugar, diabetes, and cognitive decline in chapter 3.

Eating Too Much Sugar Leads to Formation of Harmful AGEs

Consumption of excess glucose, fructose, and chronic high blood sugar leads to formation of advanced glycation end-products (AGEs), which are inflammatory substances that can damage virtually every cell type and tissue. Accumulation of AGEs can lead to complications of diabetes, high blood pressure, heart disease, asthma and other pulmonary diseases, chronic kidney disease, neurodegenerative disorders (Cepas 2020), gout (Gugliucci 2019), and non-alcoholic fatty liver disease (Jensen 2018) (see side box on advanced glycation end-products).

Few human studies of AGEs have been performed, and levels of AGEs in blood and urine vary considerably from person to person. An elevated level could simply reflect AGEs eaten with the most recent meal (Adams 2016). Hopefully, a quality blood test will come along soon to evaluate what effect dietary changes and supplements make on AGE buildup in the body.

More on Advanced Glycation End-Products (AGEs)

AGEs are sticky, toxic, inflammatory compounds that combine a sugar and a protein, lipid, or nucleic acid (RNA or DNA) molecule. This chemical reaction can take place during food processing and cooking (such as caramelizing), especially when the foods contain fructose. Therefore, AGEs can find their way into our bodies in food. AGEs do not leave our bodies easily and tend to accumulate throughout our lives (Guilbaud 2016). AGEs are also produced within our bodies when we eat foods high in simple sugar, fructose, and high-fructose corn syrup. Formation of AGEs from fructose is 7.5 to 10 times more reactive than glucose (Cepas 2020), and fructose may be more inflammatory than glucose within certain immune cells (Jaiswal 2019).

Proteins and fats that have undergone glycation are not shaped normally and may not function normally. AGEs can link together and attach to many different types of cells, interfere with molecular and cellular functions, and cause release of damaging substances, such as hydrogen peroxide, faster than the body can detoxify them (called oxidative stress). AGEs increase inflammation, promote leaking of blood vessels, and entrap and oxidize LDL in the lining of blood vessels, resulting in stiffening and decreased elasticity, called atherosclerosis, or hardening of the arteries. This process can ultimately lead to heart disease, heart attacks, strokes, asthma, kidney disease, Alzheimer's disease, cataracts, peripheral neuropathy (burning, tingling, numbness, and loss of sensation in hands or feet), arthritis, and complications of diabetes, specifically nephropathy, retinopathy, and neuropathy. AGEs can harm collagen, which is important in blood-vessel walls, joints, tendons, bones, corneas, and skin, and may also harm fibrinogen, which is involved in blood clotting. AGEs can attack myelin, the protective covering on nerves. AGEs have been implicated as carcinogens, which can cause normal cells to convert to cancer cells. The damage caused by excessive accumulation of AGEs hastens aging of the body and brain, which is further accelerated in people with diabetes.

The best way to stop accumulating AGEs is to stop eating processed and caramelized foods that contain AGEs, as well as foods with added sugars that promote AGE formation, like sucrose, fructose, and HFCS. Certain nutrients appear to slow down production of AGEs, specifically vitamin B1 (studied as benfotiamine), vitamin B6 (pyridoxamine), trans resveratrol, and hesperitin (from citrus), though more confirmatory studies are needed (Guilbaud 2016).

Cancer Cells Love Sugar

Most cancer cell types thrive on sugar. In fact, this is the basis for using PET imaging to monitor cancer and look for metastases. Cancer cells require at least eighteen times—and often much more—glucose than a normal cell to produce the same amount of ATP. Insulin resistance is associated with an increased risk of cancer (Arcidiacono 2012). Chronic high blood sugar promotes inflammation, which sets up an environment favorable for insulin resistance, cancer, and spread of cancer (Amin 2019). The ketogenic diet reduces blood sugar while providing ketones as fuel to normal cells. Most cancer cells cannot use ketones as fuel. Thus, depriving cancer cells of sugar could slow down cancer growth or even kill off the tumors and metastases. In the United States alone, more than forty clinical trials are completed, in progress, or recruiting to study the ketogenic diet combined with standard-of-care treatments for various cancers.

High Serum Triglyceride Levels Can Come from Eating Too Much Sugar

It is a common misconception that high triglyceride levels come from eating too much fat. However, eating too much sugar, eating too many calories, and especially eating too much fructose can increase your serum triglyceride level. More than 90 percent of fructose is converted to triglycerides in its first pass through the liver (Gugliucci 2019). Cutting down on sugar intake can bring the triglyceride level down dramatically in a matter of weeks.

The enormous PURE Study was conducted in eighteen countries on five continents with 135,335 participants studied for an average of 7.4 years (Dehghan 2017). People with the highest intake of carbohydrate had 1.28 times the risk of premature death compared to those with the lowest intake. Higher intake of total fat and each type of fat, including saturated fat, was associated with lower-than-average risk of dying prematurely and was not associated with a higher risk of heart disease, heart attacks, or heart-related deaths. Higher saturated fat intake was associated with a lower risk of stroke as well (Dehghan 2017).

Sugar-Sweetened Drinks Increase Dementia Risk

The next time you crave Coca Cola or Mountain Dew, or a glass of fresh-squeezed orange juice, consider this. Matthew Pase, PhD, and others studied people ages 53 to 56 in the Framingham Heart Study to determine if consuming sugary drinks was associated with signs of pre-clinical Alzheimer's (Alzheimer's is underway but symptoms are not yet obvious) and vascular injury. "Sugary drinks" were defined as sugar-sweetened soft drinks, fruit drinks with added sugar, and 100 percent fruit juice. Intake of diet soft drinks was documented for comparison. Every two years, an MRI (n=4276) and/or neuropsychological testing (n=3846) were performed. The brain normally shrinks a little bit each year as we age, but the process was accelerated in people who consumed sugary drinks. Compared to people who did not drink sugary beverages, consumption of one or more sugary drinks per day resulted in lower total brain volume, lower hippocampal volume (the hippocampus is an important area of the brain for memory, and the process of Alzheimer's disease starts there), and worse scores on delayed-recall memory testing (the ability to remember something, such as a list of words after a distraction):

- Consuming one to two sugary drinks per day led to an average of 1.6 years of accelerated brain shrinkage and 5.8 years of brain aging for delayed memory recall.
- Consuming more than two sugary drinks per day led to an average of 2.0 years of accelerated brain shrinkage and 11 years of brain aging for delayed memory recall.
- Consuming three or more sugary drinks per day led to an average of 2.6 years of accelerated brain shrinkage and 13 years of brain aging for delayed memory recall (Pase 2017).

The Bottom Line

The best way to control blood sugar and stop accumulating harmful AGEs is to stop eating processed and caramelized foods that contain AGEs and the sugars, like fructose and HFCS, that promote AGE formation. Clearly, adopting a whole-food Mediterranean-style low-carb keto diet is a perfect way to make this happen.

AVOID FOODS MADE WITH TRANS FATS AND REUSED OILS, AND REDUCE LINOLEIC ACID IN THE DIET

Trans fats are manmade fats produced during hydrogenation, a process used to make natural liquid fats more solid and stable at room temperatures to prolong shelf life. Wilhelm Normann patented the hydrogenation of fats in 1902. During hydrogenation, a polyunsaturated oil is subjected to high heat and pressure while hydrogen is introduced into the oil, which adds hydrogen atoms at sites of double bonds in the fatty acids. With full hydrogenation, all double bonds are replaced by hydrogen atoms. The transformed fatty acids may be identical to natural saturated fatty acids. However, food manufacturers found that interrupting the process, called partial hydrogenation, produced a fat with a melting point, solidity, and other properties that significantly extended shelf life and otherwise worked better than fully hydrogenated fats for use with certain foods. However, chronically eating man-made hydrogenated oils has serious health consequences. The big problem with partial hydrogenation is the transformation of the natural cis double bond found in polyunsaturated fatty acids to a trans double bond. They are like mirror images, except that the trans fatty acid is deformed from a gently curved, fluid shape to a nearly straight shape with a more rigid structure, and the fatty acid has a higher melting point.

The partially hydrogenated forms of soybean and canola oil have the added impact of raising cholesterol, particularly LDL, due to higher levels of trans fatty acids. During partial hydrogenation, the omega-3 fatty acids disappear first, then the omega-6s, followed by the monounsaturated fatty acids, like oleic and palmitoleic acids. Therefore, partial hydrogenation tends to remove the essential omega-3 and omega-6 fatty acids.

Human cells and cell membranes are not programmed through evolution to use these altered trans fats. All cell membranes and about 60 to 70 percent of the brain are made up of lipids (fats), and many cell functions take place within the cell membrane. Normally, in the cell membranes, the lipid molecules line up like tiny magnets end to end and side to side, called lipid bilayers (figure 9.3). They repel water on the inside, which keeps the contents of the cell inside the cell, and they repel the watery fluids on the outside of the cell, which keeps the outside world from entering the cell. When a cell membrane tries to incorporate a trans fatty acid, which is differently shaped, it is like trying to put a square peg into a round hole (figure 9.4). It does not line up normally with the other lipid molecules, and it can affect the fluidity and the functioning of the cell membrane and shorten the lifespan of the cell.

Trans Fatty Acids and the Cell Membrane Lipid Bilayer

Cell membranes are made up of a double layer of lipids (fatty acids) and are normally fluid structures due to the naturally bent shape of the polyunsaturated fatty acids. However, when man-made trans fats become part of the cell membrane, the membrane becomes stiffer, transport of substances into and out of the cell is affected, and cell lifespan can be shortened. This translates into bigger problems for the tissues made up of these cells, such as the heart and the brain.

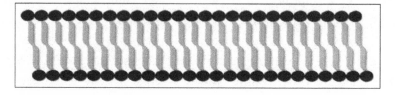

FIGURE 9.3. Lipid bilayer of cell membrane with naturally occurring fatty acids.

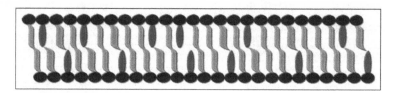

FIGURE 9.4. Lipid bilayer of cell membrane with naturally occurring fatty acids and man-made trans fatty acids. Trans fatty acids are more rigid and can interfere with the fluidity and normal function of the cell membrane.

The Nurses' Health Study, which looked at many aspects of health related to diet and other lifestyle factors, illustrates why it is very important to stay away from partially hydrogenated oils and trans fat. In 1993, Walter Willett, MD, and others collected dietary data from questionnaires completed in 1980 by 85,095 women who were not yet diagnosed with coronary heart disease, stroke, diabetes, or high cholesterol. During the next eight years, there were 431 new cases of fatal and non-fatal heart attacks. After controlling for weight and caloric intake, a higher intake of trans fatty acids was the only difference found in the diet of the affected women. Their intakes of saturated fat, mono, or polyunsaturated fat, and dietary cholesterol did not change their risk of developing heart disease (Willett 1993).

How Trans Fat Became Part of the Typical U.S. Diet

In 1911, Proctor and Gamble began to market Crisco, the first partially hydrogenated shortening, which was made from cottonseed oil. Inexpensive Crisco rapidly and steadily began to replace lard for cooking in U.S. homes through the world wars and Great Depression. Crisco and other shortenings became a staple in United States homes by the mid-twentieth century, along with margarine, another man-made partially hydrogenated fat. Crisco gave a particularly nice texture to pie crust, cake, icing, pastries, breads, cookies, and crackers. By 1985, heavily hydrogenated oils with up to 35 percent trans fats were used for deep frying in fast-food restaurants. While some animal fats contain tiny amounts of a trans fat called vaccenic acid naturally, partially hydrogenated shortening and oils used for deep-frying contained at least 30 percent and margarines about 15 to 25 percent trans fats, mainly as elaidic acid, the trans form of oleic acid, the main fatty acid found in olive and canola oils.

In the latter twentieth century, lipid researchers began to warn that consumption of trans fats could be harmful and even lead to heart attacks (Willett 1994; Enig 1999). Willett stated that "a major artificial element has been introduced into the food supply without a full understanding of all its metabolic and health implications." Compounding the problem, it became a widespread practice for restaurants and home cooks to reuse these man-made oils repeatedly at high heat, which can produce numerous other unnatural toxic lipids.

In parallel with the increasing popularity of shortenings and margarine, deaths from heart attacks were steadily and steeply on the rise in the United States, beginning in the early twentieth century. The search for the cause of this epidemic of heart disease heated up in 1955 after President Dwight Eisenhower had a heart attack while in office and the research became laser-focused on factors in the diet that might be the culprit. One study suggested that sugar could be the problem, but sugar-industry funding sources shifted the focus to fat, leading to a series of studies in North America and Europe that suggested fat, and especially saturated fat, was an issue in heart disease. Recommendations to eat less animal fat came along in 1961 and became official dogma with the first Dietary Guidelines for Americans published in 1980. Animal saturated fat was the big worry and was commonly referred to simply as "saturated fat," even though it contains mostly mono- and polyunsaturated fatty acids and less than half (35 to 45 percent) saturated fatty acids. These early guidelines have not wavered in 2021, and many Americans have replaced fat with sugar for decades. Lower fat consumption and consequent higher carbohydrate consumption, coupled with the rise of trans fats and high-fructose corn syrup in the American diet, have occurred in parallel with epidemics of obesity, diabetes, and dementia in the United States. These epidemics have spread around the world as other populations have adopted more Western foods and poorer eating habits.

High cholesterol was deemed a risk for heart disease in the 1960s, and some (but not all) studies suggested that saturated fat increased cholesterol. I clearly recall, as a teenager, being told to eat margarine instead of butter, drink skim milk, eat lean meats, to remove fat from meat and the skin and fat from chicken, and to forget about eggs altogether. A serious flaw in this organizational advice on diet at that time was the ignorance of the dangers of trans fats. Another flaw was the failure to recognize that high-trans-fat shortenings and margarines made up a substantial percentage of fats in the diets (estimated at 15 to 50 percent) of the U.S. and European populations they had studied in the 1950s and 1960s (Jensen 2012). It is conceivable that the study results reflected the effect of trans fat, not high fat, or high saturated fat, in the diet.

In 1953, Ancel Keys, plotting results from just six countries, reported that a higher percent of fat in the diet strongly correlated with a greater risk of cardiac death in men (Keys 1953). However, this study left out data from fifteen other countries; and when another researcher named Mann plotted all the available data in a critique, it showed a random pattern (see figures 9.5 and 9.6). Despite the flaws, Keys's and other mid-twentieth-century studies were the basis for the recommended limits, first on saturated fat, and then on all fat intake, by the American Heart Association (AHA) sixty years ago. These old studies are still used as core evidence in the AHA's latest advisory on dietary fats, published in 2017, to justify the continued vilification of fat, saturated fat, and coconut oil (Sacks 2017). Coconut oil was not listed as a fat used by the populations in these core studies, and the coconut oil used in small animal and human studies at that time to evaluate effects on cholesterol used partially hydrogenated or highly processed oil, rather than the virgin cold-pressed coconut oil more available today (Astrup 2020). Much research has demonstrated that partially hydrogenated oils with trans fats increase total cholesterol and LDL cholesterol levels, and have no health benefits (Institute of Medicine: Dietary Reference Intakes, 2006, page 423; Ascherio 2010; Mensink 1990; Willett 1993).

With the focus on fat, the marked steady increase in smoking, which paralleled the increase in heart attacks throughout the twentieth century, was largely ignored until the evidence that tobacco use causes lung cancer became overwhelming. Public health initiatives on smoking cessation instituted around 1970 led to a substantial drop in tobacco use by 1980, followed by a parallel reduction in heart-attack deaths (see figures 9.7 and 9.8). Deaths from lung cancer began to plummet about fifteen years after tobacco use dropped off (see figure 9.7). Lovastatin, the first statin drug approved by the FDA to lower LDL-cholesterol,

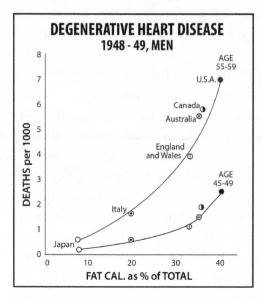

FIGURE 9.5. Ancel Keys data from six countries on dietary fat and heart deaths. In a 1953 study by Ancel Keys, data for six countries from a 1949 report by the Food and Agriculture Organization (FAO) appeared to show that the risk of death from degenerative heart disease in men increased as the percentage of fat increased in the diet. There were actually twenty-two data points available. Data adapted by Joanna Newport from Keys 1953.

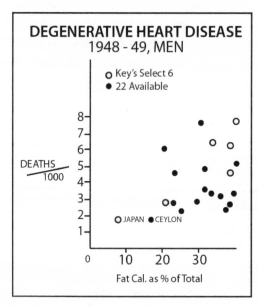

FIGURE 9.6. Data from twenty-two countries disputed Keys's hypothesis that a high-fat diet causes degenerative heart disease. George Mann plotted data for all twenty-two countries available from the FAO report showing that there was no correlation between percent of fat intake and heart disease. Data adapted by Joanna Newport from Mann 1959.

did not come on the market until 1987, and the rate of deaths from coronary heart disease had already declined to pre-1960 levels.

Simultaneously, pressure created by government guidelines on the American public to reduce saturated fat in the diet resulted in greater consumption of trans fatty acids, since partially hydrogenated oils were thought to be the most suitable alternatives to lard and other animal fat for use in processed foods. Consumption of margarine, a partially hydrogenated oil with trans fat, steadily replaced butter throughout the twentieth century, following a similar pattern to smoking and coronary artery disease mortality (figure 9.9). The combination of smoking and eating partially hydrogenated oils with trans fats is a particularly unhealthy combination for the heart and other organs.

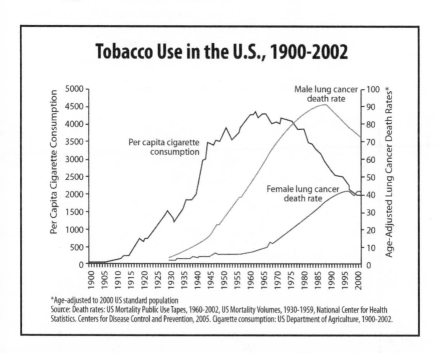

FIGURE 9.7. Trends in tobacco use in the United States, 1900 to 2002. Deaths from lung cancer about fifteen years after tobacco use plummeted. Data sources: U.S. Mortality Data, National Center for Health Statistics, CDC, USDA. Adapted by Joanna Newport.

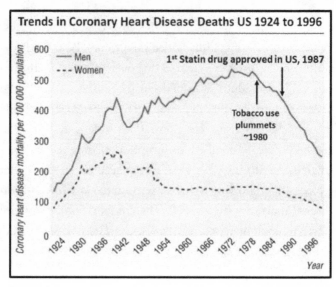

FIGURE 9.8. Trends in coronary-heart-disease deaths in the United States, 1924 to 1996. Deaths from coronary heart disease began to drop off several years after tobacco use plummeted around 1980 and well before statins were available. Adapted from CDC and other U.S. data sources.

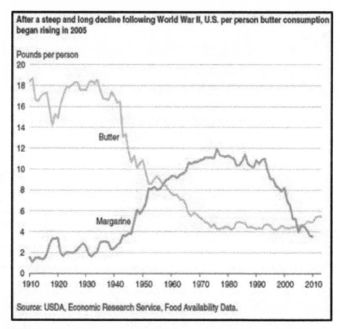

FIGURE 9.9. Trends in margarine and butter consumption from 1910 to 2010. The trend in margarine (trans fat) consumption in place of butter followed a similar pattern to tobacco use and coronary artery deaths during the 20th century. Data from USDA, Economic Research Service, Food Availability Data https://USDA.gov.

In 2002, the FDA required food manufacturers to report grams of trans fat per serving in their nutrition information and on nutrient labels, which led to a big switch in the types of fats used in many processed foods and in restaurants. In the fall of 2013, the FDA proclaimed that partially hydrogenated fats are no longer considered "generally recognized as safe" (GRAS) and would be phased out from foods in the United States within two years. At that time, FDA commissioner Margaret Hamburg said that there is no safe level of consumption of trans fat and no known benefit from consuming trans fat, and that "further reduction in the amount of trans fat in the American diet could prevent an additional 20,000 heart attacks and 7,000 deaths from heart disease each year—a critical step in the protection of Americans' health." The deadline was extended for five more years to permit food manufacturers to adjust and allow trans fat foods with long shelf lives produced before 2018 to work through the market.

Unfortunately, food manufacturers are not required to reveal trans fat in products with less than 0.5 grams per serving, and some have adjusted the "serving size" to avoid reporting trans fat. Therefore, it is important to look for trans fat content, "hydrogenated," or "partially hydrogenated" as ingredients on food labels. Ask restaurants you frequent whether they re-use their oils for frying; or, better yet, avoid deep-frying and eat a healthy whole-food diet.

Saturated Fat Is Not Trans Fat

Saturated fat is often lumped together with trans fat in WHO and other dietary guidelines as if they were equally harmful. However, saturated fatty acids and trans fatty acids are very different. Saturated fat is not structured like, and does not behave metabolically like, trans fat. The presence of the trans double bond, and the orientation of hydrogen atoms around that bond, changes how the fatty acid behaves biologically, and saturated fatty acids have no double bonds.

Stearic acid, oleic acid, and elaidic acid are all fatty acids with 18 carbons in the chain (figure 9.11). The only differences in structure are that the saturated fatty acid called stearic acid has no double bond, oleic acid (the main fatty acid in olive oil) has a natural cis double bond at the ninth carbon, and elaidic acid has a trans double bond at the ninth carbon. This does not change elaidic acid into a saturated fatty acid. The trans double bond causes the elaidic acid molecule to straighten and become more rigid, changing its biochemical properties and functions compared to oleic acid. Elaidic acid is an unnatural man-made fatty acid with no known necessary or beneficial role in human metabolism.

Stearic acid also has eighteen carbons but has no double bonds and has different biochemical properties and functions than elaidic acid. Stearic acid is synthesized naturally in the human body and can be metabolized to oleic acid as needed. Stearic acid appears to have a beneficial effect on mitochondria regulation, and white blood cell mitochondria become fragmented when stearic acid is deficient in the diet (Senyilmaz-Tiebe 2018). Stearic and oleic acid are found together with palmitic acid, another saturated fatty acid, in virtually all natural fats and oils, including common vegetable oils like soybean, corn, olive, sunflower, and coconut oil.

Studies: Compared to cells exposed to the naturally occurring stearic and oleic acids, exposure to man-made trans fat elaidic acid resulted in a more rigid cell membrane, profoundly changed the fatty acid profile of the important phospholipids in the cell membrane (see figure 9.10), decreased the lifespan of the cells, decreased cell proliferation (multiplication), allowed more influx of calcium, decreased permeability of the cell, and upregulated all proteins related to cholesterol synthesis (Vendel Nielsen 2013). In other studies, elaidic acid but not oleic increased inflammation and drastically enhanced extracellular ATP-induced cell death (Hirata 2017; Hirata 2020).

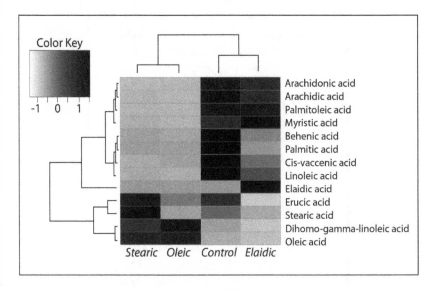

FIGURE 9.10. Heat-map representation of distribution of fatty acids in phospholipids of the HepG2-SF [liver] cells after supplementation. The FA composition of HepG2-SF phospholipids changes depending on the different supplemented fatty acids. Stearic and oleic profiles are alike, whereas the elaidic fatty acid phospholipid profile differs from all the other groups. Control samples had no free fatty acid added. Open access permission through Creative Commons License with citation: Vendel Nielsen L, TP Krogager, C Young, et al. "Effects of elaidic acid on lipid metabolism in HepG2 cells, investigated by an integrated approach of lipidomics, transcriptomics and proteomics." PLoS One V. 8 No. 9 (2013):e74283. Adapted to grayscale by Joanna Newport.

REDUCE LINOLEIC ACID IN THE DIET

In the past century, advances in the field of lipid biochemistry—analysis of oils and fats and what individual fatty acids do—led to the recognition that humans (and other mammals) have a requirement for two classes of essential polyunsaturated fatty acids: first omega-6, and, much more recently, omega-3. We cannot produce enough and must consume them to grow and develop normally and maintain physical and cognitive health. However, we require a very small amount of the essential fatty acids compared to the total amount of food we eat. For example, the recommended daily allowance for the omega-3, alpha-linoleic acid, is just 1.1 grams (1100 mg) for women and 1.6 grams (1600 mg) for men, around ¼ teaspoon.

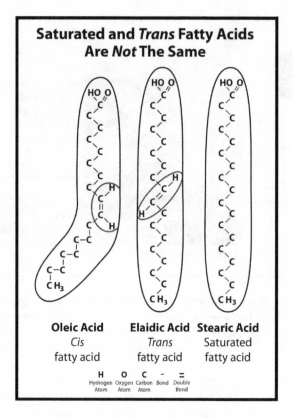

FIGURE 9.11. Saturated and trans fatty acids are not the same. Saturated fatty acids do not have a double bond like trans fatty acids, which significantly changes the biological effects of a fatty acid. The cis fatty acid oleic acid has the same basic structure the trans fatty acid elaidic acid has. Stearic acid is a saturated fatty acid with the same chain length as oleic and elaidic acids, but has no double bond.

Dietary essential fatty acids mainly come from fish, animal-meat fat, dairy fats, and plant oils but can also come from supplements. In non-marine fats and oils, nearly all omega-6 is linoleic acid, and the omega-3 is alpha-linolenic acid. By way of different biochemical pathways, these two distinct fatty acids give rise to numerous longer-chain metabolites, each of which has important but opposing functions in the brain and body (see figure 9.12). For example, some omega-6 metabolites increase acute inflammation, a function of our immune system necessary

Opposing effects of omega-6 and omega-3 fatty acids on obesity

Fatty Acid	omega-6	omega-3
Adipose cells (tissue)	▲	▼
White adipose tissues	▲	▼
Brown adipose tissues	▼	▲
Inflammation	▲	▼
Triglycerides	▲	▼
Muscle glycogen synthesis		▲
Endogenous antioxidants	▼	▲
Oxidation		
Endocannabinoid tone	▲	▼
Protein synthesis	▲	▲
Mitochondrial Biogenesis		▲
AMPK		▲
Akt (Protein kinase B)		▲
Telomeres	▼	▲
NF-kB (Nuclear factor kB)	▲	▼
PPARα	▼	▲
Leptin resistance	▲	▼
Insulin resistance	▲	▼
Adiponectin		▲
Waist circumference	▲	▼

▲ increase, ▼ decrease.
AMPK, 5' adenosine monophosphate-activated protein kinase;
PPARα, peroxisome proliferator-activated receptor α

FIGURE 9.12. Opposing effects of omega-6 and omega-3 fatty acids on obesity. Adapted by Joanna Newport from table 1 in Simopoulos AP, JJ DiNicolantonio. "The importance of a balanced ω-6 to ω-3 ratio in the prevention and management of obesity." Open Heart V. 3 No. 2 (2016):e000385. Open Access permission under Creative Commons Attribution Non-Commercial license (CC BY-NC 4.0). See: http://creativecommons.org/licenses/by-nc/4.0/.

to fight infection. Omega-3 fatty acids give rise to metabolites that are anti-inflammatory and help us recover from the infection-fighting inflammation and return to our normal pre-infection state. Omega-6 fatty acids give rise to metabolites that promote blood clotting and constrict blood vessels, whereas certain omega-3 fatty acid metabolites inhibit blood clotting and dilate blood vessels (Lands 2005).

As discussed in chapter 5, there is a complex and delicate balance between the functions of omega-6 and omega-3 fatty acids that runs smoothly when they are consumed in about the same amount, ideally in a 1:1 ratio of grams of omega-6 to grams of omega-3. For decades, the American Heart Association has encouraged replacing saturated fat with polyunsaturated fat to reduce the risk of cardiovascular disease without guidance on how much is safe. Is it possible to eat too much polyunsaturated fat? The answer is yes! Even though the requirement for omega-6 is less than 0.5 percent of our caloric intake, many Americans eat 10 to 15 percent of their total calories as linoleic acid. Eating too much linoleic acid (omega-6) can upset that delicate balance of essential fatty acids, which may increase the degree of and prolong the state of inflammation, which can promote blood clotting and constrict blood vessels.

Linoleic acid, eaten in excess, produces high blood levels of inflammatory oxylipins (oxidized lipids). Chronic inflammation is a major factor in neurological and other chronic diseases, such as rheumatoid arthritis, inflammatory bowel disease, asthma, autism, and Alzheimer's. Recent studies in animals and humans have shown that eating excessive linoleic acid increases the risks of obesity and insulin resistance, a core feature of type 2 diabetes and Alzheimer's (sometimes, as is mentioned earlier in this book, called diabetes of the brain or type 3 diabetes).

Excessive linoleic acid intake increases the number of fat cells, increases the amount of fat tissue, and keeps white fat from becoming brown fat, which provides heat and appears to keep body weight in check by controlling energy balance (Simopoulos 2016). Since 1965, the amount of dietary linoleic acid has more than doubled, and the amount of linoleic acid in fat tissue has increased by 137 percent (Guyenet 2016), which may explain the increase in blood biomarkers of inflammation found in obese people.

For most of human history, the ratio of omega-6 to omega-3 was likely close to 1:1. However, abandonment of traditional fats and oils and widespread use of mass-produced vegetable oils, especially soybean and corn oil, has greatly increased the average amount of linoleic acid we consume. These days, even our beef cows eat much more omega-6 fatty acids, since grains are used to fatten them up, unlike grass-fed pasture-raised cows. Hence, we get more omega-6 from their fat as well. By 2005, the ratio of omega-6 to omega-3 had increased to about 17:1 in the

LINOLEIC (LA) AND ALPHA-LINOLENIC ACID (ALA) IN ANIMAL FATS AND PLANT OILS

OIL OR FAT	OMEGA-6 AS LA %	LA (gm/15ml*)	OMEGA-3 AS ALA %
Coconut oil	2	0.3	0
Butter	2	0.3	0.3
Beef tallow	3	0.4	0.6
Lard	10	1.4	1
Olive	10	1.4	0.8
Avocado	12	1.7	1
Canola	13-19	2 to 3	2.5
Peanut	20	3	0.3
Soybean	50	7	6.6
Cottonseed	51	7	0.1
Corn	53	7.4	1
Sunflower	65	9	0.16
Safflower	75	11	0

*15 ml = 1 tablespoon
USDA FoodData Central - https://fdc.nal.usda.gov/

TABLE 9.1. Percent linoleic (omega-6) and alpha-linolenic acid (omega-3) found in common animal fats and plant oil. Genetically modified canola, sunflower, and safflower oils may contain lower amounts of linoleic acid than shown. Modern mass-produced plant oils contain much higher levels of linoleic acid than ancestral fats used for cooking. Excess linoleic acid promotes inflammation and increases risk for obesity and insulin resistance. All fats and oils shown have 1 gram or less of omega-3 fatty acids per tablespoon. It is easy to see how the ideal omega-6 to omega-3 ratio of 1:1 is difficult to achieve with the typical modern diet. Data source: USDA Food Data Central https://fdc.nal.usda.gov/.

United States, 15:1 in Europe, and as high as 50:1 in some urban areas of India. In Japan, where the incidence of obesity, diabetes, and Alzheimer's are much lower, the omega-6 to omega-3 ratio is a much more reasonable 4:1. Eating too much linoleic acid decreases the blood level of DHA, a long-chain omega-3 fatty acid that is critical to overall brain health, vision, and cognitive function (Simopoulos 2016). While omega-6 is overly abundant in today's foods, getting enough of the right kind of omega-3 fatty acids can be more of a challenge. We previously discussed omega-3 and DHA in more detail in chapter 5.

What are the best oils and fats to eat to avoid excessive intake of linoleic acid? Before soybean, corn oil, shortening (hydrogenated cottonseed oil), and margarine became popular in the twentieth century, lard, beef tallow, and butter were the go-to fats for cooking in the United States. Olive oil, an important component of the Mediterranean-style diet, has less than 10 percent linoleic acid. Butter and coconut oil are even lower at about 2 percent. The linoleic and oleic acid content of avocado oil are similar to olive oil. Soybean, corn, sunflower, and safflower oils are off the charts with more than 50 percent linoleic acid. Manufacturers of canola oil have genetically modified some of their oil products to contain more oleic acid and much less linoleic acid (13 to 19 percent). Look to table 9.1 on the percent of linoleic and alpha-linolenic acid in oils and fats.

AVOID NITROSAMINE COMPOUNDS, PROCESSED MEATS, AND OTHER OVERLY PROCESSED FOODS

As previously mentioned, advances in food manufacturing and delivery have made it possible to feed more than 7 billion people worldwide. The downside is that mass-produced processed foods often contain artificial substances. For example, ice cream that is not made from real cream, and a long list of synthetic chemicals are used to enhance color and taste, inhibit the growth of bacteria and mold, and increase shelf life. When we eat overly processed and artificial foods, our metabolisms may miss out on the natural forms of vitamins and other substances needed to help us function at our full potential.

Nitrosamines are food additives that have been studied extensively by Dr. Suzanne de la Monte and group at Brown University, who also coined the term "type 3 diabetes" to denote Alzheimer's (De la Monte 2005). Chronic low-level exposure to nitrosamines through tobacco use, diet, and fertilizers promote fatty liver disease that can lead to insulin resistance in the liver. Streptozotocin is a nitrosamine compound and toxic antibiotic used to treat pancreatic islet cell cancer and is similar enough to glucose that GLUT 2 will transport it into islet cells. Streptozotocin has been used to cause insulin resistance in animal models of disease for decades. The De la Monte group has found that, like excess alcohol, nitrosamines produce toxic ceramides that cross the blood–brain barrier, where they can cause insulin deficiency and insulin resistance, along with inflammation, energy failure, and further production of toxic ceramides. Therefore, chronic exposure to nitrates and nitrites could contribute to the process of neurodegeneration (De la Monte 2009; Tong 2009).

Nitrosamines are commonly used as preservatives or fortifiers in processed foods, including anything that contains white flour, processed cheeses, most bacons, sausages, deli meats, other processed meats, and even some formulas and foods made for infants and toddlers. Look on food labels for "nitrites" or "nitrates," or any words that contain "nitrite" or "nitrate." A common example is "thiamin mononitrate," a synthetic form of vitamin B1, used to fortify white flour, white rice, and many other foods. Certain vegetables naturally contain small amounts of nitrates, but the nitrate levels may be much higher if vegetables are grown in the conventional manner using nitrogen fertilizers. Therefore, organically grown vegetables are a better choice.

Many beers and some hard liquors like scotch are made with a process involving nitrosamines and may contain high levels of these compounds. The combination of alcohol and nitrosamines could greatly increase the risk of damage from toxic ceramides. There is no requirement for alcohol-containing beverages to list nitrosamine content on the label.

A great many people in the United States consume foods with nitrosamine compounds at virtually every meal, and this may even begin in infancy. Overconsumption of processed foods with nitrosamines could partly explain the simultaneous growing epidemics of Alzheimer's, obesity, and other diseases that involve insulin deficiency and/or insulin resistance.

To study the effects of high blood levels of ceramides, the Women's

Health and Aging Study II followed 100 women between ages seventy and seventy-nine for nine years who had received extensive testing for their memory, cognitive functioning, and ability to carry out activities of daily living. The women did not have dementia at baseline and received a neurologic examination and blood analysis with each visit. Over nine years, 27 of the women developed dementia, of which 18 were diagnosed with probable Alzheimer's dementia. Women with the highest levels of specific ceramides in their blood were much more likely to develop Alzheimer's than those with the lowest levels. The researchers also found that high ceramide levels in people with mild cognitive impairment appeared to predict further cognitive decline (Mielke 2012).

Dietary guidelines often warn us to limit eating all red meat, but processed meat may be the real problem. Meat and processed meat are often lumped together on dietary questionnaires used in studies, but there is a real distinction between meat from pasture-raised animals fed their natural diet and processed bacon, sausage, and deli meats made from animals raised on grains containing antibiotics, hormones, preservatives, and pesticides. An animal's fat can store these chemicals, which may end up in us when we eat the meat from animals that were raised this way. More chemicals like nitrosamine compounds may be added during processing.

The important distinction between meat and processed meat was demonstrated by Zhang and group. The UK Biobank Cohort of 493,888 participants were followed for an average of eight years, during which 2,896 people developed dementia from all causes. Of these, 1,006 cases were further diagnosed as Alzheimer's and 490 cases as vascular dementia. There was an increased risk by 1.44 times for each 25 grams (just under 1 ounce) per day of processed meats eaten. A typical piece of sausage or a hot dog could easily weigh 75 grams (2½ ounces). On the other hand, for each 50 grams per day of unprocessed meat, there was a significant reduction in the risk of developing dementia from all causes (Zhang 2021), quite unexpected results given the current thinking about red meat going into dietary guidelines.

Virtually all foods are processed in some way to bring them to market, such as picking, washing, and packaging. The point of further processing and ultra-processing foods is to create convenient tasty drinks, foods, and snacks with a long shelf life that are ready to eat or ready to heat and eat. "Ultra-processed foods" contain virtually no whole food and do contain additives such as preservatives, sweeteners, sensory enhancers, colorants, flavors, and processing aids. Ultra-processing can include extruding (pressing substances out of food), molding, re-shaping, hydrogenation (as explained in the section on trans fats), and hydrolysis (chemical breakdown of food). Ultra-processed foods may also contain contaminants from plastics and other processing exposures. Ultra-processed foods include carbonated soft drinks, many types of snacks, candies, breads, buns, cookies, pastries, cake mixes, instant soups, noodles, packaged meats, hot dogs, burgers, chicken nuggets and fish sticks, and much more.

In NHANES surveys, ultra-processed foods account for almost 60 percent of total calories consumed and about 90 percent of calories from added sugar in the United States. For people with the highest intake of ultra-processed foods, nearly 20 percent of the total calorie intake is from added sugar (Martínez Steele 2016). The prevalence of obesity and diabetes in the United States is not surprising.

Bonaccio and group studied the effects of ultra-processed food consumption on mortality in 22,475 men and women in Italy who were followed for eight years. The participants were divided into four groups based on the percent of the total calories they consumed as ultra-processed foods. Adherence to a Mediterranean-style diet was also determined from food surveys. People who reported the highest intake of ultra-processed foods compared to the lowest intake had 1.58 times the risk of death due to cardiovascular disease, 1.52 times the risk of death from ischemic heart or cerebrovascular disease, and 1.26 times the number of deaths from all causes. Sugar in ultra-processed foods had the greatest effect on mortality. The effect of ultra-processed foods on kidney function was also a significant factor in mortality. The health benefits of the Mediterranean-style diet were largely erased by a diet that was also high in ultra-processed food (Bonaccio 2021). Bonaccio's findings were consistent with another study in France of more than 100,000 people (Srour 2019).

AVOID TAKING ANTICHOLINERGIC PRESCRIPTION AND OVER-THE-COUNTER MEDICATIONS

Many different types of prescribed and over-the-counter medications are anticholinergic. Many decongestants and medications for sleep, allergies, vomiting, motion sickness, dizziness, bowel control, bladder control, and depression can block acetylcholine. Most of the medications commonly prescribed to people with Alzheimer's and other memory impairments work by increasing the availability of acetylcholine. So taking a medication that blocks the production of acetylcholine is counterproductive and may cause or worsen symptoms of confusion and cognitive impairment. It is common for people to take several anticholinergic medications on a regular basis.

For caregivers and physicians, deciding whether to treat a condition with an anticholinergic medication is quite a dilemma, since a good alternative medication may not exist. For someone who is elderly and/or has memory problems, ask the doctor or pharmacist, before using any prescribed and over-the-counter medication, whether it is anticholinergic. If the answer is yes, ask for an alternative that is not anticholinergic, if available. For example, Lomotil®, used for diarrhea, contains atropine, which is anticholinergic; but there is an alternative, Imodium®, which has little anticholinergic effect. See chapter 8 for more information on anticholinergics for sleep and bladder control.

AVOID INFECTIONS LIKE COVID-19, AND GET VACCINATED

Many different types of organisms have been found in the brains of older people and implicated as possible causes, triggers, or accelerants of Alzheimer's disease. Some of the suspects are herpes simplex, which causes "fever blisters" on the mouth and other body parts; herpes zoster, which causes chicken pox, then shingles later in life; the fungus Candida albicans; Chlamydia pneumoniae; spirochetes such as Borrelia burgdorferi, the cause of Lyme disease; and Treponema denticola, which causes gum disease. Treponema pallidum, which causes syphilis, is well known to cause dementia when untreated. Many other microbes might cause or contribute to dementia, but herpes simplex is the most studied (Itzhaki 2016).

Viruses like herpes simplex are much smaller than bacteria, at 20 to 400 nm, and can only be seen with a powerful electron microscope. It is stunning that a particle so small can take down a human being. Viruses cannot replicate (multiply) unless they find their way into a living cell of a human, animal, or plant; but when they do invade, they take over the cell's machinery to rapidly make thousands of identical copies of themselves. When the cell is packed full of virus particles, the particles rupture out of the cell and find their way to other nearby living cells. Certain variants of the SARS CoV-2 virus that causes COVID-19 fuse adjoining cell membranes together to make transmission to the next cell easier and avoid exposure to antibodies.

Viruses can infect a human, or specific animals or plants, with or without crossover between species. A virus particle is not alive per se, but can exist outside of a cell in a sort of suspended animation. The virus particle itself is a string of DNA or RNA genetic material that provides the code for the proteins it needs to multiply. The virus particle is surrounded by a protein coat (capsid) to protect the genetic material. Some viruses also are encapsulated by an envelope or capsule made of lipids.

Plaques and tangles are characteristics of Alzheimer's disease and certain other dementias, and we will discuss these in detail in chapter 10. We still do not know exactly why tangles form in the brain, but could infection be a trigger? Ruth Itzhaki and her associates in the UK have studied the herpes simplex virus 1 (HSV1) and Alzheimer's for three decades and have reported that mice infected with HSV1 develop plaques and tangles in the brain. People with an ApoE4 gene have higher rates of HSV1 infection, which may have no obvious outward evidence, though many people have recurrent fever blisters caused by

HSV1. HSV1 encephalitis (inflammation of the brain) usually begins in the same location as Alzheimer's and spreads along the same pathways through the brain. The antiviral drug valacyclovir blocks the formation of these plaques and tangles in mice (Itzhaki 2016).

Several recent large-population studies have shown a lower incidence of Alzheimer's in people who received antiviral medication (acyclovir, cidofovir, famcyclovir, gancyclovir, valacyclovir, or valgancyclovir) for herpes simplex or herpes zoster infection (Chen 2018; Tzeng 2018; Bae 2020; Schnier 2021). In a Swedish study of more than a quarter of a million people, those with untreated herpes simplex or herpes zoster infection had 1.5 times the risk of dementia, compared to those who were treated. The longer the duration of treatment was beyond thirty days, the greater the protection against dementia (Lopatko Lindman 2021).

Other studies have reported that dementia is most common in people who have a history of herpes simplex and the ApoE4 gene or other genes associated with Alzheimer's (Lopatko Lindman 2019). People who have had shingles involving the eye, which is caused by herpes zoster (the chicken pox virus), have three times the risk of dementia compared to those who have not (Tsai 2017). The eye is part of the brain, and infection of the eye allows the virus more direct access to the areas affected by dementias like Alzheimer's.

Chris Carter in the UK reported amino acid sequences in HSV1 that are identical to those on tau and other proteins involved in tangle formation. Antibodies that recognize these sequences in the virus also appear to attack the same amino acid sequences in proteins, such as tau, that are important to our neurons. Inflammatory substances of our immune defense system against microbes are also found at the sites of destruction. Therefore, the immune response to a herpes virus infection could explain the damage that occurs. In one article, Carter stated that "amyloid plaques and tangles represent cemeteries for a battle between the virus and the host's defense network" (Carter 2010).

As a neonatologist, I repeatedly experienced the tragic consequences of herpes simplex 2 virus (HSV2) infection in the newborn. This virus is one of the most common causes of seizures in newborns, and a mother is most likely to pass it to her newborn when her first herpes infection occurs near the time of delivery. This infection can reach the baby's brain, and it can be fatal or result in severe brain damage and developmental delays in babies who survive. I will never forget a baby who was delivered emergently by C-section after she began to have seizures in the womb. At birth she had a blistery rash on her face and was barely responsive. An ultrasound study showed that her brain was almost entirely replaced by fluid, with only the brain stem still intact. A sample of her spinal fluid revealed that HSV2 had destroyed her brain. I often wonder whether some children with autism are exposed to this virus or another virus in the herpes family, such as cytomegalovirus, at birth and only manifest symptoms later, perhaps when the virus is reactivated by inflammation.

My husband Steve, who had one copy of the ApoE4 gene, struggled with frequent large fever blisters on his mouth from herpes simplex virus 1 and experienced an infection with this virus around his eye when he was twenty-nine years old. He told me he had not felt the same cognitively or functioned as well at his accounting job after that. I came across Dr. Itzhaki's work on the virus and Alzheimer's in 2009, and Steve received valacyclovir thereafter, a treatment that helps prevent replication of the virus. Dr. Itzhaki and others have tried for years to get funding for clinical trials of valacyclovir to control this infection in people with Alzheimer's. One feasibility study of valacyclovir has finally been conducted, without published results yet, and another is recruiting as of late 2021.

I met Leslie Norins, MD, and his wife Rainey at the Alzheimer's Association International Conference 2018 in Chicago at their AlzGerm.org foundation booth in the exhibit hall. Dr. Norins is formerly of the U.S. Center for Disease Control and points out that Alzheimer's has all the features of an epidemic and, like most other epidemics, is almost certainly caused by a microbe. On his website, he discusses the many other brain diseases known to be caused by microbes (Norins 2018). Norins points out that viruses can remain in the body following childhood diseases: for example, the chicken pox virus (Varicella-Zoster) can lie dormant in nerves for decades, then erupt as shingles. Untreated syphilis can result in dementia many years later in 30 percent of those infected. Spouses of people with dementia have greater risk of developing dementia themselves. Neurosurgeons who are exposed repeatedly to the brain tissue of people with dementia and other brain diseases are much more likely than the average person to develop Alzheimer's (Lollis 2010).

There was an epidemic of viral parkinsonism (symptoms like Parkinson's disease—tremors, rigidity, impaired balance) a century ago in people who had had the Spanish flu of 1918. Viral parkinsonism can also occur following infection with HIV, dengue fever, and West Nile virus (Eldeeb 2020).

Given its steady rise and spread to countries throughout the world over the past few decades, I would venture to say that Alzheimer's is a slow pandemic, as opposed to the rapidly evolving pandemic caused by SARS CoV-2 (COVID-19) that was recognized in late 2019. SARS CoV-2 attaches to angiotensin-converting enzyme 2 (ACE2) receptors on cell membranes that are present in the lungs, kidneys, heart, and other tissues. The damage that occurs is due to an exaggerated immune response, called a "cytokine storm," that goes well beyond attacking and containing the virus, leading to severe prolonged illness and death in some people. A great mystery is why so many people have very mild symptoms and others have no symptoms at all.

SARS CoV-2 can also directly infect the brain by infecting cells lining blood vessels at the blood–brain barrier and causes neurological manifestations in many people, ranging from mild to severe, from loss of taste and smell to paralysis. It makes sense, then, that viruses or other microbes could cause Alzheimer's disease. Deaths in the United States from dementia have increased from about 84,000 in 2000 to 262,000 deaths in 2017, according to the CDC, of which 120,400 were from Alzheimer's (Kramarow 2019). Like Alzheimer's, diabetes is a major risk factor for serious and fatal infection in SARS CoV-2. Tissue damage and inflammation from chronically elevated blood-sugar levels could make those tissues easy targets for SARS CoV-2 and "the Alzheimer's germ" or germs.

Some infections that cause dementia or dementia-like symptoms, like the spirochetes that cause syphilis, gum disease, and Lyme disease, can be treated with antibiotics. Therefore, it is quite conceivable that one or more antimicrobial or antiviral medications could be "the cure(s)" for some people with Alzheimer's. The CDC estimates that there are an average of 476,000 cases of Lyme disease per year (CDC 2021). Lyme disease is not a small problem and may be underrecognized as a potentially treatable cause of dementia symptoms.

Kris Kristofferson's (photo 1) Lyme Disease Misdiagnosed as Alzheimer's

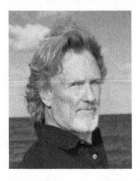

PHOTO 1. Kris Kristofferson.

Handsome young singer and songwriter Kris Kristofferson's career took off when he starred with Barbra Streisand in the movie *A Star Is Born* in 1976. When he was approaching his late seventies, he experienced progressive, debilitating memory loss and was diagnosed with Alzheimer's, versus dementia from an earlier head injury from contact sports. In 2016, a test came back positive for Lyme disease, an infection that comes from the bite of a tick carrying the Borrelia burgdoferi spirochete. The early symptoms of Lyme may or may not include redness resembling a bull's-eye around the bite, fever, and joint pain, and may evolve months to years later to include cardiac and neurological symptoms mimicking Alzheimer's. After three weeks of treatment with an antibiotic, Kristofferson's memory and other symptoms gradually improved, and he retired in 2020 at age eighty-four after a fifty-five-year career.

The Kristoferitsch group in Germany has published three case reports of people with dementia symptoms who improved dramatically after treatment of Borrelia burgdorferi for three weeks with the antibiotic ceftriaxone (Kristoferitsch 2018). The spirochete that causes syphilis is well known to cause dementia years after the initial infection if not treated.

Source: https://www.cbsnews.com/news/kris-kristofferson-misdiagnosed-alzheimers-has-lyme-disease/.

For Dr. Leslie Norins, the Alzheimer's epidemic is an emergency, and he finds it difficult to understand why it has not been treated this way. Where are the research dollars to search for the Alzheimer's germ? After all, in the United States alone, Alzheimer's kills 332 people per day and is the fifth leading cause of death. In Australia, Alzheimer's is the second leading cause of death overall and the leading cause of death for women. Thanks to the efforts of Dr. Norins and others, the Alzheimer's Association International Conference 2019 in Los Angeles included the first-ever two-hour session on infection and Alzheimer's. Other sessions discussed the connection between the microbiome in the gut and the brain, called the "gut-brain connection," as related to Alzheimer's disease—another area that is just recently gaining greater awareness. There is more on the gut microbiome and the brain in chapters 4 and 6.

Dr. Norins has focused his recent efforts on encouraging funding to test existing antiviral and antimicrobial drugs that are effective against "the six top infectious suspects" to determine if such treatment could prevent, delay, or reverse the progression of Alzheimer's disease. These suspicious microbes include herpes viruses (cause of fever blisters, shingles, and other blistery rashes), spirochetes (like Lyme and syphilis), Porphyromonas gingivalis (a cause of gum disease and dental decay), mycobacteria (a cause of tuberculosis and leprosy), and toxoplasma parasites (Norins 2021). Hopefully, Norins's "contagious" efforts will influence those who control the funding dollars for clinical trials to support the study of infection and Alzheimer's very soon.

Infections Outside the Brain Can Cause Confusion and Accelerate Cognitive Decline

When I began to perform hospice care in 2014, I quickly learned about a common phenomenon in older people, with or without known dementia: that an infection outside the brain can give rise to confusion and agitation, sometimes extreme (called delirium). A urinary-tract infection was the most common culprit in our patients and, once diagnosed and treated, the confusion would subside or completely resolve. I witnessed this change in mental status repeatedly in my own patients. Lopez-Rodriguez and group have learned from studying mouse and human brains that infection outside the brain can trigger delirium but can also accelerate cognitive decline. These changes are associated with signs of increased neuroinflammation as evidenced by elevated brain cytokine levels produced by brain cells called astrocytes and microglia (Lopez-Rodriguez 2021).

Vaccinations Could Prevent Dementia Related to Infection

Smallpox was a highly contagious and deadly infection with a 30 percent mortality rate that left most survivors with severe scarring and some with blindness and other serious neurological complications. Fortunately, due to intense global vaccination efforts in the mid-twentieth century, after plaguing humanity for at least 3,000 years, smallpox has been nearly eradicated from the Earth since about 1979. These days, only people who work in virology labs with smallpox receive the vaccine (WHO 2014).

Smallpox is one of many epidemic and pandemic microbes that cause inflammation of the brain, called meningitis (when the protective membranes around the brain are involved), or encephalitis (when brain tissue is involved). The inflammation is called encephalomyelitis when the spinal cord is affected, causing loss of the protective myelin around nerves. Brain and/or nerve inflammation can occur with the "childhood diseases" poliomyelitis, measles (rubella and rubeola), mumps, tetanus, pertussis (whooping cough), and Hemophilus influenzae, for which infants and children are immunized in the United States. Brain inflammation can also occur with AIDS, flu, yellow fever, malaria, dengue fever, bubonic plague, cholera, zika, Japanese encephalitis, West Nile virus, and the coronaviruses, including SARS CoV-1, MERS-CoV, and SARS CoV-2, the virus that causes COVID-19, our most recent pandemic

(Valerio 2020). Diphtheria does not affect the brain directly but causes damage to nerves outside the brain in 20 percent of cases, leading to peripheral neuropathy (pain and numbness in the hands and feet). Seizures are a common complication of fever and brain inflammation related to infection, especially in young children.

Some people worry about possible long-term effects of vaccination due to brain inflammation, but this is a very rare complication, occurring in less than one per million for the measles-mumps-rubella vaccine and zero to ten per million for the diphtheria-pertussis-tetanus vaccine, for example (CDC 1996).

Viruses can only survive and multiply if they find their way into living cells. These microbes invade cells in mucus membranes, which are the moist surfaces of our mouth, nose, nasopharynx (the cavities behind our nose that connect with the mouth), eyes, and gastrointestinal tract. Viruses can find their way into our brains by way of the cranial nerves that have their roots in the brain. These include, notably, the ophthalmic nerves that provide us with vision, olfactory nerves that give us our sense of smell, and the trigeminal, glossopharyngeal, and facial nerves that control various senses like taste, and facial, throat, and tongue movement. About 30 percent of people with the COVID-19 infection have reported loss of smell and taste as early symptoms, but these can become very long-lasting symptoms. Many have reported a sensation of "rotten meat" or other obnoxious smell or taste during the recovery period months later. Microbes can also enter the brain from blood by way of the endothelial cells lining blood vessels.

People can continue to harbor certain viruses in the brain or other organs after seeming to fully recover from an infection. For example, varicella, the virus that causes chicken pox, can become dormant in nerves, and can cause shingles decades later nearly anywhere on the body in the pathway of a nerve. The vagus (or vagal) nerve is the longest of the cranial nerves, traveling from the brain throughout the mouth, throat, esophagus, and stomach, then throughout the rest of the gastrointestinal tract to the anus. Markus Glatzel and his group in Germany have found at least one sign of brain inflammation in 86 percent of

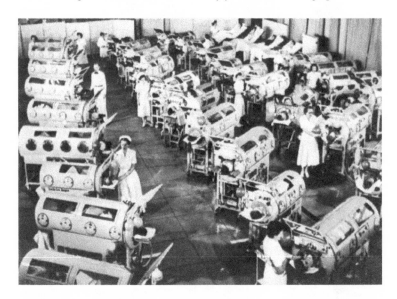

PHOTO 2. A polio ward with people in iron lungs from the 1950s. The people who were paralyzed from polio infection required iron lungs to breathe. Many did not survive (republished in numerous newspapers).

brains they studied of people who died from COVID-19 and the actual SARS CoV-2 in 53 percent of the brains (Matschke 2020). Dr. Glatzel communicated to me that they have also found RNA of the virus in the vagus nerve in 40 percent of the people who died from the COVID-19 infection. They are trying to determine whether the virus persists in a dormant state in the vagus nerve by studying people who died of other causes months after having the COVID-19 infection.

Poliomyelitis is another example of a highly contagious viral infection that caused inflammation in the brain and can remain dormant in nerves, leading to unexpected decline many years later, called post-polio syndrome. My own mother, Josephine Schell Bredestege, was a victim of polio at age thirteen during an epidemic in the United States. She could not walk for nearly a year and suffered lifelong weakness in her legs, back, and diaphragm, with symptoms of post-polio syndrome, and serious decline in her forties. She made sure that my sisters and I were first in line to receive the polio vaccine as soon as it was available, and this infection is very rare in 2020. Her mother Rose and older sister Rosemary both died with Alzheimer's in

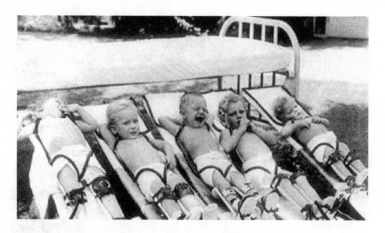

PHOTO 3. Babies with polio. Source: "How Dallas dealt polio a massive blow by vaccinating 900,000 people in two days." The Dallas Morning News, David Tarrant, July 30, 2017.

their eighties, and I have often wondered if they might have been asymptomatic carriers who harbored the virus with later consequences. Dr. Norins states that less than one-half of one percent of polio virus infections resulted in visible paralysis, and most infections were asymptomatic ("silent infections") or no worse than the common cold (see photos 2 and 3) (Norins 2018).

The Flu and Pneumonia Vaccines Could Reduce Your Risk of Dementia

A press release from the virtual Alzheimer's Association International Conference 2020 reported that the flu and pneumonia vaccines could prevent dementia. Results of three studies presented at the conference suggested that (AAIC 2020):

- "At least one flu vaccination was associated with a 17 percent reduction in Alzheimer's incidence."
- "More frequent flu vaccination was associated with another 13 percent reduction in Alzheimer's incidence."

- "Vaccination against pneumonia between ages 65 and 75 reduced Alzheimer's risk by up to 40 percent depending on individual genes."
- "Individuals with dementia have a higher risk of dying (sixfold) after infections than those without dementia (threefold)."

I suggest asking for preservative-free vaccines to avoid exposure to a mercury-containing compound called thimerosal (more on mercury shortly).

It is understandable that many people are concerned about possible long-term and serious side effects of vaccination. If you or your child are one of the unfortunate but rare people to suffer a serious adverse effect, it is devastating. However, for those who are trying to decide whether to vaccinate or not, it is a matter of weighing the much, much greater risk of poor outcome from a battle with infection, including the possibility of death or permanent damage to the brain, heart, and other organs, compared to the relatively remote chance of serious consequences from the vaccine itself.

An alternative strategy to taking flu and other vaccinations for those who are dead set against them is to take measures to prevent infection, such as avoiding people who are known to be ill and crowds where infection is likely to spread, wearing a mask in crowded situations and on public transportation, keeping a distance from others, and washing hands frequently for at least twenty seconds, or using hand sanitizer with at least 60 percent alcohol. Now that many of us are accustomed to wearing masks, I hope this will become a regular practice during flu season when we shop or cannot avoid a crowd. Between 16,000 and 60,000 people die each year from the flu in the United States, a truly astounding number of potentially preventable deaths. The CDC reported that deaths from the flu in the United States were down 98 percent for March through May 2020, compared to the previous three months through February 2020 after strict guidelines were instituted to fight COVID-19. Other countries also reported reductions in flu-related deaths (Olsen 2020).

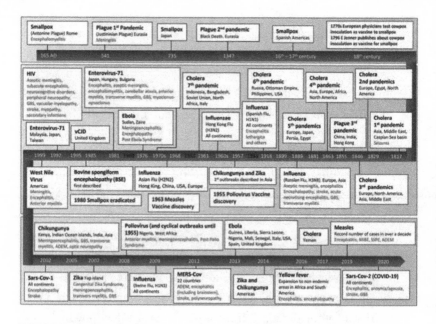

FIGURE 9.13. Timeline of important pandemics including key neurological complications. From Valerio F, DP Whitehouse, DK Menon, VFJ Newcombe. "The neurological sequelae of pandemics and epidemics." J Neurol 2020:1–27. Open access permission through Creative Commons Attribution 4.0 International License.

There is an epidemic somewhere in the world nearly every year, as well as a pandemic of flu that cycles between the lower and upper hemispheres with the seasons. Many deaths and long-term complications, such as dementia, could be prevented with vaccinations and infection-prevention strategies. The current COVID-19 pandemic is more widespread, contagious, and deadly than most. SARS CoV-2, the virus that causes COVID-19, has resulted in serious and prolonged neurological symptoms in very many people, and sometimes severe apparently permanent neurological damage. Brain hemorrhage related to COVID-19 is one of the most common causes of death, especially in people under age sixty-five. Neurological complications have been a feature of most pandemics in the past two millennia (see figure 9.13).

Given the frequency of deaths and serious complications of seasonal flu, I wonder why we have not been using the preventive measures drummed into us in 2020 all along (see figure 9.14).

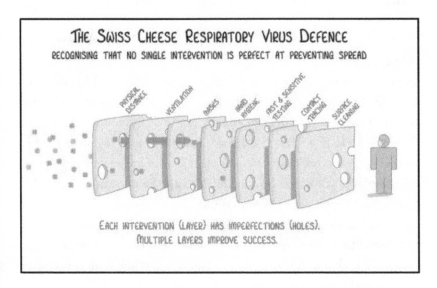

FIGURE 9.14. The Swiss Cheese Respiratory Virus Pandemic Defense. Figure created by Mackay, Ian M. "https://virologydownunder.com/the-swiss-cheese-infographic-that-went-viral. Derived from @sketchplanator based on the Swiss Cheese Model of accident causation by James T. Reason 1990. Open permission through Figshare. Figure at https://doi.org/10.6084/m9.figshare.13082618.v7.

AVOID ACTIVITIES WITH SIGNIFICANT RISK OF HEAD INJURY

More than 50 million traumatic brain injuries (TBI) occur worldwide each year (Eiden 2019). A TBI involves an insult to the head serious enough to cause loss of consciousness, confusion, or other physical or neurological impairment, which is usually temporary but can be permanent. A single episode of significant TBI increases the risk for dementia later in life and can also trigger Parkinson's and other neurodegenerative conditions. Autopsy studies report that a single TBI can cause amyloid plaque formation, and repeated injuries can lead to tangle formation. Abnormal proteins found in neurodegenerative diseases like Lewy body dementia, frontotemporal lobe dementia, Pick's disease, ALS, and Parkinson's disease, can also show up in the brain following

TBI. A mixture of such protein abnormalities is called polypathology (Washington 2016).

Forensic pathologist Bennet Omalu, MD, first described chronic traumatic encephalopathy (CTE) after performing an autopsy on famous fifty-year-old NFL football player Mike Webster in 2002. Omalu found neurofibrillary tangles (discussed in chapter 10) like those present in Alzheimer's but in a different distribution. Over the next few years, he found identical brain lesions in other football players, including twenty such lesions in a twenty-year-old college player who died by suicide. Not all the players suffered unconsciousness with their concussions, but "subconcussive" injuries are common in contact sports like football. The symptoms of CTE and dementia are similar and can include confusion, memory loss, personality changes, depression, erratic behavior, and sometimes balance and coordination issues.

Several large studies of armed-services veterans have reported that skull fractures and intracranial injuries (within the brain) led to three to six times greater risk of frontotemporal lobe dementia within the next four years, compared to uninjured age-matched controls (Washington 2016). There was greater risk with increasing age.

Apparently, helmets do not adequately protect football players from CTE related to traumatic brain injuries. Dr. Omalu's research presents a dilemma for parents of teenagers who want to play football or other sports like boxing with a high risk of head injuries. Clearly, engaging in contact sports is a choice, and there are many other options.

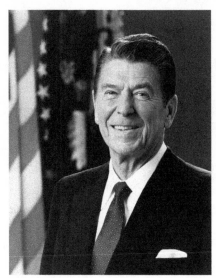

PHOTO 4. President Ronald Reagan. Months after leaving the White House in 1989, President Ronald Reagan required surgery for a subdural hematoma (blood clot on the brain) due to a head injury from falling off a bucking horse two months earlier. Some years later, his son Ron stated, looking back, that Reagan may have had early signs of cognitive impairment during his final years in office, but his cognition clearly deteriorated after the brain injury. Reagan was formally diagnosed with Alzheimer's just five years later in 1994, and died in 2004 at age ninety-three.

Ketones Could Help with Recovery from a Traumatic Brain Injury

When there is an injury to the brain, the cells in the affected area rapidly take up glucose, but the glucose transporters (GLUTs) become depleted and take several days to regenerate, depriving injured tissues of glucose. Swelling, inadequate uptake of oxygen in the injured tissue, and seizures may also occur. Transport of ketones into the injured cells is not affected. So, ketones could provide alternative fuel until glucose is usable again and help repair the injury by reducing inflammation and stimulating multiplication of mitochondria. Ketogenic diets and supplements can provide nutritional support for athletes and could aid recovery from TBI.

Two studies were conducted in Switzerland of thirty-eight people with severe TBIs requiring ICU care. Cerebral microdialysis-monitoring of intracranial pressure (pressure within the skull) allowed frequent collection of cerebrospinal fluid samples, which were analyzed using a process called metabolomics. The patients progressed through two phases with distinctly different metabolite patterns. One pattern had higher levels of glucose and other substances related to glucose and glutamate metabolism, whereas another pattern contained higher levels of certain compounds related to ketone metabolism. The duration of each phase varied substantially between individuals, with the early phase lasting for hours to several days, and the later pattern sometimes lasting for numerous days. Blood betahydroxybutyrate (BHB) levels correlated with brain BHB levels. Eiden and others concluded that ketogenic therapies could potentially help in recovery from TBI by boosting blood BHB levels (Eiden 2019).

A ketogenic formula devised by European researchers showed good results in mice with TBIs. The formulation has a 2:1 ratio of grams of fat to grams of protein plus carbohydrate; it contains coconut oil, palm oil, medium-chain triglyceride oil, tuna oil for DHA (an omega-3 fatty acid), rapeseed oil, low glycemic index carbohydrate, fiber, vitamins, minerals, and proteins, including the ketogenic amino acid leucine. Compared to the non-ketogenic low-fat control diet, the ketogenic formula markedly increased blood BHB levels, significantly reduced sensorimotor impairment, corrected defects in spatial memory, reduced the size of the injury and swelling, and increased proliferation of cells around the injury site. The formula also reduced the loss of oligodendrocytes involved in myelin formation (protection around nerve fibers). There was less evidence of oxidative damage, and there were increased markers of enhanced anti-epileptic pathways (Thau-Zuchman 2021). Hyperglycemia (high blood sugar) after a TBI correlates with poorer outcomes. Ketogenic intravenous fluids and oral formulas could be used to control blood-glucose levels as part of the treatment process. The next step is to test this ketogenic formula in humans with TBI.

REDUCE EXPOSURE TO AIR POLLUTION, IF POSSIBLE

Exposure to indoor and outdoor air pollution is the fourth leading risk factor for death (4.9 million) worldwide behind high blood pressure, smoking, and high blood sugar (Our World in Data 2017). Outdoor air pollution includes inhalation of particulate matter and metals from motor vehicles, industrial exhaust (iron-rich and magnetite nanoparticles, black carbon), and ozone, a toxic gas from electrical discharges and ultraviolet light that causes oxidative damage. Indoor pollution includes cigarette smoke, and toxic fumes in factories, laboratories, maintenance shops, and other workplace settings. Chronic exposure to outdoor and indoor pollution is associated with higher rates of cognitive deficits, dementia in general, Alzheimer's, and accelerated cognitive decline. Air pollution can provoke inflammation and an exaggerated immune response in the brain (and other organs), as well as metabolic and structural changes in brain white and gray matter (Calderón-Garcidueñas 2017; Delgado-Saborit 2021).

Control of outdoor pollution mainly requires governmental interventions and regulations, whereas some types of indoor air pollution, such as tobacco smoke, can be completely avoided. Your job may dictate that you live and/or work in a polluted environment, but, if you have a choice, it is much better for your long-term health to live and work in a location with clean air. If you have a job that subjects you to toxic air, such as welding or spraying pesticides, and you have no other choice, it is important to follow government and employer regulations to protect yourself, such as wearing eye protection and a respiratory protective device.

AVOID EXCESSIVE INTAKE OF IRON AND OTHER HEAVY METALS

Humans have a small dietary requirement for certain metals, such as iron, copper, and zinc, that are needed for normal function of numerous enzymes and more than 300 proteins. However, there is a fine line between getting the necessary amount of a metal and getting too much, which could lead to neurological damage. Other non-essential metals like mercury, aluminum, and cadmium can accumulate in and damage the brain and other organs. A U.S. public health statement (ATSDR 2008) declared that "the effects of exposure to any hazardous substance depend on the dose, the duration, how you are exposed, personal traits and habits, and whether other chemicals are present."

Industrialization and technological advances have greatly increased our potential exposure to toxic levels of essential and non-essential metals in our air, water, soil, and food supplies. In NIH studies, cumulative exposure to mixtures of heavy metals (such as industrial exposure or air pollution) were associated with greater risk of obesity and related conditions such as high blood pressure and diabetes, which are then risk factors for Alzheimer's and other dementias (Wang 2018).

In this era of food fortification and supplementation with vitamins, minerals, and other micronutrients, we can get too much of a good thing in our quest for good health and longevity. For example, true zinc deficiency is rare because it's easy to meet 100 percent of the recommended daily allowance with diet. If you routinely take a multivitamin with zinc, a supplement for "bone health" with zinc, and a nutritional shake with zinc, you might accumulate too much zinc. Excess zinc intake can cause diarrhea, abdominal cramps, and vomiting, and longer-term problems like copper or iron deficiency. While the RDA of zinc is 8 mg per day for women and 11 mg per day for men, the Upper Tolerable Limit is just 40 mg.

Essential metals like zinc, iron (including elemental iron), copper (including elemental copper), calcium carbonate, and other forms of calcium have been found within beta amyloid plaques and tau tangles (Lipinski 2013; Everett 2021). Iron and copper have also been found in alpha-synuclein deposits in Lewy body and Parkinson's disease (Lermyte 2019). Various bacteria, fungi, and plants produce minute clusters of metals, including elemental iron and elemental copper, which impart resistance to metal toxicity. Since bacteria, fungi, and other organisms are found within beta amyloid plaques, it is possible that elemental iron and copper arrive in the beta amyloid core in microbes (Everett 2021).

Non-essential metals, like aluminum, lead, cadmium, and mercury also appear to play a role in formation of beta amyloid plaques and tau tangles, and may promote inflammation in the brain (Wallin 2019; Huat 2019). It is still uncertain whether the metals discussed in this section cause, trigger, or accelerate Alzheimer's, or whether their presence in plaques and tangles is merely a downstream effect of the Alzheimer's disease process.

A LITTLE IRON IS NECESSARY, BUT TOO MUCH IRON CAN BE HARMFUL

Inhaling iron particles and consuming excessive iron are dangerous to our health. Iron tends to oxidize (think of rust on a wrought-iron gate), giving rise to oxygen-free radicals. In Alzheimer's disease, iron-induced free radicals generate fibers that do not easily dissolve. Such fibers can irreversibly trap red blood cells and obstruct oxygen delivery to the brain.

Maintaining normal iron stores requires just 1 mg daily for men and older women, and 1.5 mg for menstruating women. Many iron-rich foods are staples of a healthy Mediterranean-style diet. Animal foods contain a form of iron that is well-absorbed, whereas only 10 percent of the plant form of iron is absorbed (see table 9.2). To overcome poor absorption, the recommended daily intakes of iron are:

- Adult men and postmenopausal women: 8 mg/day, ideally in food.
- Menstruating women: 18 mg/day, ideally in food.
- Upper Tolerable Limit: 49 mg/day

The IOM recommends that men and postmenopausal women not take iron supplements or highly fortified foods, unless they have a diagnosis of iron-deficiency anemia, to avoid iron overload, which can damage the central nervous system, cardiovascular system, kidneys, liver, and blood.

Older people will remember hearing commercials for Geritol, a "cure for iron-poor blood" that claimed to provide twice as much iron as a pound of calf liver. Some Geritol products contained 50 to 100 mg of iron per serving and 12 percent alcohol. Remember I Love Lucy and the hilarious Vita-Meata-Vegamen commercial? Geritol left the market around 1979 after receiving heavy government fines for false claims.

Magnesium could undo some of the damage from excess iron by dissolving the fibers that trap red blood cells. Many people are deficient in magnesium, and vegetables are a good source of a natural, bioavailable form of magnesium (discussed in chapter 6). Polyphenols found in

IRON CONTENT

RDA*: Women: Menstruating -18 mg | Postmenopausal – 8 mg | Men - 8 mg
Upper Tolerable Limit – 49 mg | Supplement only if iron deficient

Food	Milligrams (mg)	% RDA
Breakfast cereals, fortified at 100% RDA, 1 serving	18	100
Oysters, eastern, cooked with moist heat, 3 oz	8	44
White beans, canned, 1 cup	8	44
Chocolate, dark, 45%-69%, cacao solids, 3 oz	7	39
Beef liver, pan fried, 3 oz	5	28
Lentils, boiled and drained, ½ cup	3	17
Spinach, boiled and drained, ½ cup	3	17
Tofu, firm, ½ cup	3	17
Kidney beans, canned, ½ cup	2	11
Sardines, Atlantic, in oil, drained, with bone, 3 oz	2	11
Chickpeas, boiled and drained, ½ cup	2	11
Tomatoes, canned, stewed, ½ cup	2	11
Beef, braised bottom round, trimmed to 1/8" fat, 3 oz	2	11
Potato, baked, flesh and skin, 1 med potato	2	11
Cashew nuts, oil roasted, 1 oz (18 nuts)	2	11
Green peas, boiled, ½ cup	1	6
Chicken, roasted, meat and skin, 3 oz	1	6
Rice, white, long grain, enriched, ½ cup	1	6
Bread, whole wheat, 1 slice	1	6

*Recommended Daily Allowance from Dietary Reference Intakes, Institute of Medicine, 2006
Source: Iron - Health Professional Fact Sheet https://ods.od.nih.gov/factsheets/Iron-HealthProfessional

TABLE 9.2. Iron Content of Selected Foods. Source: Iron - Health Professional Fact Sheet https://ods.od.nih.gov/factsheets/Iron-HealthProfessional. Adapted by Joanna Newport.

fruits, vegetables, dark chocolate, teas, coconut oil, olive oil, herbs, and spices could also undo some of the damage from excessive iron. Magnesium and polyphenols are two more good reasons to eat a whole-food Mediterranean-style diet.

COPPER

Copper, in the cuprous Cu+ form, is a metal found in solid foods. We need a tiny amount for normal brain function, bone growth, immune function, normal use of iron, and energy metabolism. However, excessive copper can accumulate, for example from drinking tap water delivered through old copper pipes, from foods sprayed with copper to inhibit bacterial growth, and from air pollution. Environmental copper can come in the more oxidized cupric Cu2+ form, which is neurotoxic and not useful in our metabolism. Copper must be transported into the brain, distributed correctly, and removed normally to carry out its

COPPER CONTENT

RDA*: 900 micrograms (adults) | Upper Tolerable Limit: 10,000 micrograms

Food	Micrograms (mcg)	% RDA
Beef, liver, pan fried, 3 oz	12,400	1,378
Oysters, eastern, wild, cooked, 3 oz	4,850	539
Baking chocolate, unsweetened, 1 oz	938	104
Potatoes, cooked, flesh and skin, 1 med potato	675	75
Mushrooms, shitake, cooked, cut pieces, ½ cup	650	72
Cashew nuts, dry roasted, 1 oz	629	70
Crab, dungeness, cooked, 3 oz	624	69
Sunflower seed kernels, toasted, ¼ cup	615	68
Turkey, giblets, simmered, 3 oz	588	65
Chocolate, dark, 70-85% cacao solids, 1 oz	501	56
Tofu, raw, firm, ½ cup	476	53
Chickpeas, mature seeds, ½ cup	289	32
Millet, cooked, 1 cup	280	31
Salmon, Atlantic, wild, cooked, 3 oz	273	30
Pasta, whole wheat, cooked, 1 cup (not packed)	263	29
Avocado, raw, ½ cup	219	24
Figs, dried, ½ cup	214	24
Spinach, boiled, drained, ½ cup	157	17
Asparagus, cooked, drained, ½ cup	149	17
Sesame seeds, ¼ cup	147	16
Turkey, ground, cooked, 3 oz	128	14
Cream of Wheat, cooked in water, 1 cup	104	12
Tomatoes, raw, chopped, ½ cup	53	6
Yogurt, Greek, plain, lowfat, 7-oz container	42	5
Milk, nonfat, 1 cup	27	3
Apples, raw, with skin, ½ cup slices	17	2

* Recommended Daily Allowance from Dietary Reference Intakes, Institute of Medicine, 2006. Source: Copper - Health Professional Fact Sheet. https://ods.od.nih.gov/factsheets/Copper-HealthProfessional.

TABLE 9.3. Copper Content of Selected Foods. Source: Copper - Health Professional Fact Sheet. https://ods.od.nih.gov/factsheets/Copper-HealthProfessional. Adapted by Joanna Newport.

functions, but the wrong form of copper in excess can disrupt these normal processes.

Wilson's disease is a genetic mutation in which excessive copper accumulation causes cognitive decline, along with other neurological and neuropsychiatric impairments. The genetic mutation found in Wilson's disease also confers a higher risk of Alzheimer's disease. Copper appears to be involved in the formation of the hallmark beta amyloid plaques. High "free" copper levels in the blood correlate with poorer cognitive function and indicate a greater risk of progression from mild cognitive impairment to Alzheimer's (Hsu 2018; Lermyte 2019).

The use of metal chelation (clioquinol) to remove excess copper from the brain reduced beta amyloid plaques in mice but, unfortunately, did not improve cognition in human clinical trials. Removal of copper through detoxification is thought to interfere with the normal distribution of copper in the brain (Hsu 2018). On the other hand, copper levels are abnormally low in the brains of some people with Alzheimer's, making the case for needing to find a happy medium between taking enough, but not too much, copper.

The recommended daily allowance for copper is 900 micrograms per day (less than 1 mg) for adults. See table 9.3 for the copper content of common foods.

ZINC

Zinc is most concentrated in the brain and is present in 70 percent of brain proteins, either as a structural or catalytic component. Zinc is also involved in the function of more than 300 enzymes and 2,000 transcription factors (proteins that turn genes on and off), in immune function, wound healing, regulation of certain other metals, neurotransmission (communication between brain cells), repair and remodeling of the brain, cognitive function, and much, much more. A certain amount of zinc is critical to the human brain and to normal phosphorylation of tau (explained in chapter 10), but excessive levels in the brain appear

ZINC CONTENT

RDA*: Women 8 mg | Men 11 mg | Upper Tolerable Limit - 40 mg

Food	Milligrams(mg)	% RDA
Oysters, cooked, breaded and fried, 3 oz	74.0	673
Beef chuck roast, braised, 3 oz	7.0	64
Crab, Alaska king, cooked, 3 oz	6.5	59
Beef patty, broiled, 3 oz	5.3	48
Lobster, cooked, 3 oz	3.4	31
Pork chop, loin, cooked, 3 oz	2.9	26
Baked beans, canned, plain or vegetarian, ½ cup	2.9	26
Breakfast cereal, fortified at 25% RDA, 1 serving	2.8	25
Chicken, dark meat, cooked, 3 oz	2.4	22
Pumpkin seeds, dried, 1 oz	2.2	20
Yogurt, fruit, low fat, 8 oz	1.7	15
Cashews, dry roasted, 1 oz	1.6	15
Chickpeas, cooked, ½ cup	1.3	12
Cheese, Swiss, 1 oz	1.2	11
Oatmeal, instant, plain, cooked in water, 1 packet	1.1	10
Milk, low-fat or non fat, 1 cup	1.0	9
Almonds, dry roasted, 1 oz	0.9	8
Kidney beans, cooked, ½ cup	0.9	8
Chicken breast, roasted, skinless, ½ breast	0.9	8
Cheese, cheddar or mozarella, 1 oz	0.9	8
Peas, green, frozen, cooked, ½ cup	0.5	5
Flounder or sole, cooked, 3 oz	0.3	3

*Recommended Daily Allowance from Dietary Reference Intakes, Institute of Medicine, 2006
Source: Zinc - Health Professional Fact Sheet https://ods.od.nih.gov/factsheets/Zinc-HealthProfessional.

TABLE 9.4. Zinc Content of Selected Foods. Source: Zinc - Health Professional Fact Sheet https://ods.od.nih.gov/factsheets/Zinc-HealthProfessional. Adapted by Joanna Newport.

to promote formation of beta amyloid plaques and neurofibrillary tau tangles, inflammation, and oxidative stress (damage to mitochondria). Zinc has been found within beta amyloid plaques and bound to tau tangles. Abnormally high and low zinc levels have been reported in the brains of people who died with Alzheimer's. Removal of zinc through chelation can deplete the brain of zinc with detrimental consequences. Though we need zinc to regulate the senses of smell and taste, using nasal sprays and gels containing zinc can cause loss of the sense of smell (Huat 2019; Wojtunik-Kulesza 2019).

As mentioned at the opening of this section on metals, while the RDA of zinc is 8 mg per day for women and 11 mg per day for men, the Upper Tolerable Limit is just 40 mg. So, taking too many supplements and foods fortified with zinc is not a good idea for brain health. Zinc deficiency is rare, but zinc levels can be low in people who consume excess alcohol due to poor absorption, in which case, taking more zinc would be warranted. Like iron and copper, the best way to get the right amount of zinc is by eating a healthy Mediterranean-style diet, which contains foods to deliver enough zinc. The zinc content of common foods is found in table 9.4.

CALCIUM AND CALCIUM CARBONATE

Calcium is a perfect example of a nutrient that is better to acquire in its natural forms from food than from supplements. Calcium is the most abundant mineral (also called a metal) in the human body and is vital to many biological processes throughout the body and brain. Adult human bodies contain roughly two pounds (one kilogram) of calcium. About 99 percent of calcium in humans and animals is stored in bone and teeth, where it is found mostly as calcium phosphates in a complex called hydroxyapatite, which is interspersed in collagen. The other 1 percent of calcium, mainly as free ionized calcium, is involved in critical functions such as contraction of the heart, blood vessels, and muscles, communication between neurons, signaling between cells, and hormone secretion.

Are calcium supplements a good idea for the average person? Perhaps not, in my opinion, unless you are at risk for bone fractures or osteoporosis and cannot get enough calcium from food, for example, due to severe lactose intolerance. Using calcium carbonate is a cheap and easy way to make calcium into a pill and to fortify foods. However, calcium carbonate is a major component of the core of beta amyloid plaques in the brains of people with Alzheimer's, along with other forms of calcium not yet identified with certainty. My concern is how calcium carbonate found its way into these plaques since it is not one of the natural forms of calcium commonly found in the human body or in animal flesh. The study authors did not speculate (Everett 2018). I personally quit using antacids and supplements with calcium carbonate after reading this study.

Also, several large studies in women testing the effect of calcium supplements, with and without vitamin D, on reduction of fractures, consistently reported a greater risk of heart attacks (26 to 31 percent) and strokes (19 to 20 percent) in women taking the supplements compared to controls who did not. By the same token, numerous studies have reported no increased risk of heart attack or stroke for women at any level of calcium intake from food (Bolland 2013). For this reason, experts from the Johns Hopkins School of Medicine recommend that we meet our calcium requirement directly from foods that are rich in calcium, rather than from calcium supplements, or calcium-fortified foods (Heravi 2019).

Calcium carbonate is mostly found in rocks, limestone, sediment in the sea (due to its presence in the shells of sea creatures), and in eggshells, none of which humans normally eat, except in supplements or fortified foods. Calcium carbonate may appear in tiny quantities in plant-based foods due to absorption from the soil. I have not been able to find information on whether calcium carbonate is absorbed as such from the intestine into the bloodstream, and if it crosses the blood–brain barrier.

Absorption of calcium from the gut into the bloodstream from a food or supplement is complicated. The amount absorbed depends on what form the calcium takes, whether it is eaten with food, what specific foods it is eaten with, the pH in the gut, and the vitamin D status of the individual, since factors related to Vitamin D are required for transport of calcium from the intestine into the bloodstream. Consuming dairy is the most efficient way to get calcium from food. In milk, calcium phosphate is bound to casein protein along with magnesium, zinc, and citrate in a sort of gel (called colloid), and the lactose found in milk also promotes calcium absorption. Milk products that are especially high in calcium include milk itself, ricotta cheese, yogurt, cottage cheese, mozzarella, and hard cheeses. For people who are lactose-intolerant, Lactaid® milk, dairy products, and tablets (Lactaid® and generic brands) contain the deficient lactase enzyme. Calcium in animal flesh is also bound to proteins and is relatively well-absorbed. Salmon and sardines are moderately high in calcium, whereas beef, pork, and chicken contain much less.

Vegetables and nuts contain calcium mainly as calcium hydroxide, calcium chloride, calcium sulfate, calcium carbonate, and calcium oxalate (the latter two forms are often present in kidney stones and gallstones). Some plant foods that are relatively rich in absorbable calcium include kale, mustard greens, collard greens, turnip greens, Chinese cabbage (napa cabbage), bok-choy, broccoli, cashews, walnuts, and peanuts. Some plant-based foods are high in phytates and oxalates that can bind to calcium and interfere with absorption (see side box). Calcium can form soaps with certain fatty acids during digestion and simply pass out in the stool rather than being absorbed into the bloodstream (Bronner 1999).

Oxalates and Phytates in Certain Vegetables Decrease Calcium Absorption

Many plants contain oxalates and phytates that significantly reduce calcium absorption, including spinach, beets, navy beans, soybeans, raspberries, and dates. These foods contain other important nutrients but should not be relied on for adequate calcium intake.

Raw and dried soybeans and certain other types of beans, nuts (especially Brazil nuts and almonds), seeds, and grains can contain high levels of phytates that interfere with calcium absorption. Soaking raw or dried beans, nuts (removed from the shell), and seeds in pure water removes much of the phytates and makes calcium and certain other nutrients, such as iron, more available. The amount of soaking time for maximum benefit varies from a few hours to twenty-four hours, after which the water should be drained off and discarded. Nuts and seeds are usually dehydrated after soaking for better taste and texture. Soaking beans has the added benefit of removing much of the liposaccharides that cause gas and tends to soften the beans, which may be more appealing. For more information on how and how long to soak and dehydrate beans and nuts, see the online article "Soaking Nuts & Seeds" (Soaking Nuts and Seeds 2022).

If a food is fortified with calcium, try to find out what form it takes. Cereals, breads, corn flour, wheat flour, ready-to-drink soy, coconut, almond, and other nut milks are often fortified with calcium, usually calcium carbonate. Consuming soybeans soaked before cooking would be a much better choice to meet your calcium requirement than soy milk fortified with calcium carbonate.

Excessive calcium supplementation runs the risk of calcifying non-bone tissues such as the kidneys, causing kidney stones and renal insufficiency, and can impede absorption of other important minerals. A mid-forties male friend found himself in the ICU in kidney failure due to very high blood calcium levels because of his habit of popping chewable calcium carbonate antacids throughout the day for heartburn. Values for daily recommended intake (DRI) are based on the consideration that not all the calcium in a food or supplement will be absorbed from the gut. For adults ages nineteen to fifty, the DRI for calcium is 1,000 mg, and 1,200 mg for over age fifty. The Upper Tolerable Limit is set at 2,500 mg, and chewable antacids typically contain 1,000 mg per tablet. So, it is easy to exceed 2,500 mg with calcium supplementation.

If you have true calcium deficiency, eat more calcium-rich foods, and take the smallest amount necessary of a natural form of calcium supplement, such as calcium citrate or calcium from hydroxyapatite, the form found in bone and teeth. Please see table 9.5 for calcium content of common foods.

CALCIUM CONTENT

RDA*: Adults ages 19 to 50 - 1000 mg | Adults ages >50 - 1200 mg
Upper Tolerable Limit - 2500 mg

Food	Milligrams (mg)	% RDA
Yogurt, plain, low fat, 8 oz	415	32
Mozzarella, part skim, 1.5 oz	333	26
Sardines, canned in oil, with bones, 3 oz	325	25
Cheddar cheese, 1.5 oz	307	24
Soymilk, calcium fortified, 1 cup	299	23
Milk, reduced fat (2% milk fat), 1 cup	293	23
Milk, buttermilk, lowfat, 1 cup	284	22
Milk, whole (3.25% milk fat), 1 cup	276	21
Tofu, firm, made with calcium sulfate, ½ cup	253	19
Salmon, pink, canned, solids with bone, 3 oz	181	14
Cottage cheese, 1% milk fat, 1 cup	138	11
Tofu, soft, made with calcium sulfate, ½ cup	138	11
Frozen yogurt, vanilla, soft serve, ½ cup	103	8
Turnip greens, fresh, boiled, ½ cup	99	8
Kale, fresh, cooked, 1 cup	94	7
Ice cream, vanilla, ½ cup	84	6
Chia seeds, 1 tbsp	76	6
Chinese cabbage (bok choi), raw, shredded, 1 cup	74	6
Bread, white, 1 slice	73	6
Tortilla, corn, one, 6" diameter	46	4
Tortilla, flour, one, 6" diameter	32	2
Bread, whole-wheat, 1 slice	30	2
Kale, raw, chopped, 1 cup	24	2
Broccoli, raw, ½ cup	21	2

*Recommended Daily Allowance from Dietary Reference Intakes, Institute of Medicine, 2006
Source: Calcium - Health Professional Fact Sheet https://ods.od.nih.gov/factsheets/
Calcium-HealthProfessional.

TABLE 9.5. Calcium Content of Selected Foods. Source: Calcium - Health Professional Fact Sheet https://ods.od.nih.gov/factsheets/Calcium-HealthProfessional. Adapted by Joanna Newport.

MERCURY

Do you remember playing with little balls of mercury that came out of a broken thermometer or fluorescent bulb? Did your parent spread mercurochrome on every scrape? Do you have silver dental fillings that contain mercury? Have you ever eaten lots of canned tuna when you were trying to lose weight? Unfortunately, many older people, myself included, can check off all these boxes.

Remember the Mad Hatter in Alice in Wonderland? Hat-making in the 18th and 19th centuries often used mercury-based compounds in the production of felt hats, and the common occurrence of dementia in hatters is linked to mercury poisoning. People with dementia symptoms were sometimes called "mad as a hatter" in that era.

An estimated 9,000 metric tons of mercury is released annually into the air, water, and land. Environmental and occupational exposures can occur from mercury mining, from decorative gilding with a gold-mercury amalgam, production of non-iron metals, seed and pesticide packaging, cement production, coal combustion, and from use of certain types of laboratory equipment. Release of mercury into the air can occur with cremation of people with mercury in dental fillings, accounting for about 1 percent of mercury emissions (Making Mercury History 2017). In the past, mercury was used as an ineffective treatment for medical conditions like syphilis and to promote "health" and "longevity." Large population exposures have occurred from consumption of seafood exposed to massive dumps of industrial waste containing mercury compounds. Mercury is sometimes used in cosmetics and skin-whitening products and can be absorbed directly into the bloodstream from the skin. Wastewater containing mercury from dental offices has been implicated as a source of mercury in public sewer systems.

A mercury-containing compound called thimerosal is a preservative that was commonly used in childhood and adult vaccines in the United States and Europe (and likely many other localities) until its use in vaccines was phased out around 1999, though it is still allowed in some influenza vaccines. For this reason, I always request a preservative-free flu vaccine, which most pharmacies can acquire. Thimerosal has also been used as a preservative in medications and contact lens-cleaning solutions.

Whether thimerosal in childhood vaccines might have caused cases of autism is a source of controversy. Considering the number of vaccines infants and young children receive, and that the rate of autism has been steadily increasing, it is understandable that parents would worry about mercury in vaccines. The official word from the Institute of Medicine (IOM) is that no research evidence supports the idea that vaccines cause autism, and the IOM points to the unabated increase in the rate of autism since thimerosal was removed from vaccines.

Another contentious question is whether exposure to mercury may cause or contribute to Alzheimer's disease. Studies over several decades have demonstrated the presence of mercury in beta amyloid plaques, while others have failed to confirm this. Measurement of mercury in brain tissue is particularly difficult. A lab study using two different techniques showed that mercury appeared to inhibit rather than promote the formation of beta amyloid plaques, but this has not been confirmed in living humans or in human brain tissue (Wallin 2019). This information is certainly not reason to stop worrying about mercury exposure, as other unknown harmful effects of mercury could be involved in the dementia process.

Inhalation of mercury and accumulation of mercury in the body and brain can cause neurological and other symptoms, including memory/cognitive impairment, paranoia, irritability, headaches, tremors, muscle twitching, wide emotional swings, loss of sensation in hands, and general weakness. Heavy or prolonged exposure to mercury can be irreversible and fatal. Currently, the FDA has only approved use of chelation to remove mercury following acute inorganic mercury poisoning and with just one chelation agent called DMSA (2,3-dimercapto-1-propanesulfonic acid). Some chelation agents remove other unintended metals like calcium, leading to symptoms of acute deficiency. So if you are considering chelation to remove mercury or other heavy metal, research the provider and the treatment carefully.

Similarly, many have considered whether dental amalgams containing mercury should be removed and replaced. Studies have detected release of mercury vapor from dental fillings after 30 minutes of chewing, especially when chewing nicotine gum. However, drilling out the amalgams releases much more mercury vapor than prolonged chewing (Lorscheider 1995), and the total amount released may depend on how many mercury fillings an individual has. So, the risk of mercury exposure may far outweigh the benefits of having fillings removed. If you are

Best Choices - LOWEST MERCURY LEVELS			
Anchovy	Flounder	Perch, freshwater and ocean	Skate
Atlantic croaker	Haddock	Pickerel	Smelt
Atlantic mackerel	Hake	Plaice	Sole
Black sea bass	Herring	Pollock	Squid
Butterfish	Lobster, American and spiny	Salmon	Tilapia
Catfish	Mullet	Sardine	Trout, freshwater
Clam	Oyster	Scallop	Tuna, canned light (includes skipjack)
Cod	Pacific chub mackerel	Shad	Whitefish
Crab		Shrimp	Whiting
Crawfish			

Good Choices to Eat			
Bluefish	Halibut	Snapper	Tuna, yellowfin
Buffalofish	Mahi mahi/dolphinfish	Spanish mackerel	Weakfish/seatrout
Carp	Monkfish	Striped bass (ocean)	White croaker/ Pacific croaker
Chilean sea bass/ Patagonian toothfish	Rockfish	Tilefish (Atlantic)	
Grouper	Sablefish	Tuna, Albacore/ white tuna, canned and fresh/frozen	
	Sheepshead		

Choices to Avoid - HIGHEST MERCURY LEVELS			
King Mackerel	Orange roughy	Swordfish	Tuna, bigeye
Marlin	Shark	Tilefish (Gulf of Mexico)	

Source: FDA: Advice About Eating Fish, October 2021. https://www.fda.gov/media/102331/download

FIGURE 9.15. Advice about Eating Fish. Eat fish with the lowest mercury levels. Source: "Advice About Eating Fish": https://www.fda.gov/media/102331/download. Adapted by Joanna Newport.

determined to replace your fillings, do your homework to find a dentist with extensive experience. During removal of fillings, it is important that the dentist have you wear a breathing apparatus to reduce inhalation of mercury vapor, position a rubber dam around the tooth to prevent contact of the material with oral tissues, and use a high-volume aspirator to remove the material quickly to avoid absorption into the bloodstream.

Humans don't need to consume mercury in any quantity. There are many reports of mercury poisoning in infants through adults from exposures to mercury vapors and other mercury compounds. The use of mercury in industrial applications is heavily regulated by government agencies.

Industrial air pollution and wastewater have contaminated the oceans, and consuming seafood is another potential source of mercury exposure. Fish and other sea creatures eat bacteria and smaller sea creatures that may be contaminated with mercury. The oldest and largest fish, such as whales, sharks, and tuna, tend to have the largest concentrations of mercury. Therefore, it is better to choose fish and other types of seafood that are younger and smaller. If you like to eat canned tuna, avoid bigeye tuna, and look for tuna varieties listed as "best choices" or "good choices" in figure 9.15.

ALUMINUM

Aluminum is everywhere in our natural environment—rocks, soil, water, air—but most of the aluminum that finds its way into our bodies arrives in processed foods, foods and beverages packaged in aluminum cans, foods cooked in aluminum pots and pans, flour, baking powder, food coloring and anticaking agents, cosmetics, antiperspirants, buffered aspirin, and pharmaceuticals. Substantial amounts of aluminum are found in certain antacids—one serving could contain up to 200 mg of elemental aluminum. Aluminum quickly leaves our bodies in feces and in urine but can accumulate to high levels in people who have kidney disease (ATSDR 2008).

The average U.S. adult consumes 7 to 9 mg of aluminum per day in food and drink, which is roughly the recommended daily amount of iron. There is no human biological requirement for aluminum, but aluminum crosses the blood–brain barrier and can accumulate in the brain. Aluminum can interfere with more than 200 human biochemical reactions and can damage the brain in the process.

The idea of aluminum as a cause of Alzheimer's first came on the radar in the 1960s when rabbits treated with an aluminum compound developed Alzheimer's-like abnormalities in the brain (Zhang 2021). Many studies have demonstrated that excess aluminum in the brain can promote formation of beta amyloid plaques, promote hyperphosphorylation of tau, and promote formation of tau tangles. Even worse, the combination of aluminum and beta amyloid in plaques is more neurotoxic than beta amyloid plaques without aluminum, because it damages cell membranes and mitochondria and interferes with the normal function of calcium. Aluminum can form strong bonds with DNA, RNA, and ATP, which can affect energy metabolism and gene expression (whether genes are turned on or off), and it can cause death of neurons and glial cells (other types of brain cells). Aluminum provokes an inflammatory response when taken up by glial cells. The presence of aluminum can affect the function of many enzymes, including those involved in making neurotransmitters. A high level of aluminum in the drinking water in a population is associated with a higher rate of Alzheimer's and deaths from Alzheimer's (Huat 2020).

Working in an Aluminum Mine Can Be Hazardous to Your Brain

Zhang and group in China performed the Mini-Mental Status Exam (MMSE) and other cognitive testing on 539 men and women who worked in aluminum mines and 1,720 people who did not. Even though the aluminum miners were on average 13 years younger than the non-miners (57 years old versus 70 years old), the miners were 6.77 times more likely to have cognitive impairment. While working in an aluminum mine represents extreme exposure to aluminum, this study demonstrates the neurotoxic nature of excessive accumulation of aluminum and gives us good reason to avoid consuming it (Zhang 2021).

LEAD

During the summer between college and medical school, I had an unusual seasonal job in the lab of the U.S. Bureau of Alcohol, Tobacco, and Firearms at the John W. Peck Federal Building in downtown Cincinnati, where I worked on a forensics project with chemists. My job was to study methods that might allow matching soil samples from a boot or tire, for example, to the scene of a crime. We collected soil samples from various neighborhoods in and around Cincinnati. One method we used to find a soil "fingerprint" was to identify levels of metals in the samples using mass spectrometry. Soil samples in the inner city and surrounding traffic-congested areas were loaded with lead and iron and were nearly black compared to lighter-brown samples from the suburbs. The next summer, after my freshman year of medical school, I worked in the Baby's Milk Fund Clinic in downtown Cincinnati, and many of the patients were in a special program for children with high lead levels. These children suffered from cognitive disabilities and behavioral disturbances.

The possibility of lead toxicity has been known for thousands of years but came into focus around 1892 in Australia with the recognition that eating white lead paint on porches and rails was a serious health threat to children. A century later in Cincinnati (and many other places), children would develop lead toxicity from eating old paint, exposure to high lead levels in the air from automotive vehicle exhaust, playing in soil with high lead content, and exposure to lead in house dust. Removing lead from gasoline, banning cans with lead-soldered seams, and removal of lead-based paints have substantially reduced environmental lead exposures in the United States.

Lead can bind to red blood cells and circulate throughout the body, creating havoc in many different organs, including the brain. Lead can accumulate in bone, where it stays for decades. Lead interferes biologically with vitamin D and calcium metabolism and competes with calcium, zinc, and iron for binding sites on many molecules. Anemia related to replacement of iron with lead in heme found in red blood cells is common in children with abnormal lead levels.

Lead rapidly crosses the blood–brain barrier by substituting for calcium ions and can cause extensive damage by many different mechanisms. Lead promotes formation of beta amyloid plaques, tau tangles, inflammation, and brain-cell death. Lead can interfere with protective myelination and formation of new synapses and brain cells. Lead disrupts the normal function of neurotransmitter systems related to acetylcholine, dopamine, and gamma-Aminobutyric acid (GABA), and it inhibits N-methyl-d-aspartate (NMDA) receptors. Lead can also inactivate the important antioxidant glutathione. There is no biological requirement of lead for humans, and any amount could be harmful.

Chelation therapy, usually with dimercaptosuccinic acid (DMSA), to remove lead when there is acute lead toxicity, is used to successfully reduce lead levels in the blood, but the neurological damage from lead may be permanent. Chelation that removed lead in more than 700 patients did not result in cognitive improvement. Some of the chelating agent may stay behind in tissues, where it binds to the lead; or the agent with lead attached may find its way into other tissues. Also, chelation therapy tends to drop blood lead levels very rapidly but only temporarily. Lead then leaks back into the blood from bone, other organs, and blood compartments and redistributes, resulting in higher blood lead levels once again. Studies in rhesus monkeys exposed to lead showed that chelation did not remove lead from the brain. It would seem, then, that the best way to deal with lead is to avoid further exposure (Lowry 2010).

CADMIUM

Cadmium is a cancer-causing heavy metal that is naturally present in soil, and its presence in the environment has increased greatly due to coal and fossil fuel combustion, and the mining and refining of cadmium and other metals that it tends to associate with. Cadmium in soil can turn up in agriculturally produced foods, such as rice, grains used to make flours, root plants, and vegetables. Cadmium can enter the brain and body from chewing or smoking tobacco, which may have high concentrations of cadmium, or from inhaling second-hand tobacco smoke.

Like mercury and lead, there is no biological requirement for cadmium; but once cadmium finds its way into the body, it can become concentrated in the liver and kidneys, and it can cross the blood–brain barrier. Accumulation of cadmium can lead to high blood pressure, abnormal kidney function, loss of calcium and other minerals from bone, and neurological disease. With regard to Alzheimer's, studies have demonstrated that cadmium appears to contribute to the formation of beta amyloid plaques, promote inflammation, damage mitochondria, interfere with normal energy metabolism, and cause death of brain cells. Several studies have associated elevated blood cadmium levels with higher risk of death from Alzheimer's (Huat 2019).

The half-life (time it takes for half of a substance to leave the body) of cadmium in the body is decades, and there is no effective way to get rid of it. So, staying away from smoking and chewing tobacco and avoiding secondhand tobacco smoke are good practices to accumulate as little cadmium as possible.

Pick Your Poison Carefully: Tips to Avoid Heavy Metal Toxicities

While we may be stuck with the lead, mercury, aluminum, and cadmium we have accumulated for decades, here are some strategies to avoid further accumulation to toxic levels of some essential and non-essential metals:

- Get essential metals like iron, zinc, copper, and calcium from whole foods like organically grown vegetables and fruits.
- Eat fish and seafood for their many health benefits, but choose smaller, younger fish with low mercury levels (see figure 9.15).
- Avoid eating overly processed and highly fortified foods that may contain aluminum and excessive levels of iron, copper, calcium, and zinc.
- Avoid over-supplementation of iron, zinc, copper, and calcium (especially calcium carbonate). Take an iron supplement only if prescribed for iron deficiency anemia.
- Avoid drinking unfiltered tap water. Consider installing a reverse osmosis filtration system.
- Ask for thimerosal-free vaccines, medications, and contact lens solution to avoid mercury exposure.
- Avoid chewing gum (especially gum with nicotine) if you have dental fillings with mercury.
- Avoid using zinc nasal sprays and gels.

- Avoid chewing or smoking tobacco or inhaling tobacco smoke, to reduce cadmium exposure.
- Avoid cooking in aluminum pots and pans and avoid eating food and beverages from aluminum cans.
- Avoid taking antacids that are high in aluminum and calcium carbonate.
- Before growing food in your yard, have soil and water used for watering analyzed for lead, other heavy metals, and toxic substances, especially if you live in an area where there is exposure to motor vehicle or industrial exhaust.
- Avoid living in a polluted home or work environment, if feasible (easier said than done).
- Remove lead-based paint from your older home.
- Consider that cosmetics and skin-whitening products imported from other countries might not meet United States manufacturing standards and could contain mercury, lead, or other toxic metals.
- Research the risks, benefits, and practitioners carefully if you're considering removing dental fillings with mercury or using chelation therapy. These procedures could do more harm than good, especially in the wrong hands.

Each lifestyle change you make could add another layer of protection to your brain to enjoy healthier aging and reduce your risk of dementia. It is possible to institute all these changes with some thought and planning and little, if any, impact on your wallet.

PART **THREE**

What Happens to the Brain in Aging and Diseases Like Alzheimer's: How Ketogenic Strategies Can Help

CHAPTER TEN

WHAT GOES WRONG IN ALZHEIMER'S AND OTHER BRAIN DISEASES: HOW DIET, KETONES, MCT OIL, AND COCONUT OIL CAN HELP

"Alzheimer's isn't mysterious. It's just complicated."
—Peter Dredge, author

In 1906, Dr. Alois Alzheimer reported that the brain of a fifty-three-year-old woman, Auguste Deter, who died with the type of dementia now named for him, contained large deposits of plaques and tangles, as well as abnormal lipid deposits. What he saw in her brain was the end result of a complex process that likely unfolded over many years.

While Alzheimer's lipid deposits were largely forgotten until recently, the plaques and tangles have been the primary focus for research and drug development for decades. Numerous oral medications and vaccines have been studied in clinical trials that aim to remove beta amyloid plaques from the brain. None of these drugs have significantly improved cognition or day-to-day functioning in people with Alzheimer's, and some of them increased the inflammation and edema in the brain or even accelerated the disease.

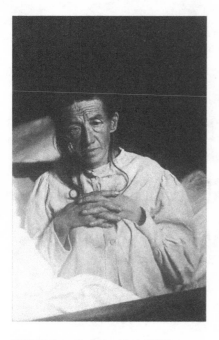

PHOTO 1. Auguste Deter (died 1906) was the first patient reported by Dr. Alois Alzheimer with the disease bearing his name. Photographer unknown, public domain.

For decades, many researchers believed that Alzheimer's has a single cause and could have a single cure that would undo the damage and might improve or even restore a person back to normal. There are very few complete cures, in the religious sense, that fully return a person to the pre-disease condition. Webster's Dictionary lists the first definition of cure as "a method or course of remedial treatment." A cardiac surgeon can prevent or treat a heart attack and buy time by inserting a stent in a blocked artery. However, the underlying heart disease is still there, and, eventually, more stents or bypass surgery might be required to buy even more time. Insulin is surely a "cure" for type 1 diabetes, since people can enjoy extra decades of life that were not possible before insulin was available. However, despite injecting insulin, the diabetes is still there, and years of inadequately controlled blood sugar can evolve into disabling complications. The right antibiotic for the right bacteria can cure pneumonia and save life, but the lung will be weaker, scarred, and more prone to infection in the future.

What I am getting at here is that there will likely never be a silver-bullet miracle cure for Alzheimer's disease. After my husband Steve was diagnosed with Alzheimer's in 2004, year after year we saw Alzheimer's Association commercials declaring that our contributions could lead to a cure within five years. We believed, if Steve could just hang in there long enough, he might be one of the first to receive "the cure," but the five-year mark came and went repeatedly.

Beta amyloid plaques are toxic and can cause damage but are not "the cause" of Alzheimer's and are more likely a downstream effect of the real cause or causes. Most pharmaceutical research is aimed at finding a single target, an enzyme-inhibitor or other substance that will interrupt the cascade of neurodegeneration that ultimately leads to death. A major problem with drugs is that the enzyme or substance targeted is likely involved in other metabolic processes, and interfering with them could lead to adverse effects in many people. Like any other drug, the benefits of a drug to treat Alzheimer's must outweigh the risks.

I want to make it clear that I am not "anti-pharma." I have no doubt that surgery and an antibiotic saved my life twenty years ago. As a neonatologist, antibiotics, and other medications like lung surfactant, saved thousands of my tiny patients. When I began to care for older patients in hospice, some were taking up to twenty-five different prescribed medications that could include three or four oral diabetes medications and two forms of insulin. Diabetic patients often did not recall receiving advice from their medical providers to cut out sugary drinks and sweets. Many people take medication to treat the adverse effects of their other medications. We call this polypharmacy or "throwing the kitchen sink" at the patient and hoping it will stick.

Drugs often fail in clinical trials because they miss the intended target and/or hit too many other targets that were unexpected before the drug was trialed in people. Pre-clinical animal research is conducted before human testing, but it is well known in the research community that "mice are not men." While there are many similarities, there are many more important dissimilarities. I have been following Alzheimer's research since 2004 and can attest that numerous new and exciting up-and-coming Alzheimer's drugs that looked so promising in animal trials failed every time in human trials—at least four hundred drugs so far.

No new Alzheimer's drugs were authorized by the FDA for fifteen years, apart from combinations of the older drugs. Then, in 2021, the drug aducanumab (Aduhelm®) was authorized through an accelerated process by the FDA which was justified on the basis that Alzheimer's is a lethal disease with no curative treatment. Three members of the FDA advisory committee resigned in protest. The initial authorization was for all people with Alzheimer's, but was scaled back to include only people with mild cognitive impairment or mild Alzheimer's. Aducanumab is an intravenous monoclonal antibody given every four weeks at an estimated cost of more than $37,000 per year and, like so many other drugs, targets beta amyloid plaque for removal. Aducanumab was previously shelved due to "futility analysis" in two phase 3 randomized placebo-controlled trials of people with mild or prodromal symptoms of Alzheimer's, but was resurrected in early 2020 for another phase 3 trial of 2,400 people that will last for three years. One of the two previous phase 3 trials of aducanumab reported reduction of beta amyloid plaque and a trend toward slower cognitive decline in a subset of people, but not improvement in cognition. Two trials of 6,000 people in the United States are now planned and must be completed by 2029. The FDA will remove authorization if the new trials fail to show clinical benefit (Athar 2021; Ferrero 2016). The company's prescribing information reports more than 10 percent of study participants experienced adverse reactions, more than with placebo, including headaches, falls, microhemorrhages, brain edema, and siderosis (abnormal deposition of iron) found on brain-imaging studies.

Eating a healthier diet and adopting other healthy lifestyle choices could allow us to enjoy high-quality survival to a ripe old age. A greater understanding of the complexity of our brains and what can go wrong can help us more fully appreciate why and how lifestyle choices have such an impact. It is difficult to explain what goes wrong in brain diseases without explaining the anatomy and functions of each type of brain cell. Therefore, a short course on brain anatomy and physiology will intertwine with the discussion of what goes wrong in Alzheimer's disease, the most studied neurodegenerative disease. I will also explain what we know about how ketogenic strategies could help overcome or prevent certain abnormalities.

After reviewing hundreds of research articles with thousands of pages on this incredibly complex subject, I hope to clearly convey how the normal anatomy and physiology of the brain is disrupted in aging and in diseases like Alzheimer's. A set of experiments that took months or years to conduct is typically written up into a scientific article fifteen to fifty pages long. My goal is to condense the massive and complex information on each topic into a few sentences in plain language. References are included for the specific studies and reviews that are discussed, but numerous research groups study each aspect of this disease, and it is impossible to include references for all of them.

As I read information about Alzheimer's and listen to hours and hours of presentations at the Alzheimer's Association International Conference each year, I am continuously humbled by how little I learned about all of this in medical school in the 1970s, even though the information I was given seemed so complex and complete at the time. I hope other physicians will open their minds to the possibility that they do not know it all and that there is so much more to learn to help their patients. The type of research conveyed here is conducted

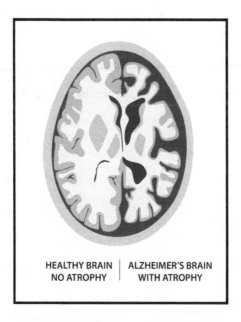

HEALTHY BRAIN | ALZHEIMER'S BRAIN
NO ATROPHY | WITH ATROPHY

FIGURE 10.1. Healthy adult brain without atrophy versus severe brain atrophy in later stages of Alzheimer's disease.

primarily by PhDs, who become experts in their field of interest, which they come to know inside-and-out and in great depth. I greatly admire their tenacity as they patiently proceed step by step to learn every detail of extremely complex processes. I apologize in advance to any researcher or reviewer if I missed something important or did not get it quite right in the translation.

The brain gradually shrinks as we age, but that process is greatly accelerated in Alzheimer's disease (see figure 10.1). The events that unfold in Alzheimer's are a silent, slow, insidious set of interlaced abnormal processes that devastate the human brain over years to decades. We will discuss the plaques, tangles, abnormal lipid deposits that Alzheimer described, as well as the roles of inflammation, insulin resistance, and metabolic dysfunction in aging and Alzheimer's disease that Dr. Alzheimer could not have known about a century ago. Since I started writing about Alzheimer's in 2008, there has been tremendous progress in what we know about the brain, and about Alzheimer's. Researchers are closing in on where the thousands of puzzle pieces fit together to answer the decades-old question—what causes Alzheimer's disease?

THE NERVOUS SYSTEM, NEURONS, AND SYNAPSES

We have neurons and nerves throughout our body, but much of the nervous system is packed into the control center, our brain, which makes up about 2 to 3 percent of our body weight but is so active and greedy for energy that it requires 20 to 25 percent of the calories we consume (Cunnane 2020). So it is easy to understand that a disturbance in the energy supply to the brain could have profound effects on how we function.

The nervous system is highly organized into the central nervous system, which consists of the brain and spinal cord, and the peripheral nervous system, which is the continuation of nerves (neurons and nerve fibers in bundles) that continue beyond the confines of the brain and spinal cord.

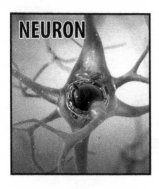

FIGURE 10.2. Healthy neuron (model). Adapted by Joanna Newport from public domain video: "How Alzheimer's Changes the Brain" at https://www.nia.nih.gov/.

Neurons (see neuron models in figures 10.2 and 10.3) are the main cell type in the central and peripheral nervous systems. Neurons connect with other brain cells by way of extensions, called axons and dendrites, that are operational in every organ and reach the very ends of our fingers and toes. Each neuron has one long slender projection, called an axon, that it uses to send signals to other neurons. An axon can be quite short or can extend up to three feet. Each neuron also has one or more, and sometimes many, short dendrites that receive signals from other neurons. There are several distinct types of support cells for neurons, called glia as a group, that nourish, repair, clean up debris, and perform many other functions to keep the brain in working order. We will discuss each type of glia shortly.

We have up to 100 billion neurons, and neurons each have an average of 7,000 connections with other neurons, called synapses (see figure 10.4). A rapidly developing three-year-old child is thought to have one quadrillion synapses; and this number declines, as we age, to a mere 100 to 500 trillion synapses. We also have up to 112,000 miles (180,000 km) of nerve fibers by age twenty (Drachman 2005). Inconceivable!

Neurons are "electrically excitable," and different types of neurons have different functions, such as responding to sensory stimuli like light, sound, touch, taste, and smell (sensory neurons), and controlling movement (motor neurons). Neurons are connected to other neurons within regions in a circuit, or between regions in a network. These networks remind me of power lines that can transmit signals for many miles through a complex system of relays and transformers. A great mystery of the brain is exactly how it is possible to create and store lifelong memories, how and where memories are stored, and what allows

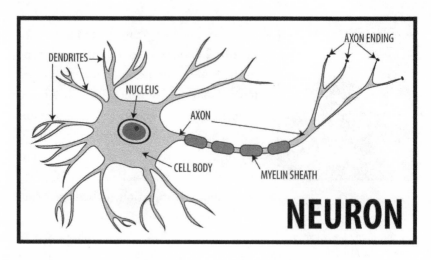

FIGURE 10.3. Parts of the neuron showing cell body, nucleus, axons, dendrites, and myelin sheath. Drawing by Joanna Newport.

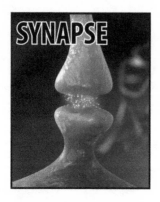

FIGURE 10.4. Synapses allow neurons to communicate (model). Adapted by Joanna Newport from public domain video: "How Alzheimer's Changes the Brain" at https://www.nia.nih.gov/.

for the consciousness we have of ourselves as separate from other people.

Direct transmissions from cell to cell occur as chemicals, called neurotransmitters, that are released through synapses at the end of axons and are taken up by dendrites. Like the insulation covering wires in power lines, axons may have a protective covering called myelin that can erode in brain diseases like Alzheimer's and multiple sclerosis, affecting the speed and other aspects of the nerve's performance and leaving the nerve vulnerable to damage. When demyelination occurs, the nerve fiber, if not repaired, can wither and die. Brain cells also secrete "signaling" substances that allow for communication within a cell and between cells, but do not go directly through synapses. I liken this process to satellites, cellphone towers, and wireless internet. Neurons also have a "cytoskeleton" that we will discuss shortly.

PLAQUES AND TANGLES

Beta amyloid plaques and tangles are the well-known hallmarks of Alzheimer's disease and the focus of billions of dollars of research to understand how they form and to find drugs that might interfere with their formation.

BETA AMYLOID AND PLAQUES

Beta amyloid is a substance that has normal functions within and outside of the brain, some of which still are not well understood. Beta amyloid (figure 10.5) is involved in activating certain enzymes, providing protection against oxidative stress (damage from reactive oxygen and reactive nitrogen species), and regulation of cholesterol transport, and it has an anti-microbial function.

Despite its beneficial activities, under the wrong conditions beta amyloid can enter and fatally injure brain cells. Excessive amounts of soluble (dissolvable) beta amyloid (specifically Aß 40 and 42) secreted from brain cells can form beta amyloid plaques, discussed in more detail shortly. Abnormal accumulation of beta amyloid can directly damage neurons (figure 10.6) and other brain cells and cause dysfunction and failure of mitochondria, where most of the energy molecule ATP is made. The mitochondria also serve as a hub in the process of making many proteins and other small molecules needed by the body. Within the cell, beta amyloid can bind to mitochondrial proteins and increase formation of harmful reactive oxygen species (ROS), leading to less production of ATP.

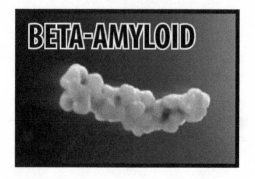

FIGURE 10.5. Beta amyloid clump that may lead to formation of a beta amyloid plaque (model). Adapted by Joanna Newport from public domain NIH video: "How Alzheimer's Changes the Brain" at https://www.nia.nih.gov/.

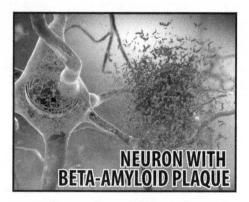

FIGURE 10.6. Neuron body with beta amyloid plaque forming nearby on dendrites (model). Adapted by Joanna Newport from public domain NIH video: "How Alzheimer's Changes the Brain" at https://www.nia.nih.gov/.

Amyloid Precursor Protein and Beta Amyloid

Amyloid precursor protein (APP) is a substance produced in the brain and many other tissues in the endoplasmic reticulum of the cell (explained later in this chapter). APP and its bioactive metabolites appear to monitor and modulate activities in the synapse from a distance through signaling, influence the growth of axons and dendrites, and regulate lipid metabolism in regeneration of the cell and mitochondrial membrane, and other important functions. APP preprocessing takes at least two different pathways using a different sequence of enzymes (α-secretase or ß-secretase plus γ-secretase) at the cell membrane where APP is cleaved into several bioactive fragments. Some of these fragments are involved in cholesterol homeostasis, transport of neurotransmitters, and synthesis and maintenance of the synapse. One type of fragment, beta amyloid, is produced continuously from APP and crosses the blood–brain barrier in both directions. Under certain conditions, beta amyloid fragments called Aß 40 and 42 can become "amyloidogenic," meaning that they form clumps (see figure 10.5) that combine to form larger plaques. Plaques can accumulate if there is overproduction of APP, such as occurs with gene mutations in familial forms of Alzheimer's, and, especially, if there is also defective removal. These sticky, toxic, accumulating plaques can damage the structure and function of neurons, the mitochondria, and other organelles in the neurons, axons, dendrites, nerve pathways and networks, synapses, and small and large blood vessels. The plaques can also damage other types of brain cells.

Beta Amyloid Is Antimicrobial

Beta amyloid can respond to the presence of microbes or accumulation of heavy metals, engulf the culprit, and, for this or another reason, form an insoluble (unable to dissolve) hard plaque. Studies show that beta amyloid has anti-microbial activity against many types of bacteria, fungi, and viruses (Soscia 2010), and thus appears to be a primitive immune response to infection and other foreign-body invasion.

Yes, beta amyloid and beta amyloid plaques can be toxic and cause damage to nearby neurons and blood vessels, but let us consider what happens when a thorn pierces the skin and the area becomes infected. If untreated, the surrounding skin will become inflamed, and pus will form as the immune system responds to attack the foreign body and bacteria. Bacteria, and toxins from the bacteria, could leak into the blood and cause life-threatening sepsis (blood poisoning). This immune response may save our life, but we might be left with a scar after the acute immune response subsides. The toxic local reaction to beta amyloid plaques could be a similar process, not necessarily the cause of Alzheimer's, but a downstream event in an inflammatory process triggered by an invasion of microbes or a heavy metal or some other invader. Perhaps a metabolic disruption, as occurs with diabetes, sets up a milieu that allows such an invasion to occur.

Viruses and other microbes are present in the brains of older people, often residing quietly in nerves. These microbes may remain dormant for many years but can reactivate at one or many points in time in response to a stress or to weakening of the immune system that occurs with aging. For example, "shingles" is a common reactivation of the Varicella-Zoster virus that lives dormant in nerves, often for decades, after a childhood chicken pox infection. Shingles lesions, often watery blisters at the beginning, appear in the distribution of a nerve pathway on the face, scalp, trunk, or extremities. Shingles can also be a reactivation of herpes simplex virus. Repeated bouts of "fever blisters" on lips or elsewhere is usually caused by herpes simplex 1 virus living in the nerves to that area. There is more discussion of infection and Alzheimer's disease in chapter 7 on "things to avoid."

For decades, there has been speculation that aluminum, lead, and mercury could trigger—or at least contribute to—Alzheimer's, supported by more recent research. Several metals have been found at higher concentrations in Alzheimer's brains, either bound to beta amyloid plaques or in the core of the plaque: zinc (Craddock 2012), iron

(Lipinski 2013), copper, calcium carbonate, and other form(s) of calcium (Everett 2018). Copper and iron have also been found in plaques formed from alpha-synuclein in Lewy body and Parkinson's disease (Lermyte 2019). There is more discussion on heavy metals and Alzheimer's risk in chapter 7.

Beta Amyloid Plaques Are Not Permanent

Beta amyloid plaques are not "insoluble," as long believed. For years, it was thought that beta amyloid plaques were permanent residents in the brain. However, formation and removal of beta amyloid plaques is a dynamic process, and this and other debris is removed from the brain through "garbage disposal" routes called glymphatics. Glymphatics are streams of lymph that flow between cells, eventually emptying into lakes of fluid deep in our brains called ventricles. The fluid continues to flow down into the spinal column, where the fluid is taken up, in the neck region, into the bloodstream to dispose of the "garbage" from the brain (Nedergaard 2013). In Alzheimer's brain, the blood–brain barrier deteriorates, and there is a decrease in low-density lipoprotein receptor-related protein 1 receptors (LRP1), which, in combination, diminish clearance of beta amyloid from the brain to the blood (Gawdi 2021).

Insulin and Beta Amyloid

There is a strong connection between insulin, beta amyloid, and amyloid plaques. Insulin is involved in the normal regulation of amyloid precursor protein (APP), which can go on to become beta amyloid (and other bioactive substances), as previously explained. Insulin can prevent the accumulation of beta amyloid plaques and the binding of beta amyloid to synapses, thus protecting neurons and their normal functions. It follows, then, that insulin resistance or insulin deficiency could allow more accumulation of beta amyloid plaques and the related collateral damage to occur. Portions of the amino-acid sequences of insulin and beta amyloid look alike to insulin receptors and insulin-degrading enzyme. Beta amyloid is known to compete with insulin for insulin receptors and can inactivate insulin receptors (Folch 2019). Insulin and beta amyloid compete for the same degrading enzyme and, when insulin is present, insulin wins the attention from this enzyme. So, in the scenario of insulin resistance with high insulin levels, degraded insulin will be removed from the brain, but beta amyloid may be left behind. Thus, beta amyloid plaques might accumulate in someone with insulin resistance who has abnormally high insulin levels.

Another factor related to sugar, insulin, and beta amyloid is overproduction of advanced glycation end-products (AGEs), which form in excess when the blood sugar level is high (more detail in chapter 9). AGEs can damage nearly every cell type, tissue, and organ and are likely responsible for many complications of diabetes and other chronic diseases. Amyloid precursor protein (APP) becomes elevated when AGEs are present, which would lead to higher levels of beta amyloid. AGEs can accelerate the formation and deposition of beta amyloid plaques. Many proteins are altered through glycation, and insulin itself can become "glycated" when blood sugar is excessive, which would affect its ability to lower blood glucose (Cepas 2020). In addition, AGEs promote the aggregation of alpha-synuclein, leading to the formation of Lewy bodies that are found in Parkinson's and Lewy body dementia (Cepas 2020).

As this book is written, amyloid PET imaging has been available for about a decade, mostly used in research. We now know that many healthy older people have plaques in their brains, sometimes quite a lot of plaque, without an obvious effect on their memory and cognition. Some people with Alzheimer's have relatively little plaque. The distinction between a healthy person with beta amyloid plaques and someone with Alzheimer's is the presence of inflammation and neurofibrillary tangles in the Alzheimer's brain.

A thrust of current research is to find biomarkers to diagnose Alzheimer's early and predict who will and will not develop Alzheimer's. People with Alzheimer's and mild cognitive impairment tend to have lower than normal levels of soluble beta amyloid in their spinal fluid. In one important study, people with higher levels of beta amyloid in spinal fluid (above 800 pg/ml) had normal cognitive and neuropsychological testing and had larger hippocampal volume, regardless of how much beta amyloid plaque was present in the brain (Sturchio 2021). The presence of insulin resistance in the impaired brain could be one explanation for the difference.

Taylor and associates used amyloid PET imaging to learn more about the connection between high sugar intake and the burden (total amount) of amyloid plaque in the brain. In a study of 138 older people, high glycemic food intake correlated with larger amounts of plaque in the whole brain as well as in most regions of the brain (Taylor 2017). The people with higher sugar intake did worse on cognitive testing for combined scores as well as on specific tests, such as the Mini-Mental Status Exam (MMSE). High-glycemic-index foods are foods high in sugar and/or other carbohydrates that spike blood glucose and insulin levels and include grains, potatoes, starchy vegetables, most fruit, and especially added sugars, like high-fructose corn syrup and table sugar.

For decades, Alzheimer's drug development has centered on the "amyloid cascade" hypothesis, the belief that the amyloid plaques are the cause of the degeneration and that using a drug to remove the plaques could restore the brain to a better cognitive state. Some of these failed drugs, like semagacestat, accelerated the disease. Unfortunately, my husband Steve received semagacestat after "crossing over" from placebo in a clinical trial. There was greater brain atrophy (shrinkage) in people who received semagacestat compared to placebo and, unexpectedly, the total amount of neurofibrillary tangles was significantly reduced in people taking semagacestat, while the placebo group had a substantial increase in tangles (Doody 2015). One might speculate that removing part of the immune system that responds to infection (beta amyloid plaques) could leave the brain wide open to attack. Despite the unwelcome news on semagacestat and similar drugs, the research in some corners has shifted focus to finding a drug that will remove the "neurofibrillary tangles"—a different silver bullet with a different target.

NEUROFIBRILLARY TANGLES

Cells each have a "cytoskeleton" that helps maintain the cell's shape, holds the cell together, allows organelles within the cell to move, and allows the cell itself to move. The cytoskeleton also allows cells to divide into two new separate cells. In brain cells, the cytoskeleton extends the length of the axons and dendrites that connect brain cells to each other. This cytoskeleton is a highly organized network of filaments, microfilaments, and microtubules. A protein called "tau" helps maintain the stability of the microtubules in the neuron.

Tau has other functions in neurons. Tau is involved in insulin signaling, cellular signaling, development of and protection of neurons, and apoptosis (programmed cell death). Phosphate groups can attach to tau protein in a normal and necessary process. However, if too many phosphate groups attach to the tau protein (called hyperphosphorylation), the hyperphosphorylated tau (P-tau) can become insoluble (unable to dissolve) and can form aggregates (clumps) that grow (figure 10.7) and become the neurofibrillary tangles (figures 10.8 and 10.9) found in Alzheimer's and in other conditions, such as traumatic brain injury. These tangles can cause the loss of synapses (connections between neurons), interfere with production of the mitochondrial ATP, disturb many cell functions, and ultimately kill the neuron (figure 10.10).

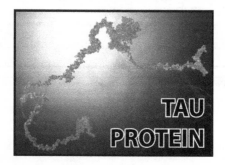

FIGURE 10.7. Tau protein forming aggregates (model). Adapted by Joanna Newport from public domain NIH video: "How Alzheimer's Changes the Brain" at https://www.nia.nih.gov/.

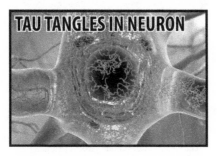

FIGURE 10.8. Tau protein forms tangles within neuron and its extensions (model). Adapted by Joanna Newport from public domain NIH video: "How Alzheimer's Changes the Brain" at https://www.nia.nih.gov/.

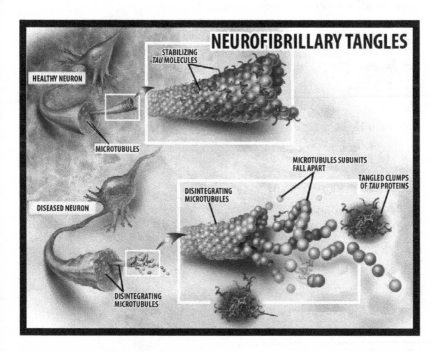

FIGURE 10.9. How neurofibrillary tangles disintegrate microtubules in extensions from the neuron (model). Public domain, source: "How Alzheimer's Changes the Brain" at https://www.nia.nih.gov/.

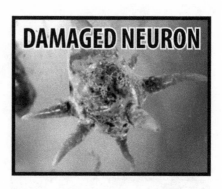

FIGURE 10.10. Neuron damaged by beta amyloid plaques and tangles has lost communication with other neurons (model). Adapted by Joanna Newport from public domain NIH video: "How Alzheimer's Changes the Brain" at https://www.nia.nih.gov/.

Insulin and Neurofibrillary Tangles

Many studies report that insulin resistance appears to promote hyperphosphorylation of tau and the formation of neurofibrillary tangles (Folch 2018). Rodriguez-Rodriguez and group demonstrated in a series of experiments that insulin accumulates as insoluble aggregates in neurons with P-tau tangles along with reduced numbers of insulin receptors on the cell membrane, reduced insulin signaling, and worsening of insulin resistance—a vicious cycle. This insulin accumulation was found in 80 percent of neurons with tangles and in 60 percent of all neurons located in the hippocampus, where Alzheimer's changes usually begin. Insulin accumulation was present in the earliest stages of Alzheimer's and progressed to other brain areas in the later stages. This insulin accumulation occurred whether or not the person with Alzheimer's had type 2 diabetes. Conversely, they did not find accumulation of insulin in brain cells in people with type 2 diabetes who did not have Alzheimer's (Rodriguez-Rodriguez 2017). Therefore, insulin accumulation in brain cells appears to be related to Alzheimer's rather than type 2 diabetes.

Spinal fluid levels of insulin are decreased in people with Alzheimer's, which could be due to increased retention of insulin and/or a problem with degradation and removal of insulin. The Rodriguez-Rodriguez group also found neuronal insulin accumulation in some other tauopathies (explained shortly), argyrophilic grain disease (AGD), progressive supranuclear palsy (PSP), and corticobasal degeneration (CBD). They recommend caution regarding the therapeutic use of insulin to treat Alzheimer's and other tauopathies until more is known about why accumulation of insulin in neurons occurs.

Neurofibrillary Tangles Are Not Exclusive to Alzheimer's Disease

Neurofibrillary tangles are not exclusive to Alzheimer's disease and may also be present following traumatic brain injuries, strokes, injury to the brain from lack of oxygen, progressive supranuclear palsy (PSP), posterior cortical atrophy (PCA), corticobasal degeneration (CBD), Pick disease, frontotemporal dementia (FTD), Lewy body dementia (LBD), syphilis, and herpes simplex 1 encephalitis, and in chronic traumatic encephalopathy, which is usually due to repeated concussions from sports injuries. Tangles are also present in about 50 percent of people with Parkinson's disease (PD) (Irwin 2013; Danics 2021). Such diseases are called "tauopathies." Advanced glycation end-products (AGEs) also contribute to hyperphosphorylation of tau, leading to formation of neurofibrillary tangles (Cepas 2020). Tangles from hyperphosphorylation of a different protein called TDP-43 are present in amyotrophic lateral sclerosis (ALS) (Hergesheimer 2019). In ALS, the tangles appear along motor nerve pathways (nerves that control movement) which can extend for as long as three feet (about one meter).

Over the past decade, tau PET imaging has become available, mainly for research purposes, to study the location and amount (burden) of tau tangles. It has become clear from long-term studies correlating tau tangle burden with cognitive testing that a significant burden of tangles is a much stronger indicator of Alzheimer's than the plaque burden. Likewise, the tangle burden correlates much more closely than the plaque burden with the degree of symptoms and stage of Alzheimer's. A tau PET scan combined with clinical history could help diagnose a specific type of dementia, due to differences in where the tangles appear initially, how the tangles progress through the brain, the presenting symptoms, and in what order symptoms unfold. There are also differences between dementias regarding what specific brain cells are affected and in the structure of tau filaments in the tangles, which cannot be seen on tau PET scans but could be studied at autopsy (Congdon 2018).

ARE PLAQUES AND TANGLES THE CAUSE, OR THE CONSEQUENCE, OF WHATEVER CAUSES ALZHEIMER'S?

Drugs aimed at removing beta amyloid plaque have failed so far to improve cognition or halt disease progression in Alzheimer's. Many "anti-tau" medications have been developed to reduce the production of tau, stop the hyperphosphorylation and aggregation of tau, or stabilize the microtubules, but they have not gotten beyond animal testing due to toxicity or lack of effect. Some anti-tau immunotherapies are still under investigation, but the jury is out, pending results of human clinical trials.

In the semagacestat study aimed at removing plaque, there was unexpected tau-tangle reduction and greater brain atrophy along with acceleration of Alzheimer's. Is it possible that neurofibrillary tangles, like beta amyloid plaques, play an important immune function in controlling infection? Perhaps plaques and tangles do not "cause" but are consequences of whatever causes Alzheimer's and other tauopathies.

For example, study results using animal models, human cell cultures, and 3D human brain models have variously reported that infection with herpes simplex virus 1 can provoke the formation of P-tau, neurofibrillary tangles, beta amyloid plaques, inflammation, cell dysfunction, and cell death (Cairns 2020; Itzhaki 2015). Similarly, introduction of the SARS CoV-2 (COVID-19 virus) into 3D human brain organoids led to redistribution of tau from its usual location in axons to the body of the neurons and induced formation of P-tau around the nucleus even though the virus did not replicate in the neurons (Ramani 2020). Could this be a protective effect of P-tau? Similar findings related to Alzheimer's disease have been reported for many other types of microbes, including other viruses, chlamydia pneumoniae, toxoplasmosis, gram-negative bacteria, dental pathogens, and spirochetes.

It is quite possible that beta amyloid plaques, which mostly form outside of brain cells, and neurofibrillary tangles, which mostly form within the cells, work together to try to stop the spread of a microbial and/or foreign-body invasion from one cell to another. Alzheimer's could be a case of the invader winning the battle, much like pneumonia, smallpox, polio, and many other infections that have shortened human lifespan throughout our history. Alzheimer's could very well be a slow pandemic. If confirmed, it would make more sense to find drugs (antibiotics or antivirals, for example) to stop the invader that causes Alzheimer's, than a silver-bullet treatment that interferes with formation of the beta amyloid plaques or neurofibrillary tangles that attempt to hold off the invader.

Effects of Ketones, Ketogenic Diet, Coconut Oil, and MCT Oil on Plaques and Tangles

- The ketone betahydroxybutyrate (BHB) increased survival of neurons in cultures exposed to toxins that cause Alzheimer's and Parkinson's. The neurons were larger and had more outgrowths than in control cultures (Kashiwaya 2000).
- Feeding the BHB ketone ester to a triple transgenic mouse model of Alzheimer's resulted in reduced amounts of beta amyloid plaques and tangles, less anxiety, and superior cognitive performance, compared to controls (Kashiwaya 2013).
- Double transgenic mouse models of Alzheimer's that received injections of BHB for 21 days, compared to controls, had better cognitive performance and less accumulation of beta amyloid plaques,

apparently by suppressing amyloid precursor protein (APP) and increasing an enzyme called neprilysin (NEP) that degrades beta amyloid. There was less overactivation of microglia, more ATP production, and other signs of neuroprotection in neurons in the hippocampus. BHB was found to regulate genes involved in aging, the immune system, nervous system, and neurodegenerative diseases (Wu 2019).

- In a series of experiments on neurons "in the dish" (in vitro) a 4:1 mixture of the ketones BHB and acetoacetate, prevented perforation of Aβ42 through the neuron cell membrane, injury to neurons from beta amyloid, membrane dysfunction, mitochondrial dysfunction, formation of reactive oxygen species (ROS), and protected synapses from Aβ42 toxicity. In live animal (in vivo) experiments, an APP mouse model and wild mice were given injections of the 4:1 ketone mixture versus saline for two months. Pyruvate dehydrogenase complex 1 activity was restored, improving mitochondrial function, and levels of Aβ42 were reduced. Memory performance was drastically improved for APP mice given ketones versus controls (Yin 2016).

- The presence of coconut oil in cultures, compared to controls, increased survival of neurons that were exposed to beta amyloid and suppressed alterations (size and shape) of mitochondria from exposure to beta amyloid. The effects were more pronounced for whole coconut oil than lauric acid (C12:0) or octanoic acid (C8:0) alone (Nafar 2014; Nafar 2017).

- A strict ketogenic diet in a transgenic Alzheimer's mouse model reduced brain beta amyloid levels by 25 percent (Van der Auwera 2005).

Studies of Ketogenic Foods That Need to Be Done:

More human clinical trials using PET imaging and monitoring changes in blood and spinal fluid biomarkers need to be performed to confirm the effects of long-term use of ketone ester, coconut oil, MCT oil, and ketogenic diets on amyloid plaque and tangle burdens, to determine if these interventions correlate with cognitive improvement and daily functioning. "Omics" studies could be useful in these investigations.

INFLAMMATION

Inflammation is a response of our immune system to defend us against microbes and other potentially harmful substances or foreign bodies. Harmful substances can come from outside or from within the body. When we think of inflammation, we might picture something obvious, like an inflamed joint that is red, hot, swollen, and tender from gout or other arthritis. However, more subtle, silent inflammation may be present: for example, in blood vessel walls of a person with untreated hypertension (high blood pressure), increasing risk for a heart attack. Smokers have inflammation in their lungs in reaction to accumulation of inhaled foreign substances. Chronically high blood sugar can cause inflammation-related damage to tissues and organs and a variety of complications, including dementia.

Chronic inflammation is a vicious cycle that becomes more and more destructive over time. For example, insulin resistance elevates blood sugar, which increases production of advanced glycation endproducts and inflammation, which damage more cells, leading to worsening insulin resistance.

Invisible, destructive neuroinflammation (affecting the brain and/or nerves) is a prominent feature of Alzheimer's and in some people with mild cognitive impairment, other dementias, autism, multiple sclerosis, ALS, Parkinson's, Huntington's, traumatic brain injury, and some psychiatric illnesses.

It was once thought that inflammation was a secondary feature of Alzheimer's, caused by the plaques and tangles. More current thinking is that inflammation may precede and drive Alzheimer's pathology. Neuroinflammation is always present in Alzheimer's. Cullen and associates measured 73 inflammatory proteins in the blood and spinal fluid of a study of 859 people at least 60 years old, ranging from cognitively normal through mild cognitive impairment, and the stages of Alzheimer's found changes in the patterns of seventy-three inflammatory proteins in blood and spinal fluid of these proteins in cerebrospinal fluid that could predict a normal person's age. The patterns could be scored and were more like people who were chronologically older in those with Alzheimer's. They called this the InflammAGE score (Cullen 2021).

Ketones Reduce Inflammation

- In cell cultures and mouse models fed ketone ester or ketogenic diet (KD), Youm et al. demonstrated that betahydroxybutyrate (BHB) has anti-inflammatory effects through inhibition of the NLRP3 inflammasome. Authors believe fasting and exercise should have similar effects (Youm 2015).

- In animal studies, caloric restriction or KD suppressed inflammation by upregulation of BHB targeting the NRLP3 inflammasome. BHB regulates nuclear proteins and acts as a histone deacetylase (HDAC) inhibitor that regulates histones and the gene p53 through beta-hydroxybutyrylation. Akt activation in microglia blocks HDAC activity, reducing neuroinflammation. Akt refers to a set of three genes (AKT 1, 2, and 3) that encode for Protein kinase B and mediates pathways involved in cell survival, growth, proliferation, cell migration, and angiogenesis by phosphorylating intracellular proteins. The short-chain fatty acid butyrate, which is produced by bacteria in the gut, inhibits HDAC even more than BHB. In animal studies, butyrate induces the expression of genes that can improve insulin sensitivity and augment energy production (Han 2020).

- Polyphenols (caffeic acid, p-coumaric acid, ferulic acid, methyl catechin, dihydrokaempferol, gallic acid, quercetin, and myricetin glycoside) in virgin coconut oil have antioxidant properties and are often added to other vegetable oils to improve their resistance to oxidation and stability. In cultures of HCT-15 cells, pre-treatment with virgin coconut oil reduced oxidant-induced oxidative stress and cell death and restored the level of glutathione to near normal, as well as the related enzymes. After induction of the inflammasome-associated gene NLRP3 through beta amyloid and a high-fat diet in an Alzheimer's rat model, addition of virgin coconut oil reduced oxidative stress and expression of NLRP3. The phenolic compound ferulic acid administered to mice that were injected with Aß42 had reduced glial fibrillary acidic protein and the pro-inflammatory cytokine IL-1beta (Chatterjee 2020).

- Look for an interesting review of the life expectancy-extending, anti-aging properties of ketones and the mechanisms involved by Richard L. Veech, MD, D.Phil., and others (Veech 2017).

ALZHEIMER'S AFFECTS ALL BRAIN CELL TYPES

There are several cell types other than neurons in the brain, called glia, including microglia, astrocytes, oligodendrocytes, and ependymal cells. In addition, neural stem cells in highly protected locations can be transformed into neurons or glia. Endothelial cells (figure 10.11) that line blood vessels provide a link between the brain and the rest of the body, called the blood–brain barrier. We will explore each of these and how they are affected by Alzheimer's disease.

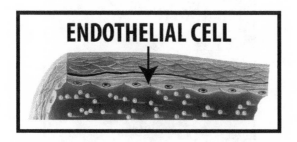

FIGURE 10.11. Endothelial cells line blood-vessel walls. Adapted by Joanna Newport from graphic purchased from iStockPhoto.com.

MICROGLIA AND ACTIVATED MICROGLIA

In Alzheimer's, neuroinflammation is most apparent in microglia, a tiny cell when compared to a neuron (see figure 10.12). You might think of a single microglia as a "jack-of-all-trades," since it can perform many different functions. Microglia can act as officers, lookouts, scouts, soldiers, messengers, reinforcements, and the clean-up crew.

Microglia are capable of morphing into various shapes and sizes and can easily move to wherever they are needed and perform whatever function is required within their armamentarium. For example, microglia can be in the "resting form," in which the body of the cell is small and remains in place but has long branches, or tentacles, that are constantly moving and surveying the area for microbes or other invaders. Substances emanating from a microbial invasion, inflammation, or damaged cell are detected by these tentacles, which then activates the microglia. Much like an amoeba, an "activated microglia" can take on different shapes large and small, move to wherever it is needed, and secrete various substances to carry out its job.

Some activated microglia greatly enlarge to become macrophages, the "garbage trucks" of the brain, that can travel to a distant site to

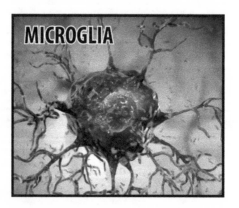

FIGURE 10.12. Microglia (model). Adapted by Joanna Newport from public domain NIH video: "How Alzheimer's Changes the Brain" at https://www.nia.nih.gov/.

consume microbes, harmful substances, and debris from dead or damaged cells. This process is called "phagocytosis." If more help is needed, these macrophages secrete a substance that signals other microglia to enlarge and join them for the cleanup. These macrophages can then "display" the foreign material they scooped up (called an antigen) in such a way that T-cells (specialized lymphocytes, a type of white cell) are called into action from afar and cross the blood–brain barrier to chop up or inactivate a virus and/or kill a virus-infected cell. When a macrophage becomes so full that it cannot take in any more debris, it becomes a "granular corpuscle."

Activated microglia that become macrophages are also triggered by beta amyloid plaques to release inflammatory substances (cytokines and others) by activating the "NLRP3 inflammasome," which then stimulates formation of more beta amyloid plaques—a vicious cycle of inflammation (Stancu 2019). Advanced glycation end-products (AGEs) are also known to activate the NLRP3 inflammasome (Cepas 2020).

In addition to providing fuel to make ATP, the ketone betahydroxybutyrate drives other pathways that suppress inflammation, including the pathway involved in the NLRP3 inflammasome (see side box). Providing fuel is an immediate process; however, reducing inflammation could take much longer and could explain more gradual improvements some people experience from adopting the keto diet and other ketogenic strategies.

Another type of microglia is the scavenger, which moves freely and mainly in the white matter of the brain, looking for garbage to discard, such as debris from dead cells related to brain development and remodeling. "Perivascular microglia" hang out near blood vessels and are involved in the repair and growth of new blood vessels.

Anti-inflammatory microglia (called M2 microglia) promote a calm atmosphere (homeostasis) and repair in areas of the brain that are not infected. M1 microglia promote inflammation in areas that are infected or damaged. Response of the brain to invasion and inflammation involves an extremely complex interplay of communication through signaling molecules between microglia, astrocytes, neurons, T-cells, and blood stem cells. The cascade leading to a massive inflammatory response is activated by release of various cytokines, nitric oxide, and reactive oxygen species from microglia. The inflammatory response further activates all nearby microglia and involves all other cell types in the area (Fan 2015; Edison 2018). Lipopolysaccharides released by bacteria and advanced glycation end-products (AGEs) are examples of substances that can set off the cascade of inflammation in the brain and other organs (Ohtsu 2017). Insulin is also involved in a complex way in regulating how microglia respond to inflammatory triggers (Arnold 2018).

In recent years, PET imaging has been developed to look for specific markers and patterns of inflammation in the brain that can be followed over time to study disease progression. Such long-term studies have reported that microglia are in "calm" anti-inflammatory mode in mild cognitive impairment but gradually switch over to pro-inflammatory mode in people with MCI who are progressing toward Alzheimer's. The rate of progression of inflammation appears to correlate with the severity of the disease and is slower for some people than for others (Hamelin 2018). A series of PET scans for inflammation could help determine if changing diet or other lifestyle factors, or adding a drug or supplement, reduces inflammation.

Inflammatory Substances Do Not Appear to Seed or Spread Tau Tangles

Experiments were conducted on mouse microglia and living human microglia retrieved shortly after death from the brains of people with Alzheimer's and frontotemporal lobe dementia (FTD). The studies reported that microglia did not contain the gene to make tau, but the microglia would pick up and carry tiny fragments of tau protein, called "tau seeds," from one cell to another, thus seeding the spread of tau tangles. Specific inflammatory substances did not appear to cause the seeding or spread of tau tangles, since the seeding of tau by microglia occurred regardless of whether these inflammatory substances were present. Also, microglia from the brains of people who had died with Alzheimer's and FTD induced more tau seeding than microglia from non-demented people. They also reported that microglia taken from the affected areas of the brain were capable of seeding tangles, whereas microglia from the unaffected or minimally affected areas were not. They concluded that microglia play an important role in seeding the spread of tau tangle pathology in the brain (Hopp 2018).

Some Inflammation May Be Beneficial . . . Out-of-Control Inflammation Is Not

A certain amount of inflammatory immune response is needed in the brain and other organs to overcome infection and control harmful substances. Some increase in brain inflammation occurs with aging but, in diseases like Alzheimer's, the inflammatory response is out of control. What we do not know at present is why. How much inflammation is the right amount of inflammation, and how do we achieve the precise balance? Neuroinflammation is an extremely complex process that can come and go in response to an acute insult to the brain, or can stay on for many years in neurodegenerative diseases.

Inflammatory substances can also find their way into the brain from infections and inflammation that occur outside of the brain, such as during a urinary tract, respiratory, or intestinal infection. Lopez-Rodriguez and group have studied this phenomenon in mice and in human brains and have learned that not only can infection outside the brain trigger delirium, but such an infection can also accelerate cognitive decline. I and other hospice nurses and doctors can attest to this phenomenon firsthand. The changes related to inflammation outside the brain are associated with signs of increased neuroinflammation, as evidenced by elevated brain cytokine levels that are produced by astrocytes and microglia (Lopez-Rodriguez 2021).

ASTROCYTES

Astrocytes are the most numerous cell type in the central nervous system (figure 10.13). These star-shaped cells are found in the brain and spinal cord. They are larger than microglia but smaller than neurons, with numerous extensions radiating from the astrocyte body. There are two basic types of astrocytes, one that exists in the gray matter and the other, in white matter, that has longer, more fibrous extensions. Astrocytes are part of the structural support for neurons and nerve fibers and are involved in control of blood flow, which is designed to protect the brain as much as possible from sudden highs and lows in blood pressure.

Astrocytes have many other functions, and there are several subtypes depending on their location and what they do. Some astrocytes provide fuel and other nutrients to neurons and nerve tissue. This type has "vascular feet" that connect the astrocyte to blood vessels and allow the astrocyte to act as a go-between to link the cells lining the blood vessels (endothelial cells) to neurons. Astrocytes help keep electrolytes and minerals, such as potassium and calcium, in balance inside and outside the cells and are involved in repair and scarring following injury. Astrocytes can produce, store, and release neurotransmitters and other substances, and their extensions wrap around synapses between neurons. A single astrocyte can interact with up to two million synapses at one time.

Astrocytes can sense glucose levels in the fluid between cells, can store glucose as glycogen, can shuttle glucose to neurons as needed, and can also make and shuttle ketones to neurons (Thevenet 2016). Astrocytes are also involved in communication between the neurons and oligodendrocytes to make myelin (which we will discuss next). Animal studies suggest that astrocytes control the circadian rhythm (the "biological clock" that regulates our sleep-awake cycles). It is also conjectured, but not proven, that astrocytes are involved in learning and memory in the hippocampus, where Alzheimer's first takes hold (Garwood 2017).

Like microglia, in Alzheimer's disease astrocytes can become "reactive," can surround beta amyloid plaques, and can release substances that promote inflammation. In the astrocytes, insulin regulates the secretion of inflammatory cytokines in response to inflammatory triggers. Like microglia, astrocytes can become phagocytic, gobbling up and breaking down the beta amyloid that forms the plaques. Until recently, researchers thought that beta amyloid comes mainly from the neurons, but a more current study demonstrated that these reactive astrocytes contain the amyloid precursor protein (APP) and the enzymes needed to secrete it from the astrocyte. One hypothesis proposes that inflammation triggers astrocytes to secrete beta amyloid (Frost 2017).

Lauric Acid from Coconut Oil Potently Stimulates Production of Ketones in Cultures of Astrocytes

Researchers at The Nisshin OilliO Group, Ltd., in Japan conducted a two-part experiment to understand how coconut oil could improve symptoms in my husband Steve and others, despite lower blood ketone levels compared to equivalent amounts of medium-chain triglyceride (MCT) oil (Nonaka 2016).

Experiment 1: Seven-week-old Sprague-Dawley rats were fed one of three oils by tube:

- Coconut oil with MCTs: lauric acid, called C12:0 (46.7 percent), C8:0 (8.3 percent), C10:0 (6.4 percent)
- High-oleic sunflower oil: no MCTs
- MCT oil: C8:0 (73.9 percent), C10:0 (35.8 percent), C12:0 (0.3 percent)

Total ketones, total triglycerides, and total free fatty acids were measured at baseline, 2 and 4 hours after the dose. MCT oil substantially and significantly increased total ketone levels as well as the area under the curve (which estimates total ketones produced), whereas there was not much difference in these measurements between coconut and sunflower oil. The total plasma triglycerides and total free fatty acid levels and areas under the curve were increased at 2 and 4 hours and were greater for sunflower oil than coconut oil, but lower than MCT oil. C8:0 and C10:0 levels were slightly but significantly higher at 2 and 4 hours for MCT oil compared to coconut and sunflower oil. Levels of C12:0 from coconut oil were substantially higher than C8:0 or C10:0 with almost no change at 2 and 4 hours (14.7 + 3.0 gm/100 gm versus 14.8 + 3.0 gm/100 gm). Therefore, lauric acid levels are sustained at high levels in the blood for several hours after consuming coconut oil.

Experiment 2: Cultures of KT-5 mouse astrocytes were treated as follows in four groups and total ketone levels were measured after four hours:

- Vehicle (non-ketogenic substance to serve as control) alone

- Vehicle plus oleic acid (C18:1) at 50 µL or 100 µL

- Vehicle plus caprylic acid (C8:0) at 50 µL or 100 µL

- Vehicle plus lauric acid (C12:0) at 50 µL or 100 µL

The difference in total ketone body levels between vehicle and oleic acid (C18:1) was significant at 100 µL but not 50 µL. However, for both C12:0 and C8:0, the total ketone bodies were significantly higher at 100 µL and at 50 µL.

Based on these and previous studies, the authors suggested that:

- Most C8:0 and C10:0 is absorbed via the portal vein to the liver and is oxidized in the liver without entering peripheral circulation and would have less availability to cross the blood–brain barrier and stimulate in vivo (in the living organism) ketogenesis in astrocytes.

- C18:1 enters the peripheral circulation when it is consumed but does not cross the blood–brain barrier well and would have low availability to astrocytes in the brain.

- C12:0 is partially absorbed by the portal vein and partly converted to ketones, but most enters peripheral circulation and stays elevated much longer than C8:0 or C10:0 in blood. It is more likely that C12:0 would produce in vivo ketogenesis in astrocytes than C8:0 or C10:0, assuming it crosses the blood–brain barrier.

The authors concluded that lauric acid (C12) "directly and potently" stimulates ketone production in vitro (in the lab) but needs to be confirmed in vivo (in the living organism). Since astrocytes supply nearby neurons with fuel, if this holds up in vivo, production of ketones in astrocytes by lauric acid could partly explain how coconut oil appears to bring about improvement in people with Alzheimer's, Parkinson's, and other disorders with insulin resistance.

OLIGODENDROCYTES

Oligodendrocytes are cells that only exist in the central nervous system (brain and spinal cord) and provide support for the neuron and its axons and dendrites. Oligodendrocytes produce myelin, forming a lipid-rich sheath that surrounds and insulates these extensions. The myelin sheath has gaps at specific intervals along the nerve fiber, looking a bit like strings of sausages. These gaps cause the electrical impulses moving along the nerve fiber to hop from one segment to the next, which increases the speed at which the impulse travels. Upon reaching the end of the axon, the impulse triggers release of a chemical neurotransmitter into the synapse, the junction between two neurons. One oligodendrocyte has numerous extensions that can provide support and myelin insulation for as many as fifty neurons. Myelin is 60 to 75 percent lipid and 15 to 25 percent protein and contains cholesterol. Myelin cannot be produced without cholesterol. Nerve fibers with myelin tend to line up parallel to form nerve tracts; this tissue appears white and, thus, is called the "white matter" of the brain.

Damage to myelin (demyelination) can occur during the aging process, in Alzheimer's, multiple sclerosis, certain other neurological diseases, and peripheral neuropathy, a complication of diabetes and certain cancer chemotherapies (see figure 10.14). While inflammation is clearly involved in the Alzheimer's process, it is not yet known whether inflammation causes white matter to deteriorate or vice versa. Perhaps this is another vicious cycle. Imaging studies show white matter hyperdensities (bright spots) in areas where there is demyelination but also in areas with decreased blood flow or inflammation (Nasrabady 2018). It is not always clear whether white matter hyperdensities are due to Alzheimer's, advancing age, or something else.

In animal studies, beta amyloid plaques appear to be harmful to oligodendrocytes. However, these plaques are rare in white matter and, therefore, may not explain why the white matter deteriorates. Demyelination can appear more than twenty years before symptoms of Alzheimer's appear, about the same timing that reduced glucose uptake appears in areas of the brain affected by Alzheimer's. This may be no coincidence. In a book chapter on this subject, Suzanne de la Monte, PhD, explains how insulin resistance, which reduces glucose uptake, could play a key role in white-matter degeneration and demyelination (de la Monte 2019).

Metabolic pathways for breakdown of both glucose and ketones are impaired in oligodendrocytes in Alzheimer's, though ketone metabolic pathways are not affected in neurons, astrocytes, or microglia (Saito 2021). However, in a dual ketone and glucose PET study, when people with mild cognitive impairment consumed MCT oil for six months, ketone uptake improved by 145 to 218 percent in 9 fascicles of interest, both in deep white matter and in fascicle cortical endpoints (where the fascicle ends in the gray matter of the cortex in the brain). The increase in ketone uptake correlated with improved processing speed in cognitive testing (Roy 2020).

Ketones Are Regenerative

In a mouse model study, a ketogenic diet (KD) induced regeneration of sciatic nerves (Liskiewicz 2016), while in another mouse model, KD restored the integrity of oligodendrocytes and increased myelination (Stumpf 2019).

An exogenous supplement of betahydroxybutyrate improved intestinal stem cell homeostasis and function through activation of Notch signaling, which is involved in tissue regeneration (Cheng 2019).

NEURAL STEM CELLS, EPENDYMAL CELLS, AND ABNORMAL LIPID DEPOSITS

Neural stem cells (see figure 10.15) are tucked into three different areas, called "niches," that are located deep in the brain near ependymal cells (figure 10.16) and are protected by and otherwise interact with endothelial cells (cells that make up walls of blood vessels). Neural stem cells require fatty acids as fuel to divide and transform into more mature types of brain and nerve cells (called neurogenesis) and to remodel the brain (called plasticity), a process that allows the brain to adapt to changes in the local environment. In adult humans, one niche is located near the hippocampus and dentate gyrus (DG), areas affected early in Alzheimer's that are involved in memory and learning. Another niche is in the superior ventricular zone (SVZ), and a third is near the

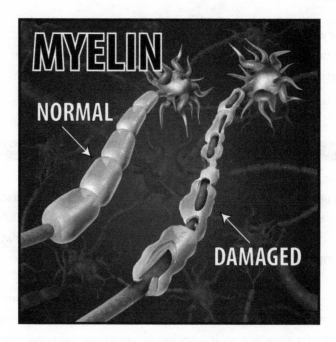

FIGURE 10.14. Myelin sheath on axon, in normal and damaged conditions. Adapted by Joanna Newport from graphic purchased on iStockPhoto.com.

hypothalamus, a part of the brain that controls hunger, thirst, temperature, and certain hormones, and has many other functions.

The study of changes in neural stem cells in Alzheimer's is relatively recent. In the past, it was the consensus that all neurons are present by early childhood and that adults do not make new neurons. Newer studies inform us that neurogenesis (the production of new neurons from neural stem cells) does occur in adults, about 1,400 new neurons per day on average, and that Alzheimer's dramatically interferes with neurogenesis and plasticity (Cosacak 2020). A mouse study suggests that, in Alzheimer's, amyloid precursor protein (APP) is normally present in the niches where neural stem cells are located. However, excessive APP in the niches decreases the growth and number of neural stem cells (Sato 2017).

There is much interest surrounding whether neural stem cells can be stimulated and used as therapy to form new brain and nerve cells in people with Alzheimer's and other neurodegenerative diseases. One might think neural stem cells could simply be injected directly into the blood or spinal fluid. However, these cells would have to find the locations in the brain where they would have the necessary support to become mature neurons. If neural stem cells were injected into a vein, they might be distributed everywhere but the brain and lack the ability to cross the blood–brain barrier. Conceivably, cell signaling could make that happen, just as T-cells are called into the brain to help fight infection. However, injecting stem cells into the fluid around the spinal cord would seem unlikely to have the desired effect, in my opinion, given that fluid in the brain flows from the ventricles downward toward the spinal column; the stem cells would need to swim against the current and pass through the ependymal lining of the ventricles to find their way into brain tissue. A substance stimulating neural stem cells to multiply and mature might be more effective than injecting neural stem cells into the blood or spinal fluid but may be pointless if all other factors related to the disease are still operational.

On the other hand, what if neural stem cells in Alzheimer's simply lack fuel to make the ATP that the stem cell needs to divide and develop into a mature cell? The answer is currently unknown.

Ependymal cells (see figure 10.16) are glia that make up the ependyma, a thin lining that separates the brain tissue from the lakes of cerebrospinal fluid called ventricles. Ependymal cells make the cerebrospinal fluid that helps remove garbage from the brain and circulates from the ventricles in the brain, like a river, down into the spinal column. Ependymal cells can also absorb this fluid. They are shaped like a column and have cilia attached to them, which look like fine hairs beating together in synchronized waves to push along the fluid. Ependymal cells are also involved in neuroregeneration, which is the regrowth and repair of nerve cells and tissues.

Ependymal cells have extensions that attach to astrocytes, and they also contain the abnormal lipid deposits described by Dr. Alzheimer in 1906. Ependymal cells normally make and store lipids in vesicles (fluid-filled sacs) as one of many functions; some of these vesicles become greatly enlarged in Alzheimer's. These abnormal lipid deposits

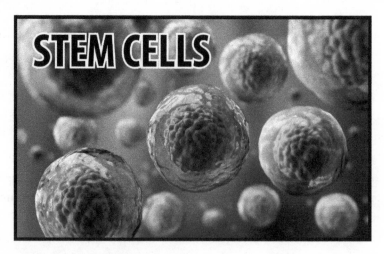

FIGURE 15. Stems cells (model). Adapted by Joanna Newport from graphic purchased on iStockPhoto.com.

have been found in the brains of certain animal models of Alzheimer's and in the brains of people who died with Alzheimer's. Compared to the vast research on plaques and tangles, abnormal lipid deposits have received relatively scant attention, and only within the last decade.

Nearly all cells have vesicles to store lipids, but these are much more prominent in certain cell types, such as ependymal cells. Cells can alter the lipids stored in their vesicles by shortening them into smaller particles (lipolysis), elongating them, or by using the smaller particles from lipolysis to make the larger fatty acids belonging to any of the three major classes, saturated (SFA), monounsaturated (MUFA), or polyunsaturated (PUFA) fatty acids. Cells can also make new fatty acids (de novo lipogenesis), as well as cholesterol and cholesterol esters starting with acetyl-CoA. These materials can be used for energy or can become part of the cell membrane and other support structure by combining with proteins or any number of other substances to make more complex molecules; these complex molecules can also act as signaling molecules for communication within a cell and between cells. The relative proportion of the three classes of fatty acids—SFA, MUFA, PUFA—in the cell membrane can affect the dynamics of the cell membrane, specifically its fluidity, and can determine what moves in and out of the cell, and how signaling occurs at the cell surface. Fatty acids can also activate factors that promote the multiplication of neural stem cells, their transformation into mature types of brain cells, and their survival (Hamilton 2018).

In Alzheimer's, lipid deposits in ependymal cells become abnormally large, as Alois Alzheimer described in 1906. In a series of experiments, these abnormal lipid deposits were found to be enriched in oleic acid (a monounsaturated fatty acid [MUFA] and the main fatty acid in olive oil and canola oil) and interfered with the proliferation (multiplication and development into more mature forms) of neural stem cells (Hamilton 2015). In one experiment, oleic acid was injected into the ventricles of wild mice and an Alzheimer's mouse model, which was found to be sufficient to cause the formation of the abnormally large lipid droplets in the Alzheimer's model. Using a radioactive label, they learned that oleic acid in the lipid droplets can be processed like other lipids in the usual way (lipolysis, desaturation, and lipogenesis). This does not suggest that people should avoid eating a high oleic oil like olive oil. Nearly all edible fats and oils, including coconut oil, contain some oleic acid. The abnormal lipid accumulation could be due to a lack of energy to process the lipids normally (the power is off in the factory) or another factor yet to be determined.

The abnormal lipid deposits also contained another MUFA, palmitoleic acid, for which higher levels may indicate greater risk of cardiovascular disease. In a study of stepwise progression from a very high saturated fat/low carb to very high carb/low saturated fat diet, palmitoleic acid blood levels increased as carbohydrate intake increased, while the proportion of saturated fat in the blood remained the same (Volk 2014). It is unknown at present what, if anything, the presence of palmitoleic acid indicates in the abnormal lipid deposits.

Periventricular (around the ventricles) hyperdensities (bright spots on imaging studies) may indicate areas of edema (swelling), possibly occurring in response to inflammation or damaged ependymal cells. This edema appears to impair removal of garbage from the brain. When ependymal cells are damaged beyond repair, they are replaced

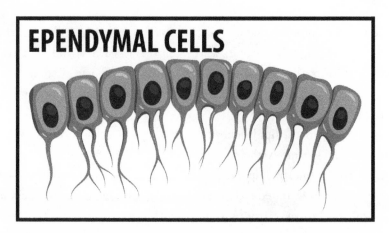

FIGURE 10.16. Ependymal cells (model). Adapted by Joanna Newport from graphic purchased from iStockPhoto.com.

by astrocyte patches, and proteins meant for disposal accumulate as well (Todd 2018), like uncollected garbage. It is not certain at present which comes first: the lipid deposits, the damaged ependymal cells, or the edema. In my opinion, it is possible that lipids accumulate because the ependymal cells are also victims of insulin resistance and/or disruption of ATP production and lack the energy to process the lipids and to provide the types of lipids that fuel division and maturation of neural stem cells require.

Hamilton's group has found 1,000 different changed genes in the SVZ niche in the Alzheimer's mice compared to wild mice, of which 14 percent are related to lipid metabolism. One of these genes upregulates (increases production of) an enzyme called SCD-1 that controls the synthesis of MUFAs from saturated fats. There is a study showing that higher levels of SCD-1 correlate with lower levels of cognition. Elevated activity of SCD-1 is also associated with insulin resistance, excess abdominal fat, and hyperlipidemia (high cholesterol and triglycerides) (Astarita 2011). Hamilton speculates that inhibiting SCD-1 would allow the neural stem cells to stay active and possibly interfere with other components of the destructive cascade that happens in Alzheimer's, though this idea is not yet confirmed.

Also noteworthy, the abnormal lipid deposits in the ependymal cells appeared before the plaques and tangles and coincided with the beginnings of brain- and nerve-related impairments in early adulthood in an Alzheimer's mouse model. In humans, this would correspond with the problem of brain-glucose uptake that occurs one or two decades before symptoms appear. A broad metabolic problem involving both sugar and lipid metabolism is at play in Alzheimer's. Lipidomic and metabolomic studies are demonstrating that insulin is intricately involved in the metabolism of glucose, proteins, and lipids, and that insulin resistance and diabetes greatly impact and disrupt the delicate balance and interaction of the many different substances involved in metabolism (Yang 2018).

Recent research using powerful microscopes and mass spectrometry have also identified abnormal lipid droplets in the core of the Lewy bodies found in Parkinson's, Lewy body dementia, and multiple system atrophy (Shamoradian 2019). Lewy bodies are abnormal aggregates mainly composed of a protein called alpha-synuclein that is normally present in the nucleus, near the synapse, in cell membranes, and in mitochondria of neurons and astrocytes.

Alpha-synuclein has several known functions related to cell membrane structure and repair of DNA, and it may be involved in the release of the neurotransmitter dopamine, which is greatly reduced in Parkinson's. Alpha-synuclein also binds to phospholipids in the cell membrane and can form tubules to connect with lipid droplets. Studies in mice have shown that excessive alpha-synuclein causes an increase in monounsaturated fatty acids (MUFAs), such as oleic acid, which makes alpha-synuclein more neurotoxic, another vicious cycle (Fanning 2020). In 2020, Nuber and group reported that inhibiting SCD-1 (the enzyme involved in MUFA synthesis) with an oral treatment called "5b" in mouse models of Parkinson's disease reduced the abnormal accumulation of alpha-synuclein and lipid droplets (Nuber 2020). This could be a promising treatment for Alzheimer's, Parkinson's, and other diseases with abnormal lipid metabolism.

PPARS IN INFLAMMATION AND ENERGY HOMEOSTASIS

There are literally hundreds of substances under study for Alzheimer's in dozens of pathways, so discussing them all is nearly impossible. A standout that is involved in disturbed lipid metabolism is a transcription factor (see side box) called "peroxisome proliferator-activated receptor α" (PPARα). PPARα regulates certain pathways affected by Alzheimer's that are involved in controlling inflammation, in production of beta amyloid, and in lipid metabolism, including cholesterol metabolism. PPARα plays a critical role in brain energy supply and is a "master regulator" of energy homeostasis, along with other PPARs. PPARα is activated by binding with various fatty acids, including some polyunsaturated fatty acids, such as palmitoleic acid, and more complex lipids. When activated, PPARα upregulates genes involved in fatty acid transport and uptake into cells and organelles, utilization of fatty acids, and burning of fatty acids as fuel. PPARα is also activated during fasting or energy deprivation and is required for the liver to generate ketones, which can be used as an alternative fuel to glucose by the brain and organs other than the liver, where they are made. PPARα is decreased in people with Alzheimer's, along with abnormal glucose uptake in cells in certain areas of the brain, though ketones are taken up normally. This is the basis for use of MCT oil (which is partly converted to ketones in the liver), exogenous ketones, and ketogenic diet for Alzheimer's and other conditions in which there is insulin resistance (Cunnane 2020).

Transcription Factor

A transcription factor is a protein that enters the nucleus and finds a pattern of DNA that marks the beginning of a gene for transcription of DNA to messenger RNA and turns genes on and off, ideally at the right time in the right cell in the right amount. Interfering with a transcription factor can disrupt the signaling cascade.

PPARα is just one member of a family of PPARs and other compounds that work in unison in many different tissues, including the brain. Other PPARs, specifically PPARγ and PPARβ/δ, regulate both lipid and carbohydrate metabolism, are anti-inflammatory, have antioxidant effects, and promote insulin sensitivity by directly activating insulin and insulin-like growth factor 1-responsive genes while bypassing insulin-resistant insulin receptors. PPARα is found in neurons and astrocytes and is highly concentrated in the hippocampus, the memory-forming area affected early in Alzheimer's disease. PPARα is involved in memory and cognition and plays a role in regulating proteins involved in neurotransmission. Researchers have found some PPARα-related gene mutations that negatively impact Alzheimer's.

PPARβ and PPARδ are found in neurons but not in glial cells. PPARδ is involved in pathways related to cognition, memory, myelination, controlling phosphorylation of tau, and regulating brain phospholipids. PPARγ is mainly found in white and brown fat tissue, the large intestine, and the spleen, and regulates the accumulation of fat, energy balance, lipid synthesis, and inflammation. PPARα and PPARβ/δ are decreased in Alzheimer's, whereas PPARγ is increased, and the function of PPARs is impaired, which may contribute to the progression of the disease pathologies.

As a reminder, insulin resistance (the opposite of insulin sensitivity) can increase oxidative stress, secretion of beta amyloid, and formation of plaques, and it can also promote formation of tau neurofibrillary tangles. So, due to opposing effects to insulin resistance, increasing levels of PPARα and PPARβ/δ could offer a treatment for Alzheimer's. Pioglitazone is a PPARγ agonist (meaning that it increases PPARγ and its effects) and is already used by people with diabetes. In one study, pioglitazone appeared to reduce dementia risk by 47 percent in diabetes, but can have adverse effects like liver toxicity and edema of the macula in the retina. Pioglitazone has shown no benefit in people who already have Alzheimer's disease, likely due to poor uptake of the drug by the brain.

An agonist of PPARβ/δ named T3D-959 has recently shown promise in animal studies, positively affecting many pathways regulated by the PPARs (De la Monte 2017). In an exploratory clinical trial, thirty-four people with mild to moderate Alzheimer's received T3D-959 at various tiny and larger daily doses for fourteen days. No one received a placebo. The drug appeared to be safe and well-tolerated. Plasma metabolomic studies of 800 chemicals showed improved blood markers for insulin sensitivity, which increased proportionately with the dose and correlated with higher glucose uptake in specific brain regions on FDG-PET imaging. There was also improvement on cognitive assessments as well as lower fasting blood-sugar levels in people taking T3D-959. There was less effect on glucose uptake at the lowest dose in people who were ApoE4+ but this difference disappeared with larger doses; oddly, for cognitive testing, the ApoE4 people had worse results at the highest dose but improved at lower doses (Chamberlain 2020). It is likely that T3D-959 will move on to larger clinical trials.

Drugs targeting PPARs have a broad range of effects, and it is possible that the beneficial effects could be offset by negative effects. For example, fibrates increase PPARα and are very effective in lowering total cholesterol and triglyceride levels. However, fenofibrate (Fenoglide®, Lipofen®, Tricor®, Triglide®) has a long list of potential severe and less serious consequences, including liver dysfunction, hepatitis, inflammation of other organs like the gallbladder, pancreas, and muscles, abnormal blood clotting, and can decrease desirable HDL-cholesterol.

Researchers cannot say with certainty whether dietary factors such as excessive intake of sugar or specific fatty acids have an impact on the abnormal lipid deposits in the brain in Alzheimer's, although it seems likely. Lipid metabolism is also disturbed in the aging process, in obesity, and in diabetes, autism, other neurodegenerative disorders, and some psychiatric illnesses. Hopefully, this area of research will continue to grow.

Ketones, MCTs, Lauric Acid, PPARγ, and Mitochondria

PPARγ regulates genes in anti-inflammatory and antioxidant pathways; and certain fatty acids bind to and activate PPARγ, thereby enhancing its functions. Medium-chain triglycerides (MCTs) cross the blood—brain barrier and provide an alternative energy source for neurons and astrocytes (reviewed in Augustin 2018), but also have other effects.

- A ketogenic diet increased PPARγ two- to fourfold in brain homogenates of wild type mice and a mouse model of epilepsy, and reduced frequency of seizures by 70 percent in the epileptic mice (Simeone 2017).

- In cell cultures and in animals, the MCT decanoic acid (also called capric acid or C10:0), directly bound to and activated PPARγ, whereas caproic (C6:0) and caprylic (C8:0) acids did not. PPARγ stimulates mitochondrial biogenesis and increases antioxidant status. C10:0 also binds weakly to PPARα and PPARβ/δ [which are decreased in Alzheimer's disease]. C10:0 was found to occupy a different "binding pocket" than long-chain fatty acids on the PPARγ molecule. Free C10:0 and its triglyceride also improved insulin sensitivity and lipid profiles without increasing fat storage or weight gain in diabetic mice (Malapaka 2012).

- A study of a drink (K.Vita) with 80 percent C10:0 and 20 percent C8:0 significantly reduced the frequency of seizures in adults and children, though the study was designed to look at tolerability and compliance and was not powered for seizure frequency (Schoeler 2021).

- C10:0 inhibits AMPA receptors of glutamate, which increases excitotoxicity and plays a role in seizures. AMPA receptor pathways are also amplified by beta amyloid in Alzheimer's (Augustin 2018). In isotope studies of the oxidation rates of C8:0 and C10:0 in human-derived neuron models, C10:0 was beta-oxidized at a 20 percent lower rate than C8:0. This was explained by a much greater dependence of C10:0 on activity of carnitine palmitoyl transferase 1 (CPT1), an enzyme involved with metabolism of fatty acids that is low in neurons. Slower oxidation allows C10:0 to be available for much longer than C8:0 to perform its other functions, and, therefore, C10:0 appears to be more responsible for anti-seizure effects than C8:0 in the MCT oil ketogenic diet for epilepsy (Khabbush 2017). Seizures are common in autism, Alzheimer's, Lewy body dementia, and some other neurodegenerative diseases.

- Macrophages play a significant role in insulin resistance. Lauric acid (C12:0) is half the fat in coconut oil. To uncover the effects of C12:0 on mitochondrial dysfunction, macrophages from THP-1 monocytes were treated with increasing doses of C12:0 from 5 to 50 micromole/L and assayed for glucose uptake, cellular reactive oxygen species, ATP production, mitochondrial content, membrane potential, and key regulators. Before treatment, the macrophages had lower glucose uptake, GLUT 1 and GLUT 3 expression, and increased markers of mitochondrial dysfunction. C12:0 increased glucose uptake and GLUT 1 and GLUT 3 expression, and restored mitochondrial biogenesis by improving ATP production, increasing oxygen consumption, mitochondrial content, and membrane potential. C12:0 also promoted expression of several regulator genes of mitochondrial biogenesis, including PPARγ. The researchers concluded that C12:0 appears to improve insulin sensitivity and mitochondrial dysregulation in insulin-resistant macrophages (Tham 2020).

- Many studies have reported that consumption of a diet high in long-chain fatty acids (LCFAs) leads to insulin resistance in muscle, liver, and adipose tissue in rodents. Mice were fed a high-fat diet for five weeks using either lard (high in LCFAs) or hydrogenated coconut oil [Note: I do not recommend hydrogenated coconut oil, which could contain trans fats]. Control mice were fed a low-fat diet for comparison. The mice receiving coconut oil had much less adipose tissue, identical to control mice, compared to the LCFA group. The MCT group had much better glucose tolerance compared to the LCFA group. Triglyceride contents of liver and muscle were much higher in the LCFA group. Changes in certain enzymes in the muscle mitochondria from feeding MCTs indicated a more potent stimulation of mitochondrial biogenesis pathways. In a separate four-week study of high-fat diet in rats, there were significantly elevated blood levels of glucose, insulin, and triglyceride levels in the LCFA group compared to the MCFA group (Turner 2009).

SYNAPSES, NEUROTRANSMITTERS, AND ALZHEIMER'S PATHOLOGIES

One prominent feature of Alzheimer's disease is the loss of synapses. As a reminder, synapses are connections between neurons and certain other brain cells that allow an electrical current, or an electrical impulse that has been converted to a chemical signal called a neurotransmitter, to pass from a neuron to another cell. This process is called neurotransmission. Neurotransmitters are stored in vesicles near the membrane at the synapse. Synapses can link an axon to a dendrite, an axon to another axon, an axon to a blood-vessel cell, or an axon to the body of a neuron or other cell. The synapse can also release a neurotransmitter into the surrounding fluid. The transmitting and receiving ends of the synapse do not touch, and there is a gap through which the electrical current or the neurotransmitter travels. The inner workings of the synapse are complex, involving machinery to produce, store, and release the neurotransmitters, a receptor at the receiving end, and then recycling of the neurotransmitter occurs. Axons can release more than one neurotransmitter at the same time.

It appears that low levels of beta amyloid are secreted normally to regulate remodeling of synapses. Beta amyloid also appears to have some normal functions related to memory. However, in Alzheimer's, excessive concentrations of beta amyloid can lead to formation of plaques in and near synapses and damage the synapses, which interfere with release of neurotransmitters and result in loss of synapses.

Likewise, hyperphosphorylated tau (P-tau) can have toxic effects, impacting transport of substances through the axons, interfering with signaling cascades, and affecting the anchoring of receptors in the synapse. Excessive P-tau may also lead to loss of synapses. In addition, advanced glycation end-products (AGEs) become excessive when blood sugar is chronically elevated as in prediabetes and diabetes type 1 and 2, and the Receptor for Advanced Glycation End-Products (RAGE) can interact with beta amyloid in neurons, in microglia, and in blood vessel cells, damaging the function of neurons and synapses and affecting cognitive functioning (Rajmohan 2017).

MITOCHONDRIA ARE ALSO DAMAGED IN ALZHEIMER'S

Excessive beta amyloid can damage mitochondria which are located throughout the neuron and its extensions and are also important in synapses. Mitochondria are tiny organelles that function as the energy-producing factories in nearly all types of cells. Mitochondria also produce numerous proteins and other metabolites, and control the cell cycle, cell growth, and cell differentiation (the process by which a cell, such as a stem cell, changes and matures to a more specific cell type). Mitochondria are also involved in cell signaling and programmed cell death.

There can be hundreds to thousands of mitochondria in a single cell, with the larger numbers occurring in very active, energy-needy cells like neurons, cardiac muscle, and skeletal muscle. Red blood cells have no mitochondria. A unique feature of mitochondria is that they have a different set of DNA than the DNA in the cell nucleus. This is called mitochondrial DNA (mtDNA) which is passed nearly always from one's mother. In contrast, the nucleus of a cell contains DNA in an equal number of chromosomes, twenty-three from each parent, except in rare occurrences like Down syndrome in which an extra chromosome can come from either parent. In mitochondrial dysfunction, errors can occur in replication of the mtDNA, leading to mutations and defective operation of those mitochondria (Bratic 2013).

While the "amyloid cascade hypothesis" of Alzheimer's has predominated for decades, the "mitochondrial cascade hypothesis" suggests that mitochondrial dysfunction may drive the accumulation of

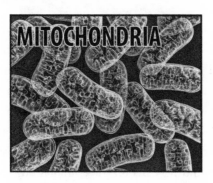

FIGURE 10.17. Mitochondria (model). There are hundreds to a thousand or so mitochondria in each neuron, including its body and extensions. ATP and many other metabolites are produced within mitochondria. Adapted by Joanna Newport from graphic purchased on iStockPhoto.com.

beta amyloid and loss of neurons and synapses (Swerdlow 2014). In Alzheimer's, the structure, size, mass, and numbers of mitochondria in brain cells are altered, along with diminished oxygen consumption and activities of enzymes located within the mitochondria. These alterations are linked to interaction of mitochondria with beta amyloid deposits in a sort of "self-propagating cycle": excess beta amyloid production appears to be a result of mitochondrial dysfunction, but also damages mitochondria (Chornenkyy 2019). Amyloid precursor protein (APP) becomes trapped in the wall of the mitochondria, affecting their function. This problem is more prominent in people with the ApoE4 gene who have cognitive impairment.

Tau tangles also appear to affect mitochondrial function, and mitochondrial dysfunction seems to promote tangle formation (Perez Ortiz 2019). There is validity to the amyloid and mitochondrial cascade hypotheses, but both appear to be downstream from more pervasive metabolic issues, such as insulin resistance and insulin deficiency and other causes of glucose hypometabolism and lower production of ATP, further exacerbated by widespread damage from AGEs and inflammation.

In a review article on mitochondria, diabetes, and insulin resistance, the authors emphasized the central role that altered mitochondria play. The authors state that both types 1 and 2 diabetes "profoundly derange fuel metabolism, including metabolism of glucose, fat, and amino acids, the main energy sources for humans" (Ruegsegger 2018). Nearly every process that occurs within the cell requires ATP. Insulin is the predominant hormone that drives production of ATP. When there is insulin resistance and/or deficiency, glucose levels can be high in the blood and glucose can be present in the fluid surrounding cells (extracellular fluid) while, at the same time, cells are starving due to the inability of adequate amounts of glucose to enter the cell. Glucose deprivation within the cell affects the ability of mitochondria to produce ATP (called cellular respiration) due to lack of fuel, unless another fuel, such as ketones, can drive the pathway to make ATP.

Damage to the mitochondria not only reduces energy production (ATP) but also interferes with the other functions of mitochondria and can result in an accumulation of reactive oxygen species (ROS), called oxidative stress. ROS can further damage mitochondria and nearby structures in the cell, as well as DNA, proteins, and lipids. Insulin resistance alters the function of mitochondria, and altered mitochondria can further impact the many important metabolic actions of insulin, such as its role in the manufacture of proteins in the cell. Heart failure is an example of a common complication of diabetes that is partly attributed to altered mitochondria in heart-muscle cells; the decrease in ATP production impedes the normal function of the affected heart-muscle cells. Ketone PET studies show that ketones from exogenous ketone salt supplements and from MCT oil are taken up avidly by the heart and kidneys (Cuenoud 2020). Therefore, ketones could be therapeutic in heart and kidney disease, and studies have shown potential for ketones to improve heart failure, help with recovery following a heart attack, and improve cardiac status in children with severe multiple acyl-CoA dehydrogenase deficiency (Kadir 2020; Byrne 2020; Fischer 2019; Nielsen 2019).

In normal healthy cells, there is expected wear-and-tear to mitochondria, and flawed mitochondria are identified, degraded, removed (called mitophagy), and replaced with new mitochondria. This process keeps the quality of mitochondria high in the healthy cell but is

defective in diabetes, Alzheimer's, Parkinson's, and some other neurodegenerative diseases, and it appears to be a key factor in aging, along
with diminishing numbers of mitochondria within the cells (Bratic
2013). Supplementation with many antioxidant substances intended to
overcome damage to mitochondria and other structures from ROS has
shown some promise in animal studies, but there are no standouts so
far in completed human clinical trials.

Ketones Could Help Mitochondrial Dysfunction

If the power goes out in a factory, production will come to a grinding halt. One can easily imagine that if mitochondria do not put out
enough energy, nearly every process that takes place in a cell—and
communications between cells—will slow down as well. If too many
mitochondria malfunction, an energy-hungry cell like a neuron might
become dormant or even die.

Studies have shown that aerobic exercise, caloric restriction, and a
ketogenic diet can decrease mitochondrial damage from oxygen-free
radicals and improve mitochondrial function while enhancing other
age-fighting pathways as well. These approaches increase insulin-like
growth factor 1 (IGF1), which improves insulin sensitivity, and result in
greater expression of brain-derived neurotrophic factor (BDNF) in neurons in the hippocampus and cortex. BDNF is important to repair and
maintenance of synapses, stimulation of neural stem cells, growth of
neurons, and stress resistance in neurons (Mattson 2018; Ruegsegger
2018). Mark Mattson, PhD, who recently retired from the National Institute of Aging, has written extensively about this and the benefits of intermittent metabolic switching from glucose to ketones, which occurs
with exercise and fasting (Mattson 2018B). Consumption of MCT oil,
exogenous ketone esters, and ketone salts could provide similar benefits related to a temporary switch to mild ketosis, but further studies are
needed to prove this one way or the other.

APOE4 GENE, CHOLESTEROL, AND
ALZHEIMER'S PATHOLOGIES

The ApoE4 gene is the most common genetic risk factor for Alzheimer's. We receive one copy of the ApoE2, 3, or 4 gene from each parent and can have any combination of ApoE2, ApoE3, or ApoE4 genes. People with an ApoE2 gene have less than average risk of Alzheimer's, two ApoE 3 genes confer average risk, and people with one ApoE4 gene have greater than average risk. About 40 percent of people with Alzheimer's have at least one ApoE4 gene, compared to 14 percent of the general population. Many people with one or even two ApoE4 genes do not develop Alzheimer's and, overall, about 14 percent of people with an ApoE4 gene develop Alzheimer's, so ApoE4 is far from a definite sentence of "death by Alzheimer's" (Jeong 2019). However, people with two copies of the ApoE4 gene have a much higher risk of early-onset Alzheimer's (before age 65).

Apolipoprotein E (ApoE) is a protein that becomes part of a larger complex lipoprotein (combination of protein and lipid) that carries lipids, cholesterol, cholesterol esters, and fat-soluble vitamins (vitamins A, D, and E) in the bloodstream. HDL and LDL are well known examples of such lipoproteins. When we hear about HDL cholesterol, called HDL-C, for example, this refers to cholesterol carried by an HDL molecule. However, HDL particles carry many other important lipids into the brain such as DHA, and how well this happens may differ between types of ApoE4 (Yassine 2017). In the brain, ApoE is produced mainly in astrocytes and microglia and is the primary carrier of cholesterol to neurons in the brain.

As a reminder, cholesterol is made in virtually every cell and is vital to the brain's support structure, cell membranes, and normal brain function. Cholesterol in the bloodstream does not cross the blood–brain barrier and, in the brain, cholesterol can be made in neurons and microglia, but most cholesterol is made in astrocytes. It has been proposed that ApoE4-mediated dysfunctional cholesterol metabolism could lead to Alzheimer's pathology. ApoE4 does not hold on to cholesterol as well as ApoE2 and ApoE3, which means that less cholesterol would be transported to neurons from astrocytes. Cholesterol might then accumulate in ApoE4 astrocytes while levels of cholesterol in neurons would be less than normal. This would affect neurotransmission at the neuron's synapse where cholesterol is required, for example. The excess cholesterol in astrocytes could then lead to increased formation of "lipid rafts," free-floating areas in the cell membrane rich in cholesterol and protective sphingolipids, where cholesterol comes together with ApoE and amyloid precursor protein (APP) along with enzymes that convert APP to beta amyloid. This could lead to excessive production of beta amyloid. A problem with cholesterol metabolism could partly explain why there is a tendency to earlier and greater accumulation of beta amyloid plaques in people who are ApoE4 (Jeong 2019).

In people with gene mutations in presenilin and amyloid precursor proteins, plaques and cognitive symptoms may appear as early as the third decade of life. The ApoE4 gene also seems to accelerate hyperphosphorylation of tau and tangle formation. ApoE is involved in clearing beta amyloid plaques, and ApoE4 is much less effective than ApoE2 or 3 at doing so.

As a reminder, GLUTs transport glucose through plasma membranes. GLUT 1 and GLUT 3 deficiency is more prominent in people with the ApoE4 gene, which translates into decreased glucose uptake into the brain and neurons decades before symptoms appear. These GLUT deficiencies resulting in decreased glucose uptake seem to be connected in some way to promoting hyperphosphorylation of tau and the resulting tau tangles (Patrick 2019).

There could be a causative link to Alzheimer's involving gene mutations, ApoE4, mitochondria, and a structure in the cell called the endoplasmic reticulum (ER) (Area-Gomez 2017). To set the stage, this structure has rough and smooth areas with different functions and looks like a complex maze with multiple pathways ultimately connecting with the membrane surrounding the nucleus of the cell. The ER serves as a transportation structure, but it is also involved in manufacturing substances like proteins, cholesterol, lipids (including complex phospholipids), hormones, and beta amyloid, and is involved in detoxification. Like the cell membrane and membranes of other organelles, the ER membrane is made of phospholipids and is supported by a cytoskeleton, which can be damaged by an excess of P-tau leading to tangle formation. Normal "folding" of proteins occurs in the ER, but "misfolding" of beta amyloid, alpha synuclein, and tau proteins can occur here as well, triggering accumulation as plaques and tangles when, for example, genetic mutations are at play (Penke 2016).

The ER is in contact with other organelles, and the connection with mitochondria is called the "mitochondrial-associated ER membrane" (MAM). Based on their studies, Area-Gomez and associates believe that the pathologies in Alzheimer's could all be explained by dysfunction in the MAM where apolipoprotein E4 (ApoE4) and Alzheimer's genetic mutations are involved in regulating operations, including formation of plaques and tangles, accumulation of lipid in droplets, altered fatty-acid and phospholipid metabolism, increased circulating cholesterol, reduced brain glucose, abnormal calcium regulation, and defective mitochondria. They also found that neurons transferred from a living brain exhibited increased lipid droplet formation when they were treated with ApoE4 lipoproteins but not with ApoE3 lipoproteins (Area-Gomez 2017).

Thus, the ApoE4 gene appears to predispose a person to the plaques, tangles, decreased glucose uptake, and abnormal lipid droplet formation that are characteristic of Alzheimer's. People with the ApoE4 gene also tend to have higher blood-cholesterol levels, are more prone to atherosclerosis (hardening of the arteries), and have a greater predilection to formation of advanced glycation end-products (AGEs) than noncarriers, which may further increase their risk for diabetes and dementia (Deo 2020).

The ApoE4 Gene and the Important Omega-3 Fatty Acid DHA

Another problem related to the ApoE4 gene involves the important brain form of omega-3 fatty acid called docosahexaenoic acid (DHA). DHA is about 30 percent of the lipids in the brain and is abundant in brain-cell and organelle membranes. One important function of DHA in the cell membrane involves regulation of GLUT 1 transport of glucose across the blood–brain barrier. However, a study by Nugent and group did show benefits of supplementation with fish oil on brain-glucose uptake using FDG-PET imaging in older people (Nugent 2011). People with Alzheimer's do not necessarily have decreased DHA. However, in some studies, a low level of DHA has been associated with increased plaques and tangles and reduced glucose uptake that are characteristic of Alzheimer's, whereas a high level of DHA can prevent or lessen these abnormalities. But simply supplementing with fish oil or concentrated DHA may not translate directly into higher levels of the preferred form of DHA in the brain, especially in people who have the ApoE4 gene.

Several studies have reported some benefits from DHA supplementation in people with ApoE3 and ApoE2 genes, but not those with ApoE4 (Patrick 2019). In her review of the subject, Dr. Rhonda Patrick explains that humans are not very efficient at converting omega-3 fatty acids in vegetable oils to the more complex DHA omega-3 needed in the brain. A study of higher dietary fish and seafood intake reported benefits on Alzheimer's pathology and cognitive symptoms in people with and without the ApoE4 gene. Patrick explains that free DHA is the primary form found in supplements, whereas DHA bound to phospholipids in fish, which are partly converted after consumption to lysophosphatidylcholine-DHA (DHA-lysoPC), appears to be the brain's preferred form of DHA. In humans, DHA in the blood is about 45 percent free DHA bound to albumin and 55 percent DHA-lysoPC. Patrick has proposed that free DHA may not be easily transported across the blood–brain barrier in ApoE4 gene carriers, due to degradation of the blood–brain barrier by ApoE4, whereas DHA-lysoPC bypasses this problem, since it enters the brain using a different transport mechanism that is not affected by ApoE4. She also states that this degradation of the blood–brain barrier occurs in aging as well as in people with genetic mutations of presenilin 1 and 2, which occur in familial forms of Alzheimer's disease (Gawdi 2021). Therefore, a marine source of DHA, such as dietary fish or fish roe (eggs) or a supplement such as krill oil, which is very rich in DHA phospholipids, could help achieve better levels of DHA in the brain. This could be especially important to consider in people who are ApoE4.

NEUROTRANSMITTERS, ALZHEIMER'S MEDICATIONS, AND MCT OIL SYNERGY

Considering how important neurotransmitters are in the brain and nervous system, there is a dearth of information on how most neurotransmitters are affected by Alzheimer's, except in the context of drug development. As previously mentioned, neurotransmitters are chemicals made within neurons that are involved in communication between neurons and other cells. Excessive beta amyloid is suspected of interfering with the actions of several major neurotransmitter pathways, but some other pathways have not been well studied. Since ATP is required in cells to carry out functions such as production and degradation of neurotransmitters, mitochondrial dysfunction is also at play, whether upstream or downstream from the beta amyloid pathology.

A study by Snowden and others reported imbalances in twelve of fifteen metabolites involved in neurotransmitter metabolism that were measured in affected areas of brain tissue taken from people with Alzheimer's pathology at autopsy, compared to normal brains. The most studied of the affected neurotransmitters in Alzheimer's are acetylcholine and glutamate, but Snowden's work demonstrated that metabolism of GABA and serotonin are affected, and dopamine is diminished as well, a core pathology in Parkinson's disease (Snowden, 2019).

Drugs have been developed to target two major dysfunctional neurotransmitter pathways involved in learning and memory, the cholinergic system centering on acetylcholine and glutamatergic systems centering on glutamate.

Insulin resistance can dampen the effects of the genes that make acetylcholine, an important brain chemical (neurotransmitter) involved in alertness, attention, learning, and memory, as well as many other functions throughout the body. Overcoming acetylcholine deficiency in Alzheimer's is the target for three of the only four medications currently recognized by the FDA for the treatment of Alzheimer's, specifically donepezil, galantamine, and rivastigmine. An enzyme that degrades acetylcholine (called acetylcholinesterase) is increased in areas where there are beta amyloid plaques, which would effectively lower the amounts of available acetylcholine in those areas. Donepezil (Aricept®), galantamine (Razadyne®), and rivastigmine (Exelon®) are inhibitors of acetylcholinesterase, which should result in increased levels of acetylcholine in the brain since less acetylcholine would be degraded. It is possible that these drugs also allow too much acetylcholine to accumulate in areas of the brain that are not affected yet by Alzheimer's, which could explain some of the drug's side effects. The cholinergic system has many other functions beyond learning and memory, and common side effects of these drugs include nausea, insomnia, nightmares, aggression, diarrhea, vomiting, fatigue, and muscle cramps. Serious side effects may include abnormal heart rhythms, frequent urge to urinate, and seizures. Ironically, many people, including some with mild cognitive impairment and Alzheimer's, take prescription and over-the-counter medications with anticholinergic effects, which interfere with the production of acetylcholine. Simply eliminating these medications could improve memory and some other symptoms of dementia. This was discussed in more detail in chapters 8 and 9.

Lin and group have used complex genetics and microscopic analyses to study neurotransmission, and they explain a possible reason why acetylcholinesterase inhibitor drugs for Alzheimer's may lack effectiveness or have temporary minimal effects on cognitive improvement, and then may result in accelerated decline after discontinuation. They believe acetylcholinesterase inhibitors may reduce the physiological precision of cholinergic transmission at the synapse. They also believe that long-term use of such drugs may upregulate acetylcholinesterase in the Alzheimer's brain and/or downregulate release of acetylcholine at the synapse, which could explain the accelerated deterioration with discontinuation (Lin 2021).

In contrast to the other two drugs that affect acetylcholine, galantamine was found in 6- and 12-month studies to also affect nicotinic acetylcholine receptors and to have more beneficial effects than donepezil and rivastigmine on improving and preserving cognition and daily functioning, as well as delaying behavioral symptoms. This translated into an improved ADAS-Cog score by an average of 3 out of 75 points after starting the drug, but unfortunately the score then declined to the baseline score by 12 months. A historical placebo group had scores that were 6 points worse than the people taking galantamine at the end of 12 months, so overall, galantamine provided a possible reprieve from decline for a year, which would be very worthwhile to most of us. Galantamine also showed fewer negative effects on sleep and other symptoms than the other two drugs. Starting early in Alzheimer's disease has shown the greatest benefit for galantamine (Lilienfeld 2002).

Huperzine A is a popular supplement made from a Chinese herb that potently inhibits acetylcholinesterase and has been used to treat Alzheimer's in China but is not recognized as a drug in the United States. People who are also taking donepezil, galantamine, or rivastigmine aren't advised to take this supplement.

Glutamate is an excitatory neurotransmitter, and levels are abnormally high in Alzheimer's, which can create neuronal excitotoxicity. The loss of insulin signaling and mitochondrial dysfunction that occurs in Alzheimer's contribute to glutamate excitotoxicity. Excess glutamate can damage and kill brain cells. The drug memantine (Namenda®) is designed to block the related receptor N-methyl-D-apartate (NMDA), which should reduce the effects of glutamate (Kandimalla 2017). Memantine can also bind to receptors in other neurotransmitter pathways, such as serotonin, dopamine, and histamine, which could explain some of the common side effects, such as worsening of cognition at the start of treatment, which some people experience. Other common adverse effects include dizziness, drowsiness, headaches, insomnia, agitation, and hallucinations. Some less common but serious effects of memantine include heart failure, blood clots, and psychosis.

Each of the four FDA-recognized drugs targets a single pathology among the many complex pathologies that occur in Alzheimer's, which likely explains the short-term beneficial effects, if any, that people experience. It is common for physicians to prescribe a combination of donepezil, galantamine, or rivastigmine with memantine.

People often ask me if they could, or should, stop taking Alzheimer's medications when they begin consuming coconut oil, MCT oil, or a ketone supplement. First, I remind them that this is a decision between patient and physician, but I encourage them to continue taking these medications as prescribed because there appears to be synergy (more benefit than either alone) between MCT oil and these medications. In a study of the MCT oil medical food AC-1202 by the Accera company, when they analyzed the data of 140 people who were taking any Alzheimer's medication, they found on day 90 that people who were taking 20 grams of MCT oil once per day and any Alzheimer's medication had significantly more improvement on the standard 75-point ADAS-Cog test than those taking MCT oil without medication or one of the medications without MCT oil. This was especially true for people taking MCT oil and galantamine (Razadyne®), who demonstrated an average 8-point improvement compared to people taking galantamine and placebo. They reported a 0.75-point improvement for people taking Aricept (donepezil) plus MCT oil compared to Aricept plus placebo, and 1.53 points for people taking Namenda (memantine) plus MCT oil compared to Namenda plus placebo. The details can be found in the patent application for the Accera MCT oil medical food that I found online on that fortunate day in May 2008 when I came across a press release on AC-1202 (Accera 2008).

INSULIN RESISTANCE COULD EXPLAIN ALZHEIMER'S AND CERTAIN OTHER NEUROLOGICAL DISEASES

If there is a single common denominator that could explain the complex and vast collection of abnormalities in the Alzheimer's brain we have discussed so far, it is insulin resistance.

There are many similarities between insulin resistance in the brain and elsewhere in the body. Outside of the brain, insulin is made in beta cells located in the "islets of Langerhans" in the pancreas. A healthy beta cell can increase its production of insulin tenfold if needed. However, constant overstimulation of beta cells to produce insulin by a continuous barrage of excessive nutrients, especially sugar, but also certain lipids and amino acids, could, through oxidative stress, damage the mitochondrial-associated ER membrane (MAM) and the mitochondrial outer membrane, thereby compromising mitochondrial function. Likewise, chronically high blood sugar level results in the formation of advanced glycation end-products (AGEs) and reactive oxygen species, which can also damage the endoplasmic reticulum and other structures within the cells. Mitochondrial damage via this route results in less production of ATP, which is needed to carry out the cell's functions; and, for beta cells, that eventually means making less insulin.

Excessive caloric intake also leads to excessive fat storage, which is orchestrated by insulin. Inflammatory substances can be released from this fat, which may also damage the structures within the mitochondria of pancreatic islet beta cells and other types of cells. Here again, there is a vicious cycle of inflammation, because oxidative stress also sets off inflammatory pathways, resulting in even more damage to the cell (Keane 2015).

HOW INSULIN AND INSULIN RESISTANCE AFFECT THE BRAIN

Brain insulin resistance could be defined as reduced sensitivity of brain cells to insulin, or a failure of brain cells to respond to insulin. This lack of response could be due to fewer insulin receptors being available on the cell membrane, and/or malfunction of the receptors such that they do not allow insulin to attach. Or perhaps insulin attaches to the receptor but fails to trigger the insulin-signaling cascades related to glucose uptake and subsequent ATP production, release of neurotransmitters, response to inflammation, growth and repair of neurons, and many other normal effects of insulin. These insulin effects, or lack thereof, appear to be at play in the Alzheimer's brain.

The "brain insulin-resistance hypothesis" of Alzheimer's was proposed by Siegfried Hoyer in 1998. Almost thirty years earlier in 1970, Hoyer first reported in a German medical journal that glucose and cerebral glucose metabolism were decreased in the brains of some people with dementia (Hoyer 1970). Dr. Hoyer also showed that brain amino acid catabolism is increased in Alzheimer's, and he continuously studied the role of glucose hypometabolism, insulin receptors, and insulin resistance in Alzheimer's until he died in 2014. Somewhat surprising is that Hoyer did not report on brain ketone metabolism. Dr. Hoyer's associates carry on the work today. Additional studies by Hoyer and group are also included in the part 2 references.

In the early 1980s, brain-imaging techniques became available that demonstrated decreased glucose uptake in specific areas of the brain in Alzheimer's. In 1991, Hoyer reported that, in Alzheimer's, there is a severe imbalance between the utilization of glucose in the cerebrum of the brain (reduced by 45 percent) versus cerebral blood flow (reduced by 17 percent) and cerebral oxygen utilization (reduced by 18 percent) (Hoyer 1991). Many other groups have confirmed this using different techniques, and a few have also reported that ketones are taken up normally in the affected areas of the brain (Lying-Tunnel 1981; Swerdlow 1989; Cunnane 2020). A study by Saito and group also reported that there was mostly no change in ketones and glucose-metabolizing enzymes (Saito 2021). In 1998, Hoyer and his associates demonstrated that there are reduced levels of insulin in the brain as well as dysfunction of insulin receptors (Riederer 2014). The Hoyer group has reported from animal studies that insulin resistance in the brain changes the fatty acid composition of the cell membrane and degrades its structure and performance (Plaschke 2010).

Hoyer and associates, as well as many other groups of researchers, have performed extensive studies of the many aspects of insulin resistance and how these factors play out in Alzheimer's disease. The problem of insulin resistance and deficiency in the brain is sometimes referred to as diabetes of the brain or type 3 diabetes, but Hoyer's associates prefer the term "insulin resistance brain state" (IRBS) (Salkovic-Petrisic 2009).

As discussed in chapter 3, it is possible to have brain insulin resistance without having type 1 or type 2 diabetes, although people with diabetes are much more likely to develop dementia, though not necessarily the Alzheimer's type. Several studies have reported that there is greater cognitive impairment associated with poorer blood sugar control, longer duration of diabetes, and in people with complications of diabetes, such as kidney failure and damage to the retina in the eyes. Cognitive impairment is also common in people with chronic diseases that are often associated with diabetes, like high blood pressure and heart disease. Brain-imaging studies show areas of decreased glucose uptake and/or accelerated atrophy (shrinkage) of the brain in some diabetics who may not yet display cognitive impairment on testing.

There are also reports of people with Alzheimer's becoming diabetic only after developing Alzheimer's (Janson 2004; Clarke 2015), but it is not clear if this is related to what they are eating and/or the change in glucose metabolism. It has been proposed that beta amyloid generated in the brain can accumulate in other organs, such as the pancreas and muscles, and attach to and damage insulin receptors, resulting in insulin resistance (Folch 2018). Each factor involved in insulin resistance—elevated insulin levels, high blood sugar, abnormal glucose tolerance, obesity, atherosclerosis, and high blood pressure—is a separate risk factor for developing Alzheimer's. Therefore, having these other factors rolled into type 2 diabetes greatly increases the risk of developing Alzheimer's and other dementias, some of which are now called "atypical Alzheimer's" (Zhao 2009).

In a study of the brains and pancreases of 100 people with Alzheimer's, compared to people who had type 2 diabetes without Alzheimer's, and controls with neither, 81 percent of the people with Alzheimer's also had type 2 diabetes or abnormal fasting glucose levels (prediabetes). Also, deposits of beta amyloid in the islets where insulin is made in the pancreas were more frequent and more extensive in the people who had Alzheimer's compared to the people who did not (Janson 2004).

In type 2 diabetes, blood insulin levels tend to be abnormally high, sometimes extremely high, and this appears to result in downregulation (fewer numbers available) of insulin receptors at the blood–brain barrier, which would lead to decreased transport of insulin across the blood–brain barrier. Also, the inflammation associated with diabetes, which is related to chronically elevated blood sugar and high insulin levels, may damage the blood–brain barrier, delicate brain cells, and other structures, such as the myelin sheath surrounding nerve fibers and small and large blood vessels. So, there seems to be a strong link between diabetes and dementia, but it is not crystal-clear which comes first in all cases. On the other hand, insulin resistance with decreased uptake in the brain has been documented in young people in their twenties who are at risk due to family history of Alzheimer's (Reiman 2004), in young women with polycystic ovary syndrome (Castellano 2015), and in case reports of young people with mutations of presenilin 1 and 2, which causes the familial form of Alzheimer's (Reiman 2012; Schöll 2011; Nikisch 2008).

People who have type 2 diabetes and the ApoE4 gene tend to have a higher burden of beta amyloid plaques, and the plaques appear earlier than in people with diabetes who are not ApoE4 carriers. Insulin receptors are normally located on the cell membrane. However, Zhao and associates were able to show in a mouse model of Alzheimer's that ApoE4 interacts with insulin receptors and traps them in endosomes, which interferes with insulin signaling, production of ATP, and metabolism of glucose (Zhao 2017). Endosomes are tiny organelles inside cells that are involved in sorting and transporting various substances to and from the cell membrane and other structures. Also, ApoE4 carriers tend to have higher levels of those toxic, sticky advanced glycation end-products (AGEs), which appear to place them at greater risk of diabetes and dementia (Deo 2020; Mooldijk 2020). So having the ApoE4 gene as well as diabetes is not a good combination if a person wants to avoid Alzheimer's.

For many years, the prevailing belief was that the brain operates independently of insulin, an idea that is not correct and has been difficult to overcome. Just over two decades ago, multiple groups began to report study results that contradict this idea. A basic well-known function of insulin is to unlock the door for glucose uptake into most cells outside the brain, but this may occur more indirectly in brain cells.

As it turns out, there are insulin receptors on neurons and all types of glial cells throughout the brain. Insulin receptors are present in cells at the blood–brain barrier and are more concentrated in areas like the cerebellum (involved in physical movement and balance), hypothalamus (controls hunger, thirst, temperature, certain hormones, and more), and olfactory bulb (involved in sense of smell). Insulin receptors

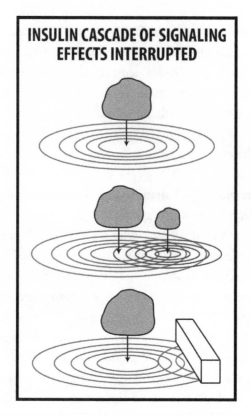

FIGURE 10.18. The insulin cascade of signaling effects. When insulin attaches to insulin receptors, its signaling effects set off an enormous cascade of chemical reactions throughout multiple biochemical pathways. This is not a one-way single chain of events but more like what happens when you drop a giant rock into a lake, which generates waves going out in a radial fashion. A second smaller rock (think of an unexpected substance like a drug) dropped near the original rock will disrupt the symmetric pattern of the ripples and introduce confusion as the ripples take off in many different directions. A dam (think of insulin resistance) near the rock will completely block the radiating pattern at that point and divert the water in a different direction.

are even more densely packed on cells located in the hippocampus and cerebral cortex, two areas important to learning and memory that are directly affected early in Alzheimer's. The available evidence has not yet drawn a complete and direct line between insulin receptors on neurons and other brain cells, nor determined if the receptors are required for transport of glucose into those cells.

Insulin regulates glucose uptake into the brain at the blood–brain barrier. Insulin affects production of neurotransmitters, such as acetylcholine and dopamine, and controls their reuptake (reabsorption) into cells after they are deployed at the synapse. Insulin regulates appetite, food intake, and reproduction by controlling hormones in the hypothalamus, and it also promotes the very survival of neurons. Given its very broad range of effects, it is logical that disruption in how much insulin is present in the brain and in how insulin functions would have many undesirable consequences (see figure 10.18).

In Alzheimer's and in some other neurodegenerative diseases, beta amyloid binds to insulin receptors and causes inactivation and migration of insulin receptors away from their normal location (Zhao 2017; Folch 2019). As previously mentioned, insulin also tends to accumulate within neurons that contain P-tau tangles; these cells also have fewer insulin receptors and exhibit insulin resistance (Rodriquez-Rodriguez 2017).

Insulin, GLUTs, and PDH Complex 1

Contrary to older assumptions, insulin crosses the blood–brain barrier, but slowly, and gains entry by binding to insulin receptors (Gawdi 2020). Insulin can be measured in the cerebrospinal fluid (CSF). Brain insulin levels are much lower than blood levels. The amount of insulin transported into the brain appears to be reduced in obesity, inflammation, high blood sugar, diabetes, brain aging, and in Alzheimer's. Current evidence, requiring further confirmation, indicates that insulin is also produced in specific areas of the brain (Arnold 2018), such as in immature and mature neurons but not in glia (Salkovic-Petrisic 2009).

Insulin appears to play a role in monitoring energy stores related to glucose uptake, and directly or indirectly activates glucose transporters, called GLUTs. There are at least eight basic types—GLUT 1 through GLUT 8—and at least three glucose "co-transporters" used in different tissues and cell types. Also, the type of sugar affects what GLUT is needed. Each brain-cell type uses at least two types of GLUTs, one for transporting glucose or other sugar through the cell membrane, and another involved in glucose metabolism within the cell. Currently, much is unknown about some of the GLUTs and co-transporters.

In Alzheimer's disease, GLUT 1 and GLUT 3 are deficient, occurring very early in the disease process (Koepsell 2020). GLUT 1 is influenced by insulin activity and is involved in glucose uptake at the blood–brain barrier, where the endothelial cells lining blood vessels form tight junctions to regulate what goes in and out of the brain. So, deficiency of GLUT 1 results in less glucose transport into the brain. GLUT 1 is also important for shuttling glucose from astrocytes to neurons. The deficiency of GLUT 1 also decreases blood flow to the brain and increases formation of beta amyloid plaques, thereby contributing to memory impairment. GLUT 1 deficiency syndrome (GLUT 1 DS) is a rare disorder that can result in severe developmental delays and seizures in infants and children. Children with GLUT 1 DS respond remarkably well to a strict ketogenic diet, since ketones, when elevated in the blood, readily cross the blood–brain barrier, and ketones can provide fuel in place of glucose to brain cells. This supports use of a keto diet and other ketogenic strategies in people with Alzheimer's, since they also suffer from GLUT 1 deficiency.

GLUT 3 is influenced by, but is not dependent on, insulin and is involved with glucose uptake directly into neurons. GLUT 3 deficiency impacts many functions of neurons, since there is inadequate fuel to make enough ATP to fully operate the cell machinery (Norwitz 2019).

GLUT 4 is dependent on insulin and is also important to neurons, where it is more directly involved in ATP production and firing of impulses by neurons to communicate with other neurons. GLUT 4 also appears to regulate whole-body glucose homeostasis (stability of glucose levels) from the brain. Elsewhere in the body, GLUT 4 is mainly found in fat cells, skeletal muscle, and heart muscle. In type 2 diabetes, reduced insulin sensitivity interferes with the circuit involving insulin, insulin receptors, and GLUT 4, resulting in decreased glucose uptake into cells (Koepsell 2020).

GLUT 5 is primarily involved with transporting fructose, the main sugar found in fruit. Standard table sugar is about half fructose, and high-fructose corn syrup has been added to a great many sugary drinks and processed foods since about 1970. Fructose induces the formation of the sticky inflammatory advanced glycation end-products (AGEs).

High consumption of fructose leads to insulin resistance in neurons and promotes memory impairment in animal models of dementia (Koepsell 2020).

In addition to deficiencies in certain GLUTs, pyruvate dehydrogenase (PDH) Complex 1 is deficient in Alzheimer's. This is a critical enzyme set used in the multi-step conversion of pyruvate (the product of glycolysis) to acetyl coenzyme A before it enters the TCA cycle in the mitochondria in the pathway to make ATP (Gray 2014). PDH Complex 1, GLUT 1, and GLUT 3 deficiencies also occur in certain other neurodegenerative diseases and following traumatic brain injury. As for GLUT 1 DS, the ketogenic diet is the first line of treatment for PDH deficiency syndrome, a genetic disease that causes neurodegeneration.

Considering PDH Complex 1 deficiency, insulin resistance, and deficiencies of GLUT 1 and 3, there seems to be a conspiracy against getting glucose into the Alzheimer's brain and brain cells. This set of deficiencies could also explain the "brain-energy gap" described in chapter 2. As a reminder, in cognitively healthy older adults, there is a 7 to 9 percent difference between how much energy the brain needs and how much is available, called the "brain-energy gap." The brain-energy gap widens to at least 10 percent in mild cognitive impairment and to at least 20 percent in mild Alzheimer's, worsening with each stage of progression (Cunnane 2020). Age is the biggest risk factor for developing Alzheimer's, affecting 3 percent of people ages sixty-five to seventy-four, 17 percent ages seventy-five to eighty-four, and 32 percent of people eighty-five and older (Alzheimer's Association 2019). The age-related brain-energy gap may be at one end of a continuum that can progress to MCI and then Alzheimer's if poor diet or other exacerbating factors come into play such as insulin resistance, inflammation, high blood pressure, air pollution, or infection.

An unanswered question for me is whether GLUT 1, GLUT 3, and PDH Complex 1 are inherently deficient in Alzheimer's, or whether levels are low due to insulin resistance since the GLUT 1 and GLUT 3 are influenced by insulin and PDH Complex 1 is at the end of glycolysis. If glucose cannot enter the cell, glycolysis will be lower within the cell and there would be less need for PDH Complex 1.

Ketones Bypass Insulin Resistance, GLUT, and PDH Complex 1 Deficiency

Ketones do not require insulin or GLUTs to cross the blood–brain barrier or to enter neurons and other cells. Ketones use monocarboxylic acid transporters, which are unimpaired in Alzheimer's, allowing ketones to easily cross the blood–brain barrier and enter neurons and other brain cells. Ketones do not require conversion to pyruvate or the use of PHD complex 1 to drive production of ATP or other metabolic pathways. It makes sense, then, to incorporate ketogenic strategies into our lifestyles to help fill the brain-energy gap, reduce brain inflammation, and benefit from the other ketone effects that could ameliorate pathologies that occur in the aging brain and certain other neurological disorders, like Alzheimer's.

Ketones Restore Pyruvate Dehydrogenase (PDH) Complex 1 Activity, Improve Mitochondrial Function, and Reduce Oxidative Stress

In in vivo experiments, APP mouse model and wild mice were given injections of a 4:1 ratio of betahydroxybutyrate to acetoacetate versus saline for two months. Mitochondrial function improved by restoring PDH complex 1 activity (Yin 2016).

Glutathione is an antioxidant that protects mitochondrial DNA (mtDNA). Mitochondria from the hippocampus of rats fed a ketogenic diet showed increased production of glutathione, decreased production of hydrogen peroxide, which in excess is toxic to mitochondria, and decreased mtDNA damage (Jarrett 2008).

Virgin coconut oil (VCO) is rich in polyphenolic compounds, including caffeic acid, coumaric acid, ferulic acid, and several others. Pretreatment of HCT-15 (colon cancer) cells with VCO reduced oxidant-induced oxidative stress and cell death by restoring glutathione and related enzymes to near-normal levels (Illam 2017).

Addition of the MCT decanoic acid (C10:0) to neuron cultures led to a marked increase in activities of catalase, an enzyme found in peroxisomes, and PDH complex 1, and increased numbers of mitochondria. Caprylic acid C8:0 did not have this effect (Hughes 2014).

Insulin Resistance Provides a Broad Explanation for What Goes Wrong in Alzheimer's Disease: Vicious Cycles Explain Why It Progresses

Glucose homeostasis (steadiness of glucose levels within a relatively narrow range) is critical to the overall health of our body and brain. In Alzheimer's disease, every cell type in the brain is affected by insulin resistance and other factors related to getting glucose into the brain and into brain cells. Insulin resistance could set up a milieu that allows propagation of the many pathologies that occur in the Alzheimer's brain. Insulin resistance could then provide a broad explanation for what goes wrong in Alzheimer's disease.

Insulin resistance is involved in several vicious cycles that cause pathologies that then promote further insulin resistance. This phenomenon could explain why Alzheimer's progresses, spreading throughout the brain, eventually leading to severe disability and death. Insulin resistance:

- Promotes formation of beta amyloid plaques and reduces clearance of plaques from the brain. Plaques further worsen insulin resistance.
- Promotes formation of P-tau leading to neurofibrillary tangles. Neurons with tangles have fewer insulin receptors and accumulate insulin.

- Promotes inflammation and mitochondrial dysfunction which, in turn, lead to greater insulin resistance.
- Leads to chronic elevation of blood sugar, thereby promoting formation of inflammatory damaging advanced glycation end-products (AGEs). AGEs promote formation of plaques and tangles, and damage insulin, leading to further insulin resistance.

Insulin is highly involved in the metabolism of sugars, lipids, and proteins, and clearly affects glucose uptake into the brain and brain cells. It is likely that insulin resistance factors into formation of abnormally large lipid droplets, deficiencies and excess accumulation of many substances, and malfunction of many metabolic pathways that occur in Alzheimer's disease.

If glucose cannot get into the brain and brain cells to make ATP due to insulin resistance and/or insulin deficiency, that cell will become energy-starved, malfunction, and eventually die unless an alternative fuel is provided, such as ketones. As discussed in part 1, a healthy ketogenic diet can help control blood sugar in type 1 diabetes, put type 2 diabetes in remission, and improve cognition in type 3 diabetes (Alzheimer's).

Unfortunately, as Alzheimer's progresses, the extent and location of dead neurons and defective synapses may determine how much recovery is possible from ketogenic strategies, or from any other therapy for that matter. On the other hand, reversing insulin resistance and providing fuel to the brain as ketones by adopting a ketogenic lifestyle could slow down or stabilize the process by allowing dormant neurons to recover and form new synapses.

What About Insulin and Other Diabetes Treatments?

We have already discussed that diabetes greatly increases the risk of developing accelerated brain atrophy, cognitive decline, and dementia. Since insulin resistance is a fundamental metabolic setup for Alzheimer's and some other dementias, couldn't we simply treat people suffering from dementia with insulin and other diabetes medications like Metformin? On the other hand, could such a treatment help control blood sugar but also cause harm? While this idea is logical, clinical trials of insulin and diabetes drugs have been disappointing.

Many studies of the effects of insulin and diabetes medications on Alzheimer's have been reported. Until recently, the most promising appeared to be intranasal insulin (Frazier 2020). Deep in the nasal cavity, perforations in the bone separate the nasal cavity from the brain, called the cribriform plate. Olfactory nerves involved in the sense of smell connect to the brain through these perforations. This presents an opportunity to give insulin direct access to the brain using an inhalation device.

In several studies, intranasal insulin appeared to improve memory in healthy people and people with insulin resistance, though not in people with the ApoE4 gene. For example, a pilot study of 100 people with Alzheimer's and mild cognitive impairment treated for 4 months with intranasal insulin (20 or 40 units) reported moderate cognitive improvement, improved ability to function, and improved glucose uptake on FDG-PET scans; these improvements continued for at least 2 months after the insulin was discontinued (Craft 2012). However, a larger 240-person, 12-month study using 40 units of insulin daily versus a placebo, showed no beneficial effect for cognition or ability to function—a very disappointing outcome (Craft 2020).

While the idea of giving insulin intranasally to enter the brain is brilliant, this method would not necessarily direct insulin to the areas with insulin deficiency or correct the problem of fewer or unresponsive insulin receptors. Accumulation of insulin within neurons that have tangles is another concern, particularly around whether intranasal insulin could promote further abnormal accumulation.

What about other diabetes medications? Metformin works by decreasing glucose production in the liver, increasing insulin sensitivity in tissues, and suppressing appetite. Sulfonylureas are drugs that increase insulin release from the pancreas, appear to decrease glucose production in the liver, and suppress breakdown of fat. Newer-generation sulfonylureas include common drugs like glipizide, glimepiride, and glyburide.

One study analyzed results from five large cohorts totaling more than 4,000 older participants who were evaluated periodically over several years with cognitive testing and MRI imaging. Outcomes were compared for people with diabetes who were and were not taking insulin, Metformin, and sulfonylureas. People with diabetes who used insulin had a 50 percent greater risk of developing dementia than those who did not, but not necessarily Alzheimer's-type dementia. People who require insulin tend to have high blood sugars despite using other diabetes medications. Sulfonylurea drugs did not appear to increase or decrease risk of dementia. Unexpectedly, there was a 42 percent increased risk of dementia in people with diabetes who used Metformin (Weinstein 2019). The Takeda Pharmaceutical Company also reported that their drug pioglitazone was not effective in preventing MCI and Alzheimer's in clinical trials.

The results for insulin and Metformin were quite the opposite of what one might expect for a glucose-lowering drug. The authors speculated that a common adverse reaction of such drugs, hypoglycemia (low blood sugar), could explain the poor results. This happens when the blood insulin level exceeds what is needed to metabolize blood glucose. Just one episode of hypoglycemia in people with diabetes appears to increase the risk of later dementia by 27 percent compared to those who do not experience hypoglycemia (Mehta 2017). Hypoglycemia can have serious consequences, beginning with tremors, sweating, weakness, and, if untreated, confusion, loss of consciousness, seizures, and even death. Hypoglycemia has sent many diabetics to the emergency room. It is unclear whether the episodes of hypoglycemia reported in the Mehta study required medical intervention. It is more likely that serious, rather than mild, episodes of hypoglycemia would have a long-term consequence like dementia.

On the other hand, repeated episodes of hypoglycemia could be very harmful to the brain. During hypoglycemia, excessive, toxic concentrations of the excitatory amino acid glutamate can accumulate around neurons. Neurotoxicity induced by amino acids (glutamate and aspartate) is a hallmark of neurodegenerative diseases, such as Alzheimer's, ALS, Parkinson's disease, and others. Glutamate-induced neurotoxicity increases intracellular calcium ion levels, which "triggers a cascade of pathological reactions that culminate in the death of nerve cells" (Blaszczyk 2020).

In my opinion, due to the possible risk of hypoglycemia, Metformin and especially insulin do not appear to be appropriate drugs to prevent or treat dementia in people who are not diabetic. However, taking MCT oil, which is partly converted to ketones, can provide fuel to the brain in place of glucose and help prevent severe symptoms related to hypoglycemia in diabetics. An important study of MCT oil was conducted in people with "intensively treated" type 1 diabetes who were prone to severe hypoglycemic attacks, between six and thirty episodes per month. Ten of the eleven participants used a continuous pump to administer insulin under the skin; the eleventh required multiple daily shots of insulin. Hypoglycemia was induced in the participants by administering insulin. Nine people were studied twice, receiving MCT oil (40 grams) on one day and placebo on another. Cognitive testing was performed before and after by people who did not know whether they had received MCT oil or placebo. Blood glucose, insulin, fatty acids, and beta-hydroxybutyrate (BHB) levels were measured. BHB levels increased to an average of 0.35 mmol/L after taking MCT oil. In contrast to placebo, MCT prevented decline in cognitive performance during the hypoglycemic episodes on five of seven cognitive tests. Their findings suggest that MCT could be used as preventive therapy for such patients to preserve brain function during hypoglycemic episodes (Page 2009).

What Causes Insulin Resistance?

As we have discussed, insulin resistance could cause, trigger, or accelerate Alzheimer's, and the vicious cycles could explain the progressive downward spiral of the disease in a "self-propagating process"

(Salkovic-Petrisic 2009). Insulin resistance, and insulin deficiency in the brain and chronic elevation of blood sugar may provide a broad underlying explanation for the pathologies that occur in Alzheimer's, but what causes insulin resistance? If we can nail down the answer to that question, we may better understand what causes Alzheimer's disease.

Since diet can reverse insulin resistance, it is likely that poor diet could be a cause of insulin resistance, though not necessarily the one and only cause. Eating too much sugar, the wrong kind of sugar or fat, or synthetic chemicals or contaminants in our food could be the simple answer, considering that a major dietary shift in our diet has coincided with the epidemics of obesity, diabetes, and dementia over the past half century. Here are some possible culprits that could lead to insulin resistance, some of which are discussed in more detail in chapter 9:

- Nitrosamine compounds in processed foods, vitamin supplements, nitrogen fertilizers, beer, hard alcohol, and tobacco
- Excessive sugar intake, and especially high-fructose corn syrup, which promote formation of advanced glycation end-products
- Trans fats, toxic fats in reheated oils, and excessive linoleic acid

Some non-dietary culprits could include:
- Metals like lead, iron, mercury, and cadmium that accumulate through environmental exposures
- Infections: Viral infections, such as hepatitis C, enteroviruses, SARS CoV-2 (COVID-19), and others have been associated with new onset of diabetes in studies and case reports. Serious infections with SARS CoV-2 are more common in people with diabetes, and deterioration in blood sugar control can occur during infection, sometimes requiring massive doses of insulin (Lim, 2021). The 2003 SARS CoV virus was found to attach to receptors and directly damage pancreatic islet cells (Yang 2010).

Guidance from the NIH, CDC, and American Diabetes Association (https://diabetes.org) all agree that the causes of insulin resistance are not clear but have identified some predisposing factors. All three organizations agree that a healthier diet and increased physical activity can prevent progression from prediabetes to diabetes. These organizations have joined together to support a special initiative to recognize programs that follow specific guidelines to promote lifestyle changes to prevent diabetes.

People with the following predisposing genetic and lifestyle risk factors are more likely to develop insulin resistance (prediabetes, diabetes) (NIH/NIDDK):

- Overweight or obesity
- Age 45 or older
- Family history of diabetes (parent or sibling)
- African American, Alaska Native, American Indian, Asian American, Hispanic/Latino, Native Hawaiian, or Pacific Islander American ethnicity
- Lack of physical activity
- Disorders such as high blood pressure and abnormal cholesterol levels
- Sleep problems, especially sleep apnea
- A history of gestational diabetes (diabetes during pregnancy)
- A history of heart disease or stroke
- Metabolic syndrome—a combination of high blood pressure, abnormal cholesterol levels, and large waist size
- Polycystic ovary syndrome
- Hormonal disorders, such as Cushing's syndrome and acromegaly
- Use of certain medications such as glucocorticoids, certain antipsychotics, and others
- Depression

Insulin resistance does not happen overnight but may take years of poor diet to unfold. Adopting a low-carb higher-fat whole-food Mediterranean-style diet could reverse insulin resistance and slow down the progression of the pathologies in Alzheimer's disease. Some biomarkers of insulin resistance could improve within a matter of weeks to months, though people with more severe, longstanding insulin resistance might require eighteen months or longer to reach full remission. The key to overcoming insulin resistance is to be consistent and persistent and to recognize that this is a lifestyle change, not a temporary diet. A digression here or there is understandable and unlikely to undo your progress. However, if a person reverts to old habits and an unhealthy sugary diet, it will not take long for insulin resistance and its consequences to return.

It is also crucial to correct the gap in brain energy by providing ketones as fuel to brain cells that have been impacted by insulin resistance. Putting "fuel in the tank" could allow dormant or poorly functioning brain cells to resume their many important functions.

We do not know yet whether neurons will be repaired and fully restored, but correcting insulin resistance and providing fuel as ketones are reasonable strategies to prevent and fight Alzheimer's and other disorders of insulin resistance.

BRAIN ENERGY: GLUCOSE, KETONES, FATTY ACIDS, AND ATP

Glucose is the predominant fuel for the brain and other organs for people on a typical higher-carbohydrate diet. A critical purpose of "fuel" is to produce the energy molecule adenosine triphosphate (ATP), which also requires oxygen. To be useful as fuel, glucose must be able to cross the cell membrane and begin the multi-step process of glycolysis mostly within the cytosol (the watery component of the cell).

Glycolysis leads to production of pyruvate, which enters the mitochondria by way of the mitochondrial pyruvate carrier in the mitochondrial membrane. Within the mitochondrial matrix, pyruvate is metabolized to acetyl coenzyme A (acetyl-CoA). Acetyl-CoA delivers the simple acetyl group ($CH3CO$) (see figure 10.19) to the tricarboxylic acid (called TCA, citric acid, or Krebs) cycle (see figure 10.20) and other biochemical pathways, such as synthesis of steroid hormones, melatonin, and acetylcholine (acetyl group + choline). The TCA cycle is a series of chemical reactions that propels electron transport, ultimately leading to formation of the end-product ATP. ATP is made

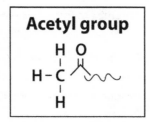

FIGURE 10.19. The simple acetyl group is important to many biochemical pathways, including production of ATP.

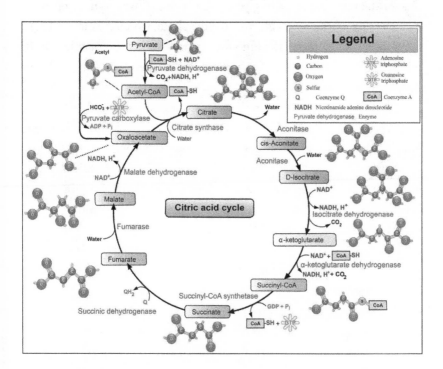

FIGURE 10.20. The tricarboxylic acid (TCA, Krebs, or citric acid) cycle in the mitochondria. Glucose is converted in several steps to pyruvate, which is transported into the mitochondria to enter the TCA cycle by way of acetyl-CoA to make ATP. Ketones and fatty acids also enter the mitochondria and enter the TCA cycle by way of acetyl-CoA. Figure from: "Citric acid cycle." Wikipedia. https://en.wikipedia.org/wiki/Citric_acid_cycle#/media/File:Citric_acid_cycle_with_aconitate_2.svg. Permission through GNU Free Documentation License – Wikipedia https://en.wikipedia.org/wiki/GNU_Free_Documentation_License

continuously through a recycling process. The other intermediate metabolites in the TCA cycle enter many other biochemical pathways as well.

Ketones and fatty acids, including medium-chain triglycerides, also enter the mitochondria and enter the TCA cycle by way of acetyl-CoA but do not require production of pyruvate through glycolysis first like glucose.

Making ATP Requires ATP

One of the required steps in glycolysis on the pathway to making ATP is conversion of glucose to glucose-6-phosphate, which requires ATP in a sort of feedback loop. The amount of energy a neuron or other brain cell needs dictates how much glucose is pulled into the brain and into the pathway to make ATP (Cunnane 2020). If glucose is available and glucose-6-phosphate levels are high due to energy demand, so long as oxygen is also available, ATP production will increase proportionately. This is referred to as "ATP-controlled glucose-oxygen metabolic synergy" (Blaszczyk 2020). If insulin resistance and/or other critical factors slow down the production of ATP (deficiencies of the vitamin NAD, GLUT 1, GLUT 3, or PDH Complex 1 deficiency or inhibition), the decreased availability of ATP will slow down glycolysis, which will further decrease ATP production. Deficiencies of the vitamin B3 (niacin), also called NAD, and its important metabolite nicotinamide riboside, are discussed in chapter 7.

The slowing of ATP production and the glycolytic pathway become a vicious cycle that intersects with the vicious cycles involving insulin resistance and other Alzheimer's pathologies, all of which contribute to the aging process and neurodegeneration. You might picture a battery-operated handheld tool that gradually slows as the battery dies and finally stops if you do not replace the battery. Energy production by compromised mitochondria within a neuron winds down and eventually takes the whole brain cell down, along with the cell's ability to communicate with other brain cells. This winding-down process may ultimately leave the neuron or glial cell in a dormant state until either the insulin resistance (or vitamin deficiency or other factor) is corrected, and an effective fuel (ketones) is provided to ramp energy production back up. Neurons can also die in the process.

In the winding-down scenario, the highest energy-consuming processes are likely to be affected first. For example, synaptic neurotransmission uses 80 percent of the energy necessary for the functioning of neuronal networks, and there are trillions of synapses engaged in constant activity. Neurogenesis, synaptogenesis, and synaptic pruning, called neuronal plasticity, are also high-energy-consuming processes that mainly rely on ATP-controlled glucose-oxygen synergy. Early on, the brain may be able to compensate; but as this self-propagating process continues and spreads, signs and symptoms of neurodegeneration will appear. Areas of the brain likely to be affected first are those with high energy requirements, the smallest numbers of neurons, and mediocre replacement of connecting neurons through neurogenesis. Neuronal plasticity is critical to learning and memory; therefore, impairments in learning and memory are some of the earliest signs of Alzheimer's disease (Blaszczyk 2020).

Ketones Bypass the Problem of Glucose Hypometabolism

Fatty acids, including medium-chain triglycerides, and ketones are transported across cell membranes and enter the mitochondria, where they are metabolized (like pyruvate from glucose metabolism) to acetyl-CoA which provides the acetyl group to the TCA cycle, ultimately leading to production of ATP. Worth noting, acetyl-CoA can also be converted to ketone bodies when acetyl-CoA levels are high, which occurs when the TCA capacity is exceeded.

Dependency on insulin, whether directly or indirectly, differentiates glucose metabolism from fatty acid and ketone metabolism in the production of ATP. Fatty acids and ketones do not require insulin, GLUTs, or PDH complex 1 and have their own specific transporters

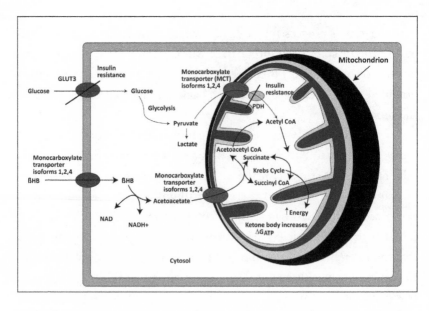

FIGURE 10.21. Ketones bypass problem of insulin resistance and gain access to cells when glucose cannot. Drawing by Joanna Newport.

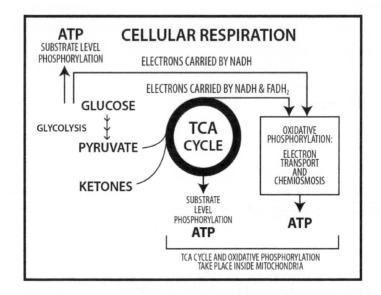

FIGURE 10.22. Aerobic cellular respiration requires oxygen to convert fuel from food (glucose, fatty acids, proteins, and ketones) to produce adenosine triphosphate (ATP), by adding a phosphate group to adenosine diphosphate (ADP), carbon dioxide, and water. Drawing by Joanna Newport.

to enter the cell. Long-chain fatty acids do not cross the blood–brain barrier easily, but medium-chain triglycerides and ketones do and, therefore, can bypass the problem of insulin resistance, allowing the mitochondria to produce ATP (see figure 10.21). Ketones are more efficient as fuel, using less oxygen to make more ATP than an equivalent amount of glucose. The process of producing ATP under the usual condition in which oxygen is available is called aerobic cellular respiration (see figure 10.22).

A downstream consequence of insulin resistance is decreased production of ATP. Numerous cell processes are highly dependent on ATP. Here are some of the important things that will not happen normally if there is not enough ATP (Salkovic-Petrisic 2009; Blaszczyk 2020):

- Conversion of glucose to glucose-6-phosphate during glycolysis leading to TCA cycle to make more ATP
- Sorting, folding, transport, and degradation of proteins
- Maintenance of a pH of 6.0 in the endoplasmic reticulum and Golgi apparatus, and heat shock-guided transport across these compartments
- Axonal transport of proteins, often over a long distance
- Regulation of the conformational state of insulin-degrading enzyme (which degrades insulin as well as beta amyloid)
- Maintenance of intracellular and extracellular ion homeostasis
- Maintenance of biophysical membrane properties
- Regulation of synaptic membrane phospholipase A2
- Maintenance of synaptic transmission
- Metabolism of tau protein and beta amyloid precursor protein

CONCLUSIONS AND FINAL WORDS

Alzheimer's disease is a complex intertwining of many derangements involving numerous biological pathways and processes affecting every type of brain cell. Many of these derangements are also at play in aging, but are exaggerated and accelerated in Alzheimer's and other brain disorders, likely exacerbated by inflammation.

Abnormal brain-glucose metabolism is the earliest known feature of Alzheimer's, appearing one or two decades before symptoms begin. A significant "brain-energy gap" between how much energy the brain requires and how much it receives is present even in cognitively healthy older adults (7 to 9 percent). The brain-energy gap widens in people with mild cognitive impairment (>10 percent) and becomes much more prominent in early Alzheimer's disease (>20 percent), worsening with each stage of the disease (Cunnane 2020). Abnormal glucose metabolism has many consequences; most fundamentally, it impairs the production of ATP in mitochondria, thereby impacting nearly every cellular function. Cellular processes include, at the very least, synthesis, recycling, transport, and disposal of thousands of proteins, lipids, and other substances; maintenance of the integrity of the cell membrane, mitochondria, and other organelles within the cell; homeostasis in metabolic processes; detection and control of foreign-body or microbial invasion; and effective communication and coordination of activities with other cells.

Insulin is a powerful signaling master hormone that directly or indirectly controls many components of numerous biological pathways, including the metabolism of glucose, lipids, and proteins, and control of inflammation. A problem with insulin would impact every function of insulin and is currently the best explanation for the brain-energy gap and the abnormal glucose uptake that precedes Alzheimer's symptoms. Damage to the insulin molecule; inactivation or sequestration of insulin; decreased responsiveness of insulin receptors; and smaller numbers of available insulin receptors could all be in play as mechanisms that lead to abnormal glucose uptake and decreased ATP production.

Insulin resistance and insulin deficiency are present in the earliest stages of Alzheimer's in the area of the brain where Alzheimer's begins, affecting all signaling pathways involving insulin and insulin growth factor. This problem with insulin spreads throughout the brain with each stage of Alzheimer's and eventually becomes widespread and severe (De la Monte 2008). Brain atrophy, along with deterioration in cognition and functionality, occurs simultaneously with the spread of insulin resistance and deficiency. It becomes quite pronounced in the last stages of Alzheimer's, when the victim becomes completely dependent for every personal need and can no longer communicate those needs.

Nearly every brain pathology in Alzheimer's has a connection to insulin and insulin resistance. In a series of self-propagating vicious cycles, insulin resistance promotes formation of and impedes removal of plaques; promotes inflammation and tangle formation; and damages mitochondria and other cell structures, all of which, in turn, further worsen insulin resistance. Energy production winds down until individual cells no longer function normally. Collectively, as massive numbers of dormant or abnormally functioning cells accumulate and become disconnected from each other, the brain can no longer compensate. Symptoms appear that herald the progressive downward spiral that will ultimately take the life of its victim unless either another fatal process intervenes, or a treatment intercedes to stop the downward spiral.

The pathologies that occur in Alzheimer's disease are almost certainly downstream effects of a broader process that causes Alzheimer's, although these pathologies contribute to the progression as part of the self-propagating cycle. Most drugs developed to treat Alzheimer's target a specific enzyme or other substance deep in a biological pathway, and are meant to interfere with a single pathological process, or remove the product of that process—such as plaques or tangles—as if what happens in Alzheimer's occurs in a straight line from beginning to end. Such drugs ignore what triggers the process and what chemical reactions precede the point of intervention in the pathway leading to that abnormal process. In addition, such drugs do not address the broader fundamental problem that could explain the complex intertwining of many derangements affecting the brain in Alzheimer's disease: a problem with insulin. By the same token, drugs are usually synthetic compounds, often analogs of natural substances, similar but not the same, and target unintended tissues and biological processes, leading to adverse and sometimes serious effects.

A problem with insulin could provide a broad explanation for what goes wrong in the Alzheimer's brain, setting up a milieu that allows propagation of the many pathologies we have discussed. There are several possible triggers or causes of insulin resistance, and nearly all of them are related to what we eat. Since a change in diet can reverse and even put insulin resistance into remission while improving cognition, it is likely that a poor diet can also cause insulin-resistance related cognitive decline.

Correcting insulin resistance and providing fuel as ketones are reasonable strategies to prevent and fight Alzheimer's and other disorders of insulin resistance. Adopting a reasonable ketogenic wholefood Mediterranean-style diet, as detailed in chapter 4, could reverse insulin resistance and slow down the progression of the pathologies in Alzheimer's disease. Overcoming insulin resistance requires a lifestyle change, not just a temporary diet, and patience, persistence, and consistency are important.

A whole-food Mediterranean-style diet and a few key supplements, like DHA, choline, and certain B vitamins, could also ensure that the brain has the nutrients it needs to produce energy, grow and maintain healthy cells, and carry out many other important cell functions.

Increasing blood ketone levels through a ketogenic diet and other ketogenic strategies, like fasting, exercise, consuming medium-chain triglycerides, and exogenous ketone supplements can provide immediate fuel to neurons and other brain cells that are affected by insulin resistance and unable to use glucose normally to make ATP. Over the longer term, ketones could help reduce inflammation and control or prevent pathologies related to aging and Alzheimer's. Ketones also mimic some signaling activities of insulin and could help address the broad fundamental problem of insulin resistance.

Correcting insulin resistance and providing ketones to the brain could provide the key to unlocking the pathway to healthier brain aging and preventing, slow down, and possibly reversing symptoms and pathologies of Alzheimer's and other dementias. Changing other lifestyle risk factors like controlling blood pressure; getting better-quality sleep; treating sleep apnea; and avoiding potentially harmful dietary exposures, polluted air and soil, infections, and activities with high risk of head injury could remove factors that can trigger or contribute to unhealthy brain aging.

Alzheimer's does not have to be your fate!

ADDENDA

KETO-FRIENDLY RECIPES

MCT AND COCONUT OIL MIXTURE

YIELD: 28 ounces

16 ounces MCT Oil
12 ounces coconut oil

DIRECTIONS: Warm coconut oil until completely liquid by placing container in a pan of hot water. Use funnel to add MCT and coconut oil to a glass quart container, such as MCT oil bottle, recap securely, and invert several times to mix the oils now and before each use. Store at room temperature.

OPTIONAL: Add 1 or more tablespoons of liquid soy lecithin to allow for easier mixing with other liquids and provide phospholipids.

COCONUT MILK

YIELD: Each 4-ounce serving provides 15 grams (about one tablespoon) of coconut oil

> 1 can of undiluted full fat coconut milk (with 11 grams fat per 2 ounces)
> ½ can of water or coconut water
> 10 drops liquid stevia OR 1 to 2 teaspoons of honey, agave syrup, or other sweetener to taste
> Pinch of salt

DIRECTIONS: Place ingredients in a container and shake well before use. Store coconut milk in the refrigerator and discard unused portion after four days. When used for children, discard after two days.

VARIATION: For a thinner version, use 1½ cans of water or coconut water.

BERRY-COCONUT MILK SMOOTHIE

YIELD: One 14- to 16-ounce serving

½ cup crushed ice
1 cup frozen blueberries or 4 large frozen strawberries
⅓ cup sliced almonds
1 teaspoon honey, agave syrup, or equivalent sweetener such as stevia
1 cup Coconut Milk (above),
  or cow or goat milk while gradually increasing your coconut oil intake
1 hard-boiled or raw egg (microwave for at least 20 seconds)
2 tablespoons vanilla or unflavored whey protein powder
Extra coconut oil (melted) or MCT/coconut oil (optional)

DIRECTIONS: Place all ingredients in a blender and blend on "liquefy" speed for about 30 seconds. If mixture is too thick, add more coconut milk as needed.

NOTE: For those who are concerned about adding raw egg, microwave the egg for about 20 seconds to kill bacteria before adding to other ingredients.

VARIATIONS: Add ½ banana and 2 large strawberries per serving, or substitute equivalent amount of apple, blueberry, or pomegranate juice for part or all of the milk.

For probiotic smoothie, substitute ½ cup kefir for part of the coconut milk.

For peanut butter smoothie, add ¼ frozen banana and 1 tablespoon fresh ground or natural peanut or almond butter in place of berries.

GREEN COCONUT SMOOTHIE

YIELD: One 14- to 16-ounce serving

½ cup crushed ice

⅓ cup sliced almonds

1 cup leafy greens, such as kale, spinach, and/or spring mix

½ cucumber cut up

1 celery stalk cut up

1 tablespoon lemon juice

1 teaspoon honey, agave syrup, or equivalent stevia or sweetener, if desired

1 cup Coconut Milk (above),

or cow or goat milk while gradually increasing your coconut oil intake

2 tablespoons vanilla or unflavored whey protein powder

⅓ cup sliced almonds (optional)

Extra coconut oil (melted) or MCT/coconut oil (optional)

DIRECTIONS: Place all ingredients in a blender and blend on "liquefy" speed for about 30 seconds. If mixture is too thick, add more coconut milk as needed.

MARY'S GREEK YOGURT BREAKFAST OR SNACK

YIELD: 1 serving

½ cup plain full fat Greek yogurt

6 to 8 drops liquid stevia

1 tablespoon MCT oil or MCT//143

1 tablespoon unsweetened grated coconut

¼ cup unsalted organic nuts (your choice), crushed or whole

Optional: 1 or 2 tablespoons peanut protein

DIRECTIONS: Mix stevia, oil, and peanut protein into yogurt thoroughly with a spoon. Sprinkle coconut and nuts on top and stir in.

MARY'S RICOTTA CONCOCTION
(BREAKFAST OR SNACK)

YIELD: 1 serving

- ½ cup full fat ricotta
- 6 to 8 drops stevia
- 2 ounces coconut milk or 1 tablespoon MCT oil or MCT//143
- ¼ cup organic seeds and/or nuts, whole, sliced, or chopped
- 1 tablespoon unsweetened grated coconut

DIRECTIONS: Mix stevia and coconut milk or oil into ricotta thoroughly with a spoon, then add nuts and grated coconut and stir again.

MARY'S NUT AND SEED GRANOLA

YIELD: About 12 half-cup servings

16 Brazil nuts, chopped

1 cup each of almonds, macadamias, pecans (or favorite nuts), chopped

¼ cup sunflower seeds

2 tablespoons each of chia seeds, flax seeds, and sesame seeds

½ cup unsweetened grated or flaked coconut

1 teaspoon cinnamon

1 teaspoon sea salt

1 tablespoon monkfruit powder (to taste)

1 teaspoon vanilla extract

½ cup macadamia oil or coconut oil, melted

2 tablespoons coconut milk, heavy cream, or half and half

DIRECTIONS: Preheat oven to 300°F (150°C). Thoroughly mix all dry ingredients together in a large bowl. Mix oil and vanilla extract together and pour over top of dry ingredients and toss thoroughly. Spread mixture on a large ungreased baking sheet. Bake for twenty minutes, remove from oven, and toss ingredients. Spread out ingredients again and place back in oven for 10 more minutes. Allow 30 minutes to cool before eating. Serve with about 2 tablespoons coconut milk, heavy cream, or half and half.

KETO EGGY PECAN PANCAKES

YIELD: 4 pancakes

2 eggs, beaten
10 drops liquid stevia or another sweetener
½ cup "keto" pancake mix (such as Birch Benders)
¼ cup pecan pieces or halves
1 tablespoon coconut oil
1 tablespoon butter

DIRECTIONS: Add sweetener and "keto" pancake mix to eggs and whisk. Preheat large skillet to low-moderate heat and add coconut oil and butter. When oils are bubbling, spoon out mixture to form 4 pancakes in the skillet. When edges of pancakes appear dry (about 3 to 4 minutes), carefully flip pancakes over and continue to cook until pancake is firm and slightly browned on both sides. Eat as is or with honey spread thinly on pancake.

MARY'S KETO OATMEAL

YIELD: About 6 servings

3 cups water

1 cup steel-cut whole grain oats

¼ cup unsweetened grated coconut

2 tablespoons chia seeds (optional)

¼ teaspoon sea salt

10 to 15 drops liquid stevia (optional)

¼ cup coconut oil

DIRECTIONS: Bring water to a boil. Stir in oats, coconut, and chia seeds. Add salt and stevia (optional). Stir every few minutes until oatmeal reaches desired consistency, about 15 to 20 minutes. Stir in coconut oil, turn off heat, and rest oatmeal for about 5 minutes. Divide into bowls to make about six servings. Serve with coconut milk, heavy cream, or half and half, if desired, to increase fat content further.

MARY'S FAVORITE OMELET

YIELD: One serving

> 1 tablespoon coconut oil
>
> 2 or 3 fresh eggs
>
> 2 pinches of salt
>
> Pepper to taste
>
> 4 cherry tomatoes, cut in half
>
> 6 pitted kalamata olives, cut in half
>
> 1½ ounces shredded cheddar cheese

DIRECTIONS: Heat coconut oil at low-medium heat in a nonstick omelet-style skillet. With a wire whisk, beat eggs, then whisk in salt and pepper and pour evenly into hot skillet. Leave undisturbed for several minutes. When the omelet is about ¾ set (some liquid egg still on top) carefully flip omelet with a spatula. Evenly distribute the tomato and olive pieces as well as about one ounce of cheese on half of the omelet and use spatula to fold omelet in half, covering the vegetables and cheese. Distribute the rest of the cheese evenly over the top of the folded omelet. When cheese on top begins to melt, the omelet is done.

VARIATIONS: Make a Greek-style omelet by using 2 to 3 large spoonfuls of Greek Salad (see below) with feta cheese in place of other vegetables and cheeses.

Add 1 cup fresh spinach leaves and 2 ounces feta cheese.

MARY'S WHATEVER FRITTATA

YIELD: 4 servings

4 tablespoons coconut oil
About two cups fresh or one bag frozen vegetables of your choice
Salt and pepper, and/or your favorite spice mix to sprinkle on vegetables
¾ cup of your choice of shredded cheese or ½ cup crumbled feta cheese
6 fresh eggs
Two to three more pinches of salt
1 tablespoon grated parmesan or Romano cheese

DIRECTIONS: Select an omelet-style skillet that can also be used in the oven. Place oven rack about five inches below broiler and preheat broiler to high temperature. Crack eggs into a bowl. Heat coconut oil in the skillet on top of the stove at low-medium heat. Sauté vegetables in the oil, stirring often, until tender, about 4 to 5 minutes. Add salt and pepper and other spices to vegetables when nearly finished, mix well, and distribute the vegetables evenly around the bottom of the skillet. While vegetables are cooking, beat eggs with a wire whisk and add salt and cheese and mix thoroughly. When vegetables are ready, pour egg mixture evenly over the vegetables, then continue to cook undisturbed for about 4 to 5 minutes until edges are dry and slightly brown; egg mixture will appear runny on the top. Sprinkle parmesan or Romano cheese evenly on top of frittata and place under broiler for at least three minutes. Be sure to set a timer to avoid burning. After three minutes, open oven and pull rack out enough to check omelet. With an oven glove on your hand, shake handle of the skillet gently; if top does not "jiggle" and appears lightly browned, the frittata is set and ready to be removed from the oven. If the top jiggles, replace under broiler for 1 to 2 more minutes, watching closely, and check again. Allow to cool for at least five minutes, then cut into quarters and serve.

VARIATION: Add leftover meat, fish, or poultry of any kind. You can add whatever you like!

SIMPLE SALAD DRESSING OR VEGETABLE TOPPING

YIELD: One or two servings

1 tablespoon of your favorite salad dressing
1 tablespoon MCT oil or coconut/MCT oil mixture

DIRECTIONS: Mix all ingredients together with a wire whisk and pour immediately onto salad or vegetables and toss. Excess can be stored in refrigerator, then rewarmed and remixed before serving.

MANY COLORS SALAD

YIELD: About 6 servings

1 cup broccoli florets

1 cup cauliflower florets

1 cup red cherry tomatoes

½ to 1 cup yellow sweet or bell peppers, cut up

2 carrots, cut up

1 cup mushrooms, cut up

½ large sweet or purple onion, cut up

About 6 cups leafy green and purple spring mix

1½ cups shredded cheddar cheese

For Simple Salad Dressing:

6 tablespoons of your favorite salad dressing

6 tablespoons MCT oil or coconut/MCT oil mixture

DIRECTIONS: Wash all vegetables and spring mix thoroughly, place in a large salad bowl with cheese, and toss. Mix together ingredients of Simple Salad Dressing with a wire whisk and pour immediately onto salad and toss again just before serving.

ALTERNATIVE: Toss all vegetables except spring mix together, and use for two or three days by storing in refrigerator. At time of serving, add about one cup of mix to one cup of spring mix, and toss with a two-tablespoon serving of "Simple Salad Dressing or Vegetable Topping" above.

CHOPPED GREEK SALAD

YIELD: 6 to 8 servings

½ cup garbanzo or cannellini beans, drained

1 large cucumber, chopped

1 large bell pepper, chopped

½ large sweet onion, chopped

24 cherry tomatoes or 1 medium tomato, chopped

25 to 30 kalamata or black olives

7-ounce block of feta cheese, cut into small pieces

About 6 cups leafy green and purple spring mix

Salad dressing:

3 tablespoons olive oil

1½ tablespoon lemon juice

¼ teaspoon sea salt

2 teaspoons Greek seasoning (salt, garlic powder, black pepper, oregano, sage)

Optional: Additional salad dressing, per serving:

Your serving of MCT oil or MCT/coconut oil mixture

DIRECTIONS: To a large bowl or storage container add garbanzo beans, chopped cucumber, onion, bell pepper, tomatoes, olives, and feta, and toss together with ingredients of salad dressing (except MCT and coconut oil mixture). This can be stored in the refrigerator for several days. When ready to serve, for each serving add leafy spring mix to medium-size salad bowls about half filled. Add 2 to 3 large serving spoons full of chopped vegetable/feta mixture. Pour MCT/coconut oil mixture evenly over salad and toss.

VARIATION: At time of serving, add fresh cooked or canned beets (not pickled), chopped. If added beforehand, the beets will discolor other vegetables.

CHICKEN OR TUNA SALAD

YIELD: 2 to 4 servings

> 2 cups cooked chicken or tuna, cut into small chunks
> ½ cup celery, chopped
> ½ cup sliced almond or chopped walnuts
> ¼ cup mayonnaise
> 2 tablespoons MCT oil or MCT//143
> Salt and pepper to taste

DIRECTIONS: Toss chicken or tuna, celery, and nuts together. In a separate bowl, use a wire whisk to thoroughly blend mayonnaise and MCT oil or coconut-MCT oil mixture, then add to chicken mixture with salt and pepper to taste, and toss again until well mixed.

OPTIONAL: Mix additional MCT oil or MCT//143 oil mixture into your serving.

VARIATIONS: Add about 8 ripe black or kalamata olives, cut up.

GARLICKY SPINACH

YIELD: 2 to 3 servings

1 bunch of fresh spinach
2 to 3 tablespoons coconut oil
Level tablespoon minced garlic
¼ teaspoon sea salt

DIRECTIONS: Heat coconut oil in a large skillet at just below medium heat. When heated, add minced garlic and use a spatula to distribute over skillet surface. Add spinach and move around with the spatula until all the leaves are just moist and slightly wilted but not soggy. Sprinkle with sea salt and stir in quickly, then remove from the skillet to avoid overcooking.

VARIATIONS: Add a heaping tablespoon of pine nuts along with the garlic.

MARY'S ROASTED ASPARAGUS, MUSHROOMS, AND BROCCOLI

YIELD: About 8 servings

1 bunch asparagus, with tough end broken off

1 head broccoli, cut into florets and stem pieces

2 cups favorite mushrooms, whole or sliced

½ teaspoon sea salt

¼ teaspoon pepper

2 tablespoons olive or avocado oil

2 tablespoons coconut oil, melted

1 tablespoon minced garlic

¼ cup parmesan or pecorino, grated

DIECTIONS: Preheat oven to 350°F (175°C). Distribute vegetables on a large baking sheet or two separate smaller baking sheets. Mix seasonings with oil and use pastry brush to coat the vegetables with the mixture. Sprinkle or grate cheese over all vegetables. Place in oven for 15 to 20 minutes.

ANGELA's HARISSA CHICKEN WITH CREAMY SAUCE

YIELD: 2 servings

1 whole boneless skinless chicken breast
4 tablespoons whole fat sour cream
2 ounces crumbled feta cheese
avocado oil or olive oil
1½ teaspoons harissa powder
salt and pepper

DIRECTIONS: Pat chicken dry with paper towels. Cut chicken breast into four long pieces, removing and discarding white cartilage down the middle. Season with 1½ teaspoons harissa powder, salt, and pepper on both sides. Cover bottom of skillet with olive oil or avocado oil. Preheat skillet on medium or medium-low. Do not overheat oil. Add chicken and cook until browned and cooked through to 165°F, about 4 to 6 minutes on each side. Mix sour cream with feta cheese, and add 1 tablespoon of olive oil or avocado oil and stir. If too thick, add water. Add salt and pepper to taste. Pour sauce over chicken and serve.

OPTIONAL: To sour cream sauce, add 1 to 2 tablespoons avocado, olive, or MCT/coconut oil mixture.

ANGELA'S BAKED SALMON WITH CREAMY DILL SAUCE

YIELD: 2 servings

¾ pound salmon
3 tablespoons whole fat sour cream
coconut oil (melted)
lemon (zested and cut)
fresh dill (finely chopped)
Za'atar spice (a pinch)
salt and pepper

DIRECTIONS: Preheat oven to 350°F. Pat salmon dry with paper towels. Place skin-side down on sheet pan. Melt coconut oil in a small bowl. Using a pastry brush, brush the tops of salmon with coconut oil. Season with pepper. Bake for 20 minutes or until the temperature is 145°F. In a small bowl, mix 3 tablespoons of whole-fat sour cream, lemon zest, a squeeze of lemon juice, and chopped dill. Salt and pepper to taste. Add a small amount of water and mix until dripping consistency. Pour sauce over salmon and season with a pinch of Za'atar spice.

OPTIONAL: For sauce, in place of water, add 1 to 2 tablespoons avocado, olive, or MCT/coconut oil mixture.

ANGELA'S EASY PORK CHOPS WITH
GREEN GODDESS SAUCE

YIELD: 2

2 medium boneless pork chops

3 tablespoons whole fat sour cream

lemon

2 teaspoons parsley (chop finely)

2 teaspoons chives (chop finely)

1 tablespoon Za'atar spice

1 clove garlic (minced)

avocado oil or olive oil

salt and pepper

DIRECTIONS: Squeeze lemon into a bowl. Hold one teaspoon back for sauce. Sprinkle in Za'atar spice, ¼ teaspoon of salt, and a pinch of pepper. Add the pork chops to the bowl, turning once to coat with spices. Let sit to marinate for about 10 minutes. Cover the bottom of a medium skillet with oil and heat on medium. Do not overheat. Add the pork chops to the skillet, turning once and cooking through to 170°F. If the chops are thick, you may need to cover loosely with a lid to trap the heat. Allow the pork chops to rest on a plate for about 5 minutes before serving. Add 3 tablespoons of sour cream to a small bowl. Add parsley, chives, a teaspoon of lemon juice, garlic to taste, salt and pepper. Stir until mixed. Add one teaspoon of water and stir again. Drop in dollops over pork chops. Optional: use a low-carbohydrate Green Goddess Dressing that has no added sugar.

CAROL'S QUICK MINESTRA

YIELD: About 12 cups.

⅓ cup extra virgin olive oil, plus extra for serving

1 large onion, chopped

8 to 10 garlic cloves (or fewer, to taste), finely chopped

1¼ pounds mushrooms, sliced

Fine sea salt

Freshly ground black pepper

1¼ pounds sliced or chopped kale

1 (24-ounce) jar Arrabiatta (spicy) pasta sauce, or other marinara sauce
  seasoned to taste with dried red hot chile flakes as desired

4 cups (32 ounces) chicken bone broth or vegetable broth, purchased or
  homemade

2 (15-ounce) cans cannellini beans, rinsed and drained,
  or about 3½ cups cooked cannellini beans

Parmigiano Reggiano or other hard cheese, for serving

DIRECTIONS: In a Dutch oven or other large pot, heat the ⅓ cup of olive oil over medium heat. Add the onion and cook, stirring occasionally, until softened but not browned, 3 to 5 minutes. Add the garlic and cook until fragrant, about 1 minute. Stir in the mushrooms and season with about ½ teaspoon of salt and a few grindings of pepper. Stir to coat the mushrooms well and cook 3 minutes longer.

Increase the heat to medium-high and stir in the kale, pasta sauce, and broth. Bring to a boil. Cover and reduce the heat to low. Cook until the kale is tender, and the flavors have blended, about 15 minutes. Stir in the beans and cook uncovered until heated through, about 5 minutes longer. Taste, adding more salt and pepper if needed. Ladle into shallow bowls and top each serving with a drizzle of olive oil and some freshly grated cheese.

COCONUT CHICKEN TENDERS OR FISH FINGERS

YIELD: 4 servings

1 whole egg, beaten

½ cup whole wheat panko or whole wheat Italian breadcrumbs

½ cup unsweetened grated coconut

¼ cup grated parmesan cheese

1 teaspoon garlic salt

¼ teaspoon pepper

3 tablespoons coconut oil

1 tablespoon olive or canola oil

12 fresh raw chicken tenders or cod fish filets, cut into strips

DIRECTIONS: Beat egg with a fork in a bowl. Combine all dry ingredients on a large plate and mix thoroughly with a fork. Place tenders or fish fingers in bowl with egg and stir until all are thoroughly coated. Heat coconut and olive or canola oil in a large skillet over medium heat. Roll each tender in dry mix until covered and set aside on another plate. When all tenders or fish fingers are coated, place in hot oil in skillet for about 3 to 4 minutes on each side until done.

SIMPLE SALMON DINNER FOR TWO

YIELD: 2 to 3 servings

10 to 12 ounces salmon fillet, any size

1 bunch fresh asparagus

2 to 3 tablespoons coconut oil, melted

Garlic and herb or other favorite seasoning

DIRECTIONS: Preheat oven to 350°F. Place aluminum foil on a large ungreased cookie sheet, or spray the cookie sheet with olive oil spray. On one side of the cookie sheet place a salmon fillet, skin side down, and on the other evenly distribute the asparagus spears. Melt about 2 to 3 tablespoons of coconut oil (or more for a very large fillet) and paint the oil onto the salmon and asparagus using a pastry brush. Sprinkle seasoning over fish and asparagus. Bake for 20 minutes. The salmon should be very moist and separate easily with a fork.

SIMPLE FISH SAUTE

YIELD: 1 fillet per serving

    1 fillet mahi, grouper, halibut, or other firm fish about ½ to ¾ inch thick
    Greek salad dressing for marinade
    2 tablespoons coconut and/or olive or avocado oil

DIRECTIONS: Marinate fish in Greek salad dressing for 30 minutes or longer. Heat skillet to low-moderate setting and add oil. When oil is hot, add fillet and cook for about 4 to 5 minutes on each side until fork-tender.

COCONUT FUDGE OR CANDIES

YIELD: About 16 ounces

1 cup coconut oil
8 ounces low carb or carb-free artificially sweetened dark chocolate bar
   or chips

DIRECTIONS: In a double boiler, melt and thoroughly mix together the oil and chocolate. Divide mixture equally into paper candy cups on a large plate, or into a plastic or silicone ice cube tray or mold, and place in the refrigerator. Chill until set. In a sixteen-cube tray, each cube will equal one tablespoon of coconut oil and will easily pop out of the tray.

VARIATION: Add about ¼ cup grated coconut to part or all of mixture and/or add nuts or nut pieces for variety. Put some mixture in bottom of candy cups or sections of ice cube, add peanut butter or creamed coconut that has been cut into pieces; then add remainder of mixture over the top of each candy piece. Chill in refrigerator until set, about 2 hours. Store in refrigerator.

RESOURCES

Suggested Reading Beyond References

Bredesen, Dale. The End of Alzheimer's. New York: Avery, 2017
———. The End of Alzheimer's Programme. London, UK: Vermilion, 2020.
———. The First Survivors of Alzheimer's. New York: Avery, 2021.
Christofferson, Travis. Ketones: The Fourth Fuel. Columbia, SC: Independently published, 2020.
Cunnane, Stephen C., Survival of the Fattest: The Key to Human Brain Evolution. Singapore: World Scientific Publishing, 2005.
Dayrit, Conrado S., Fabian M. Dayrit, and Bruce Fife. Coconut Oil from Diet to Therapy. Philippines: Anvil Publishing, 2013.
Davis, Ellen. Fight Cancer with a Ketogenic Diet. 2nd ed. www.ketogenic-diet-resource.com (digital book), 2014.
Dredge, Peter. Breakthrough: Surviving Alzheimer's and How You Can Too. Independently published, 2020.
Enig, Mary, PhD. Know Your Fats. Silver Spring, MD: Bethesda Press, 2000.
Fife, Bruce, ND. Coconut Cures. Colorado Springs, CO: Picadilly Books, 2005.
———. Coconut Lover's Cookbook. 3rd ed. Colorado Springs, CO: Picadilly Books, 2008.
Graveline, Duane, MD. Statin Drugs Side Effects and the Misguided War on Cholesterol. 4th ed. Self-published, 2008.
Guyenet, Stephan J., PhD. The Hungry Brain: Outsmarting the Instincts That Make Us Overeat. New York: Flatiron Books, 2017.
Heimowitz, Colette. The New Atkins Made Easy: A Faster, Simpler Way to Shed Weight and Feel Great—Starting Today! New York: Touchstone/Simon & Schuster, 2013.

Kalamian, Miriam, Ed.M, MS, CNS, and Thomas N. Seyfried, PhD. Keto for Cancer: Ketogenic Metabolic Therapy as a Targeted Nutritional Strategy. White River Junction, VT: Chelsea Green Publishing, 2017.

Kossoff, Eric H., MD, John M. Freeman, MD, Zahava Turner, RD, and James E. Rubenstein, MD. Ketogenic Diets: Treatments for Epilepsy and Other Disorders. 5th ed. New York: Demos Medical Publishing, 2011.

Lands, William E.M. Fish, Omega-3 and Human Health. 2nd ed. Urbana, IL: AOCS Press, 2005.

Lord, Ethelle, M.Ed., DM. Alzheimer and Dementia Coaching: Taking a Systems Approach in Creating an Alzheimer's Friendly Healthcare Workforce. Mustang, OK: Tate Publishing & Enterprises, 2016.

Lugavere, Max. Genius Foods. New York: Harper Collins, 2018.

Masino, Susan A., Ph.D. Ketogenic Diet and Metabolic Therapies. New York: Oxford University Press, 2017.

Netzer, Corinne T. The Complete Book of Food Counts: The Book that Counts It All. 9th ed. New York: Dell/Random House, 2012.

Newport, Mary, MD. Alzheimer's Disease: What If There Was a Cure? The Story of Ketones. 2nd ed. Laguna Beach, CA: Basic Health Publications, 2013.

———. The Coconut Oil and Low Carb Solution for Alzheimer's, Parkinson's, and Other Diseases. Laguna Beach, CA: Basic Health Publications, 2015.

———. The Complete Book of Ketones: A Practical Guide to Ketogenic Diets and Ketone Supplements. Nashville, TN: Turner Publishing, 2019.

Perlmutter, David, MD, and Kristin Loberg. Brain Maker: The Power of Gut Microbes to Heal and Protect Your Brain—For Life. New York: Little, Brown/Hachette Book Group, 2015.

———. Grain Brain: The Surprising Truth About Wheat, Carbs, and Sugar—Your Brain's Silent Killers. New York: Little, Brown/Hachette Book Group, 2013.

Schopick, Julia. Honest Medicine. Oak Park, IL: Innovative Health Publishing, 2011.

Seyfried, Thomas N. Cancer as a Metabolic Disease: On the Origin, Management, and Prevention of Cancer. Hoboken, NJ: John Wiley & Sons, 2012.

Sinatra, Stephen, MD. The Sinatra Solution: Metabolic Cardiology. Laguna Beach, CA: Basic Health Publications, 2008.

Volek, Jeff S., PhD, RD, and Stephen D. Phinney, MD, PhD. The Art and Science of Low Carbohydrate Living. City Not Listed: Beyond Obesity, LLC, 2011.

Wahls, Terry, MD, and Eve Adamson. The Wahls Protocol: How I Beat Progressive MS Using Paleo Principles and Functional Medicine. New York: Avery/Penguin Random House, 2014.

Westman, Eric C., MD, Stephen D. Phinney, MD, and Jeff S. Volek, PhD. The New Atkins for a New You: The Ultimate Diet for Shedding Weight and Feeling Great. New York: Touchstone/Simon & Schuster, 2010.

Wilson, Dr. Jacob, and Ryan Lowery, PhD. The Ketogenic Bible, The Authoritative Guide to Ketosis. Las Vegas, NV: Victory Belt Publishing, 2017.

Organizations

The following is a list of organizations and medical websites:

Alzheimer's Association (www.alz.org)

Alzheimer's Disease Cooperative Study (www.adcs.org)

Alzheimer's Disease International (www.alz.co.uk)

Alzheimer's Family Organization (www.alzheimersfamily.org)

Catholic Charities: https://www.catholiccharitiesusa.org/find-help/

The Charlie Foundation (https://charliefoundation.org/)

Dementia Alliance International (https://www.dementiaallianceinternational.org)

Epigenix Foundation (https://epigenixfoundation.org)

George W. Yu Foundation for Nutrition and Health, Inc. (www.YuFoundation.org)

Ketogenic.Com, Education and Recipes (https://ketogenic.com)

KetoNutrition (https://ketonutrition.org)

Ketone Technologies (https://ketonetechnologies.com/)

Keto Pet Sanctuary—Help with pet cancers (https://www.ketopetsanctuary.com)

Matthews Friends (www.matthewsfriends.org)

Michael J. Fox Foundation for Parkinson's Research (www.MichaelJFoxFoundation.org)

National Institute on Aging Alzheimer's Disease Education and Referral Center (www.nia.nih.gov/Alzheimers)

National Institutes of Health Clinical Trials Registry (www.clinicaltrials.gov)

National Institute of Neurologic Disorders and Stroke (www.ninds.nih.gov)

Forums, Websites, Blogs, Foundations, Podcasts, and Message Boards

ALS Forums (www.alsforums.com)

Alzheimer's Association Message Board (www.alz.org/living_with_alzhei mers_message_boards_lwa.asp)

Alzheimer's Research Forum (www.alzforum.org)

Coconut Research Center (www.coconutresearchcenter.org)

Dementia and Alzheimer's Weekly (www.alzheimersweekly.com)

Dr. Dominic D'Agostino's websites: KetoNutrition (https://ketonutrition .org) and Ketone Technologies (https://ketonetechnologies.com)

Dr. Mary Newport's website for Alzheimer's, dementia, other neurological disorders, diabetes, and obesity (www.coconutketones.com)

Dr. Mary Newport's website for Clearly Keto (www.clearly-keto.com)

Dr. Mary Newport's Blog (www.coconutketones.blogspot.com)

Dr. Mary Newport's Facebook page—Coconut Oil Helps Alzheimer's, De-mentia, ALS, MS (https://www.facebook.com/CoconutOilandAlzheimers /?ref=hl)

Dr. Mary Newport on TikTok @marynewportmd

Ketogenic.Com (https://ketogenic.com)

Ketogenic Diet Calculator from Beth Zupec-Kania (https://www.ketodiet calculator.org)

Miriam Kalamian –Twitter @DietaryTherapy; Facebook at Miriam Kala-mian. (www.DietaryTherapies.com)

Winning the Fight—Deanna Protocol for ALS (https://www.winningthe fight.org)

Sources for Coconut Oil, MCT Oil, MCT Foods, and Formulas

There are many good brands of virgin coconut oil, MCT oil, and MCT food products available on Amazon, in groceries, health food stores, and big box stores. Some standouts include Alpha Health Products (Canada), Barlean's Organic Oils, Carrington Farms Liquid Coconut Cooking Oil (high in lauric acid), Nutiva, Nature's Approved, Spectrum, Tropical Traditions, and Wilderness Family Naturals. Also:

Dr. Schär AG/SPA, Winkelau 9, 39014 Burgstall/Postal, Italy (www.dr schaer.com)

drMCT from Ketoscience, Singapore and elsewhere in Asia (https://mydr mct.com)

Medica Nutrition (https://medica-nutrition.com)

Pruvit Ventures: Dr. Mary Newport's formulation MCT//143 (https://mary-newport.pruvitnow.com)

The Nisshin OilliO Group, Ltd. in Asia (http://www.nisshin-oillio.com/)

Sources for Ketone Salts

Audacious Nutrition (https://audaciousnutrition.com)
Pruvit Ventures (https://marynewport.pruvitnow.com)
Real Ketones (https://realketones.com/Realenergy10

Sources for Ketone Esters

KetoneAid (https://ketoneaid.com)
TDeltaS (https://deltagketones.com)
Juvenescence (https://juvlabs.com)
Kenetik (https://drinkkenetik.com)

Ketone Monitoring Devices

Keto Mojo Blood Glucose and Ketone Monitor (https://keto-mojo.com)
Ketonix Ketone Breath Analyzer (https://ketonix.com)

Special Products for Elders

The Meal Lifter® (https://meallifter.com). Unique product that brings the meal plate closer to the mouth, invented by Ann Royer.

ACKNOWLEDGMENTS

When writing a book on the ketogenic lifestyle, it is important to share real-life stories of people whose health improved because of such changes in their lives. Joe Prata and Carol Henry Prata, William Curtis, and Dr. Andrew Koutnik have chosen a ketogenic approach to diet and lifestyle, reaping the rewards of sustained better health. I wish to thank each of them for permitting us to peek through a window into their private journeys and the active roles each has played in getting the upper hand in managing their health issues.

Many thanks go to Dr. Dominic D'Agostino, who researches "everything keto" at the University of South Florida, and his wonderful associate Dr. Milene Brownlow for writing the inspiring foreword to the book.

My deepest love and gratitude go to my daughter Joanna Newport for her countless hours and enormous patience while creating more than one hundred graphics for the book. I cannot thank Joanna and her husband, Forrest Rand, enough for the years they spent helping me take care of her father Steve in our home. They never hesitated for a second to come to our rescue when I called, day or night.

I wish to acknowledge Dr. Stephen Cunnane for reviewing and making suggestions for chapter 10 on what goes wrong in the Alzheimer's brain, and even more for the many years Cunnane and his associates at Sherbrooke University have spent working on the problem of the brain energy gap and brain energy rescue.

I also wish to thank William Curtis and Todd King for their review and input for chapter 10 and other "sciency" parts of the book, and for helping me to convey very technical information. I wish to further acknowledge Todd King for the many hours he spent proofreading the entire book with a fine-tooth comb.

I wish to thank my good friend Kaori Nakajima for inviting the readers into the world of Japan, where the food on the plate may look different to Westerners but has much in common with the "Mediterranean-style" diet.

My deep appreciation goes to my sister Angela Bertke for the countless hours she has worked to increase awareness among the older population of ketones as an alternative fuel for the brain. I also wish to thank Angela for agreeing to pose for photos of exercise, and for providing delicious recipes, proofreading, and commentary, as well as the love, encouragement, and support she and her husband, John Bertke, have given me.

Thanks to my daughter Julie DiPalo for her help with getting certain photos just right and for her love and support.

I also wish to acknowledge editor Ryan Smernoff, and many others involved in getting the book to press at Turner Publishing, thereby helping me to carry on my husband Steve Newport's legacy by sharing the message of ketones with the world.

I would also like to pay tribute to the memories of two pioneers of ketone research who became friends and mentors for me: Richard L. Veech, MD, DPhil was a driving force behind ketone research for Alzheimer's and many other disorders, inventor of the ketone ester that helped my husband, and passed away at age eighty-four in 2020, tirelessly working at the NIH until the very end. Theodore VanItallie, MD, was a great proponent of ketones as a potential therapeutic, wrote the foreword for my previous book, The Complete Book of Ketones, and died just before his one-hundredth birthday in 2019.

REFERENCES

AAIC 2020. Press release: "Flu, pneumonia vaccinations tied to lower risk of Alzheimer's dementia." https://www.alz.org/aaic/releases_2020/vaccines-dementia-risk.asp

Abbott A. "Are infections seeding some cases of Alzheimer's disease?" Nature V. 587 No. 7832 (2020): 22–25.

Abe T, et al. "Capric Acid Up-Regulates UCP3 Expression without PDK4 Induction in Mouse C2C12 Myotubes." J Nutr Sci Vitaminol (Tokyo) V. 62 No. 1 (2016):32–9.

Accera/Samuel T. Henderson. "Combinations of Medium-Chain Triglycerides and Therapeutic Agents for the Treatment and Prevention of Alzheimer's Disease and Other Diseases Resulting from Reduced Neuronal Metabolism." U.S. Patent Application Publication, Pub. No. US 2008/0009467 A1, January 10, 2008, page 29.

ADA. "Carb Counting and Diabetes." (2021) https://www.diabetes.org/healthy-living/recipes-nutrition/understanding-carbs/carb-counting-and-diabetes.

Adams JN, et al. "Analysis of advanced glycation end-products in the DHS Mind Study." J Diabetes Complications V. 30 No. 2 (2016): 262–8.

Adkins S, et al. "Growth and Production of Coconut." in Soils, Plant Growth and Crop Production, Vol III, UNESCO-Encyclopedia of Life Support Systems. (2010): http://www.eolss.net/Eolss-sampleAll Chapter.aspx

Aghaloo T, et al. "In Vitro Models, Standards, and Experimental Methods for Tobacco Products." Adv Dent Res V. 30 No. 1 (2019):16–21.

Alisi L, et al. "The relationships between vitamin K and cognition: a review of current evidence." Front Neurol V. 10 (2019):239.

Allen L, et al. "Guidelines on food fortification with micronutrients." Publication of the World Health Organization and Food and Agriculture Organization of the United Nations (2006).

Almeida CC, et al. "Bioactive Compounds in Infant Formula and Their Effects on Infant Nutrition and Health: A Systematic Literature Review." Int J Food Sci (2021):Published online.

Alzheimer disease: the Women's Health and Aging Study II." Neurology V. 79 (2012): 633–641.

Alzheimer's Association. "2019 Alzheimer's Disease Facts and Figures Report." https://www.alz.org/media/Documents/alzheimers-facts-and-figures -2019-r.pdf

Alzheimer's Association. "2020 Alzheimer's Disease Facts and Figures." Alzheimer's Dement V. 16 (2020):391–460.

Alzheimer's Association. "Alzheimer's Facts and Figures 2021." (2021) https:// www.alz.org/media/documents/alzheimers-facts-and-figures.pdf

Amin MN, et al. "How the association between obesity and inflammation may lead to insulin resistance and cancer." Diabetes Metab Syndr V. 13 No. 2 (2019):1213–1224.

Anderson HR, et al. "Passive smoking and sudden infant death syndrome: review of the epidemiological evidence." Thorax V. 52 No. 11 (1997):1003–1009.

Anderson TM, et al. "Maternal Smoking Before and During Pregnancy and the Risk of Sudden Unexpected Infant Death." Pediatrics V. 143 No. 4 (2019):e20183325.

Arcidiacono B, et al. "Insulin resistance and cancer risk: an overview of the pathogenetic mechanisms." Exp Diabetes Res 2012:789174.

Area-Gomez E, et al. "On the Pathogenesis of Alzheimer's Disease: The MAM Hypothesis." FASEB J V. 31 No. 3 (2017):864–867.

Aridi YS, et al. "Adherence to the Mediterranean diet and chronic disease in Australia: National nutrition and physical activity survey analysis." Nutrients V. 12 No. 5 (2020):1251.

Arnold SE, et al. "Brain insulin resistance in type 2 diabetes and Alzheimer disease: concepts and conundrums." Nat Rev Neurol V. 13 No. 3 (2018):168–181.

Ascherio A, et al. "Trans fatty acids and coronary heart disease." NEJM Vol 25 (1999): 1994–1998.

Assunção ML, et al. "Effects of dietary coconut oil on the biochemical and anthropometric profiles of women presenting abdominal obesity." Lipids V. 44 No. 7 (2009):593–601.

Astarita G, et al. "Elevated stearoyl-CoA desaturase in brains of patients with Alzheimer's disease." PLoS One V. 6 No. 10 (2011):e24777.

Astrup A, et al. "Saturated Fats and Health: A Reassessment and Proposal for Food-Based Recommendations." J Am Coll Cardiol V. 76 No. 7 (2020):844–857.

Athar T, et al.. "Recent advances on drug development and emerging therapeutic agents for Alzheimer's disease." Mol Biol Rep (2021): Published online ahead of print.

Athinarayanan SJ, et al. "Impact of a 2-year trial of nutritional ketosis on indices of cardiovascular disease risk in patients with type 2 diabetes." Cardiovasc Diabetol V. 19 No. 1 (2020):208.

ATSDR. "Public health statement for aluminum." https://www.atsdr.cdc.gov/ToxProfiles/tp22-c1-b.pdf (2008)

Augustin K, et al. "Mechanisms of action for the medium-chain triglyceride ketogenic diet in neurological and metabolic disorders." Lancet Neurol V. 17 No. 1 (2018):84–93.

Avgerinos KI, et al. "Ketone Ester Effects on Biomarkers of Brain Metabolism and Cognitive Performance in Cognitively Intact Adults ≥ 55 Years Old. A Study Protocol for a DoubleBlinded Randomized Controlled Clinical Trial." J Prev Alz Dis V. 1 No. 9 (2022):54–66.

Bae S, et al. "Association of herpes zoster with dementia and effect of antiviral therapy on dementia: a population-based cohort study." Eur Arch Psychiatry Clin Neurosci (2020): Epub ahead of print.

Bah TM, et al. "Sleep as a Therapeutic Target in the Aging Brain." Neurotherapeutics V. 16 No. 3 (2019):554–568.

Ball K, et al. "Effects of cognitive training interventions with older adults: A randomized controlled trial." JAMA V. 288 No. 18 (2002): 2271–81.

Basu S, et al. "The relationship of sugar to population-level diabetes prevalence: an econometric analysis of repeated cross-sectional data." PLoS One V. 8 (2013): e57873.

Baumeister A, et al. "Short-term influence of caffeine and medium-chain triglycerides on ketogenesis: A controlled double-blind intervention study." J Nutr Metab (2021):1861567.

Bernstein RK. Dr. Bernstein's Diabetes Solution. 4th Edition, Little, Brown, Spark, New York NY, 2011.

Bixel M G, et al. "Generation of ketone bodies from leucine by cultured astroglial cells." J Neurochem. V. 65 No. 6 (1995): 2450–61.

Blaszczyk JW. "Energy Metabolism Decline in the Aging Brain-Pathogenesis of Neurodegenerative Disorders." Metabolites V. 10 No. 11 (2020):450.

Boespflug EL, et al. "The Emerging Relationship Between Interstitial Fluid-Cerebrospinal Fluid Exchange, Amyloid-β, and Sleep." Biol Psychiatry V. 83 No. 4 (2018):328–336.

Bolland MJ, et al. "Calcium supplements and cardiovascular risk: 5 years on." Ther Adv Drug Saf V. 4 No. 5 (2013):199–210.

Bonaccio M, et al. "Ultra-processed food consumption is associated with increased risk of all-cause and cardiovascular mortality in the Moli-sani Study." Am J Clin Nutr V. 113 (2021):446–455.

Borges CR, et al. "Alzheimer's disease and sleep disturbances: a review." Arq Neuropsiquiatr V. 77 No. 11 (2019):815–824.

Bouxsein ML. "Determinants of skeletal fragility." Best Pract Res Clin Rheumatol V. 19 No. 6 (2005):897–911.

Brands MW, et al. "Sodium-retaining effect of insulin in diabetes." Am J Physiol Regul Integr Comp Physiol V. 303 (2012): R1101–R1109.

Bratic A, et al. "The role of mitochondria in aging." J Clin Invest V. 123 No. 3 (2013):951–957.

Bredesen DE. "Reversal of cognitive decline: a novel therapeutic program." Aging (Albany NY) V. 6 No. 9 (2014):707–17.

Bronner F, et al. "Nutritional aspects of calcium absorption." J Nutr V. 129 No. 1 (1999):9–12.

Broom GM, et al. "The ketogenic diet as a potential treatment and prevention strategy for Alzheimer's disease." Nutrition V. 20 (2019):118–121.

Brouwer IA, et al. "Effect of animal and industrial trans fatty acids on HDL and LDL cholesterol levels in humans—a quantitative review." PLoS One Vol 5, No 3 (2010): e9434.

Browne D, et al. "Vitamin E and Alzheimer's disease: what do we know so far?" Clin Interv Aging V. 14 (2019):1303–1317.

Brownlow ML, et al. "Ketogenic diet improves motor performance but not cognition in two mouse models of Alzheimer's pathology." PLoS One V. 8 No. 9 (2013):e75713.

Bubu OM, et al. "Sleep, cognitive impairment, and Alzheimer's disease: a systematic review and meta-analysis." Sleep (Basel) V. 40 No. 1 (2017):e1–18.

Butterfield DA, et al. "Oxidative stress, dysfunctional glucose metabolism and Alzheimer disease." Nat Rev Neurosci V. 20 No. 3 (2019):148–160.

Byrne NJ, et al. "Chronically elevating circulating ketones can reduce cardiac inflammation and blunt the development of heart failure." Circ Heart Fail V. 13 No. 6 (2020):e006573.

Cairns DM, et al. "A 3D human brain-like tissue model of herpes-induced Alzheimer's disease." Sci Adv V. 6 No. 19 (2020):eaay8828.

Calderón-Garcidueñas L, et al. Apolipoprotein E4, Gender, Body Mass Index, Inflammation, Insulin Resistance, and Air Pollution Interactions: Recipe for Alzheimer's Disease Development in Mexico City Young Females." J Alzheimer Dis, V. 58 N. 3 (2017):613–630.

Camargos EF, et al. "Trazodone improves sleep parameters in Alzheimer disease patients: a randomized, double-blind and placebo-controlled study." American Journal of Geriatric Psychiatry V. 22 No. 12 (2014):1565–74.

Carradori D, et al. "Retinoic acid-loaded NFL-lipid nanocapsules promote oligodendrogenesis in focal white matter lesion." Biomaterials V. 230 (2020):119653.

Carson JAS, et al. "Dietary cholesterol and cardiovascular risk: a science advisory from the American Heart Association." Circulation V. 141 No. 3 (2020):e39–e53.

Carter CJ. "Alzheimer's disease plaques and tangles: cemeteries of a pyrrhic victory of the immune defense network against herpes simplex infection at the expense of complement and inflammation-mediated neuronal destruction." Neurochem Int V. 58 No. 3 (2011):301–320.

Case DR, et al. "Synthesis and chemical and biological evaluation of a glycine tripeptide chelate of magnesium." Molecules V. 26 No. 9 (2021):2419.

Castellano C-A, et al. "Regional brain glucose hypometabolism in young women with polycystic ovary syndrome: possible link to mild insulin resistance." PLoS ONE V. 10 No. 12 (2015):e0144116.

Castellano CA, et al. "A 3-Month Aerobic Training Program Improves Brain Energy Metabolism in Mild Alzheimer's Disease: Preliminary Results from a Neuroimaging Study." J Alzheimers Dis V. 56 No. 4 (2017):1459–1468.

Castellano C-A, et al. "Lower brain 18F-fluorodeoxyglucose uptake but normal 11C-acetoacetate metabolism in mild Alzheimer's disease dementia." J Alzheim Dis V. 43 (2015): 1343–1353.

CDC. "How many people get Lyme disease?" (2021) https://www.cdc.gov/lyme/stats/humancases.html

CDC. "Know your risk for heart disease." (2021) https://www.cdc.gov/heart-disease/risk_factors.htm

CDC. "Leading causes of death." (2021) https://www.cdc.gov/nchs/fastats/leading-causes-of-death.htm

CDC. "Update: Vaccine Side Effects, Adverse Reactions, Contraindications, and Precautions Recommendations of the Advisory Committee on Immunization Practices (ACIP)." MMWR V. 45-RR-12 (1996):1–35. https://www.cdc.gov/mmwr/preview/mmwrhtml/00046738.htm

Cepas V, et al. "Redox signaling and advanced glycation end-products (AGEs) in diet-related diseases." Antioxidants (Basel) V. 9 No. 2 (2020):142.

Chamberlain S, et al. "An exploratory Phase IIa study of the PPAR delta/gamma Agonist T3D-959 assessing metabolic and cognitive function in subjects with mild to moderate Alzheimer's Disease." J Alzheim Dis V. 73 No. 3 (2020):1085–1103.

Chambers TL, et al. "Skeletal muscle size, function, and adiposity with life-long aerobic exercise." J Appl Physiol V. 128 (2020): 368–378.

Chandler J, et al. "Impact of 12-month smartphone breathing meditation program upon systolic blood pressure among non-medicated stage 1 hypertensive adults." Int J Environ Res Public Health V. 17 No. 6 (2020):1955.

Chatterjee P, et al. "Potential of coconut oil and medium chain triglycerides in the prevention and treatment of Alzheimer's disease." Mechanisms of Ageing and Development. 2020:111209.

Chen VC, et al. "Herpes Zoster and dementia: a nationwide population-based cohort study." J Clin Psychiatry V. 79 (2018):16.

Cheng CW, et al. "Ketone body signaling mediates intestinal stem cell homeostasis and adaptation to diet." Cell V. 178 (2019):1115–1131.

Chin-Yee B, et al. "Emerging trends in clinical research: With implications for population health and health policy." Milbank Q V. 96 No. 2 (2018):369–401.

Choi D, et al. "Effect of smoking cessation on the risk of dementia: A longitudinal study." Ann Clin Transl Neurol V. 5 No. 10 (2018):1192–9.

Chornenkyy Y, et al. "Alzheimer's disease and type 2 diabetes mellitus are distinct diseases with potential overlapping metabolic dysfunction upstream of observed cognitive decline." Brain Pathol V. 29 No. 1 (2019):3–17.

Clarke K, et al. "Kinetics, safety and tolerability of (R)-3-hydroxybutyl (R)-3-hydroxybutyrate in healthy adult subjects." Regul Toxicol Pharmacol V. 63 (2012): 401–8.

ClinicalTrials.gov. Search for "Ketogenic Clinical Trials." (2020) https://clinicaltrials.gov/

Congdon EE, et al. "Tau-targeting therapies for Alzheimer disease." Nat Rev Neurol V. 14 No. 7 (2018):399–415.

Conze DB, et al. "Safety assessment of nicotinamide riboside, a form of vitamin B3." Hum Exp Toxicol V. 35 No. 11 (2016):1149–1160.

Cosacak MI, et al. "Alzheimer's disease, neural stem cells and neurogenesis: cellular phase at single-cell level." Neural Regen Res V. 15 No. 5 (2020):824–827.

Courchesne-Loyer A, et al. "Inverse relationship between brain glucose and ketone metabolism in adults during short-term moderate dietary ketosis: A dual tracer quantitative positron emission tomography study." JCBFM. Open Access (2016): E1–9.

Courchesne-Loyer A, et al. "Stimulation of mild, sustained ketonemia by medium-chain triacylglycerols in healthy humans: Estimated potential contribution to brain energy metabolism." Nutrition. (2013): 1–6.

Courtice FC, et al. "The effects of prolonged muscular exercise on the metabolism." Proc R Soc Vol 119B (1936): 381–439.

Cox P J, et al. "Nutritional ketosis alters fuel preference and thereby endurance performance in athletes." Cell Metabolism. V. 24 (2016): 1–13.

Craddock TJ, et al. "The zinc dyshomeostasis hypothesis of Alzheimer's disease." PLoS One V. 7 No. 3 (2012):e33552.

Craft S, et al. "Intranasal insulin therapy for Alzheimer disease and amnestic mild cognitive impairment: a pilot clinical trial." Arch Neurol V. 69 (2012):29–38.

Craft S, et al. "Safety, efficacy, and feasibility of intranasal insulin for the treatment of mild cognitive impairment and Alzheimer disease dementia: a randomized clinical trial." JAMA Neurol V. 77 No. 9 (2020):1–11.

Crane PK, et al. "Glucose levels and risk of dementia." NEJM V. 369 No. 6 (2013):540–548.

Croteau E, et al. "Ketogenic medium chain triglycerides increase brain energy metabolism in Alzheimer's disease." J Alzheim Dis In press May 2018.

Cuenoud B, et al. "Metabolism of Exogenous D-Beta-Hydroxybutyrate, an Energy Substrate Avidly Consumed by the Heart and Kidney." Front Nutr V. 7 (2020):13.

Cullen NC, et al. "Accelerated inflammatory aging in Alzheimer's disease and its relation to amyloid, tau, and cognition." Sci Rep V. 11 No. 1 (2021):1965.

Cunnane S C, et al. "Carbon recycling into de novo lipogenesis is a major pathway in neonatal metabolism of linoleate and α-linolenate." Prostaglandins, Leukotrienes and Essential Fatty Acids. V. 60 No. 5 & 6. (1999): 387–92

Cunnane S C, et al. "Survival of the fattest: fat babies were the key to evolution of the large human brain." Comparative Biochem and Physiol Part A. V. 136 (2003): 17–26.

Cunnane SC, et al. "Brain energy rescue: an emerging therapeutic concept for neurodegenerative disorders of ageing." Nat Rev Drug Discov V. 19 No. 9 (2020):609–633.

Cunnane, Stephen C. Survival of the Fattest: The Key to Human Brain Evolution. Singapore: World Scientific Publishing Ct. Pte. Ltd., 2005.

Curtis, W, 2021. From interview with William Curtis on November 3, 2017. Updated in interview on August 10, 2021.

Curtis B. YouTube Videos. https://www.youtube.com/watch?v=riGYq5iD2SM and https://www.youtube.com/watch?v=oYaFv-8dv58

Danics K, et al. "Neurodegenerative proteinopathies associated with neuroinfections." J Neural Transm (Vienna) (2021):1–16.

Das BC, et al. "Potential therapeutic roles of retinoids for prevention of neuroinflammation and neurodegeneration in Alzheimer's disease." Neural Regen Res V. 14 No. 11 (2019):1880–1892.

Dayrit FM. "The properties of lauric acid and their significance in coconut oil." J Am Oil Chem Soc V. 92 (2015):1–15.

De Felice FG, et al. "Brain metabolic stress and neuroinflammation at the basis of cognitive impairment in Alzheimer's disease." Front Aging Neurosci V. 7 (2015):94.

De la Monte SM, et al. "Epidemiologic trends strongly suggest exposures as etiologic agents in the pathogenesis of sporadic Alzheimer's disease, diabetes mellitus, and nonalcoholic steatohepatitis." J Alzheimers Dis V. 17, No. 3 (2009): 519–529.

De la Monte SM, et al. "Alzheimer's disease is type 3 diabetes—evidence reviewed." J Diabetes Sci Technol V. 2, No. 6 (Nov 2008): 1101–1113.

De la Monte SM, et al. "Review of insulin and insulin-like growth factor expression, signaling, and malfunction in the central nervous system: relevance to Alzheimer's disease." J Alzheimer's Dis V. 7 (2005): 45–61.

De la Monte SM, et al. "The liver-brain axis of alcohol-mediated neurodegeneration: role of toxic lipids." Int J Environ Res Public Health V. 6 (2009): 2055–2075.

De la Monte SM, et al. "Improved brain insulin/IGF signaling and reduced neuroinflammation with T3D-959 in an experimental model of sporadic Alzheimer's disease." J Alzheimers Dis V. 55 No. 2 (2017):849–864.

De la Monte SM, et al. "Nitrosamine exposure exacerbates high fat diet-mediated type 2 diabetes mellitus, non-alcoholic steatohepatitis, and neurodegeneration with cognitive impairment." Mol Neurodegener V. 4, No. 54 (2009): 1–13.

De la Monte SM, et al.. "Mechanisms of ceramide-mediated neurodegeneration." J Alzheimers Dis V. 16, No. 4 (2009): 704–714.

De la Monte SM, et al. "Insulin resistance and oligodendrocyte/microvascular endothelial cell dysfunction as mediators of white matter degeneration in Alzheimer's disease." Wisniewski T, ed. Alzheimer's Disease: Chapter 8. Brisbane (AU): Codon Publications (2019).

De la Monte SM. "Brain insulin resistance and deficiency as therapeutic targets in Alzheimer's disease." Curr Alzheimer Res V. 9 No. 1 (2012):35–66.

De la Rubia Ortí JE, et al. "Improvement of main cognitive functions in patients with Alzheimer's disease after treatment with coconut oil enriched Mediterranean diet: A pilot study." J Alzheimers Dis V. 65 No. 2 (2018):577–587.

Dehghan M, et al. "Associations of fats and carbohydrate intake with cardio vascular disease and mortality in 18 countries from five continents (PURE): a prospective cohort study." Lancet V. 390 No. 10107 (2017):2050–2062.

Delgado-Saborit JM, et al. "A critical review of the epidemiological evidence of effects of air pollution on dementia, cognitive function and cognitive decline in adult population." Sci Total Environ V. 757 (2021):143734.

Deo P, et al. "APOE ε4 Carriers Have a Greater Propensity to Glycation and sRAGE Which Is Further Influenced by RAGE G82S Polymorphism." J Gerontol A Biol Sci Med Sci V. 75 No 10 (2020):1899–1905.

Dietary Guidelines for Americans 2020 to 2025. Https://dietaryguidelines .gov.

Ding J, et al. "Antihypertensive medications and risk for incident dementia and Alzheimer's disease: a meta-analysis of individual participant data from prospective cohort studies." Lancet Neurol V. 19 No. 1 (2020):61–70.

Dodge J, et al. "Antiviral and antibacterial lipids in human milk and infant formula." Arch Disease Childhood V. 66 No. 2 (1991):272.

Doody RS, et al. "Peripheral and central effects of γ-secretase inhibition by semagacestat in Alzheimer's disease." Alzheimers Res Ther V. 7 No. 1 (2015):36.

Drachman DA. "Do we have brain to spare?" Neurology V. 64 No. 12 (2005): 2004–2005.

Durazzo TC, et al. "Alzheimer's Disease Neuroimaging Initiative. Smoking and increased Alzheimer's disease risk: a review of potential mechanisms." Alzheimers Dement V. 10 Suppl. 3 (2014):S122–45.

Edison P, et al. "In vivo Imaging of Glial Activation in Alzheimer's Disease." Front Neurol V. 9 (2018):625.

Edison P, et al. "Role of Neuroinflammation in the Trajectory of Alzheimer's Disease and in vivo Quantification Using PET." J Alzheimers Dis V. 61 No. s1 (2018):S339–S351.

EFSA Panel on Dietetic Products, Nutrition, and Allergies. "Scientific opinion on dietary reference values for choline." EFSA J V. 14 No. 8 (2016):4484.

Eiden M, et al. "Discovery and validation of temporal patterns involved in human brain ketometabolism in cerebral microdialysis fluids of traumatic brain injury patients." EBioMedicine V. 44 (2019):607–617.

Elamin M, et al. "Ketone-based metabolic therapy: is increased NAD+ a primary mechanism?" Front Mol Neurosci V. 10 (2017):377.

Eldeeb MA, et al. "COVID-19 infection may increase the risk of parkinsonism - Remember the Spanish flu?" Cytokine Growth Factor Rev S1359–6101 (2020): Published online ahead of print.

Enig MG, et al. "The Oiling of America." Originally published in Nexus Magazine in two parts Nov/Dec 1998 and Feb/Mar 1999. Available online at: http://westonaprice.org/knowyour-fats/525-the-oiling-of-america.

Evangeliou A, et al. "Branched chain amino acids as adjunctive therapy to ketogenic diet in epilepsy: pilot study and hypothesis." J Child Neurol. V. 24 No. 10 (2009): 1268–72.

Everett J, et al. "Biogenic metallic elements in the human brain?" Sci Adv V. 7 No. 24 (2021):eabf6707.

Everett J, et al. "Nanoscale synchrotron X-ray speciation of iron and calcium compounds in amyloid plaque cores from Alzheimer's disease subjects." Nanoscale V. 10 V. 25 (2018):11782–11796.

Fan Z, et al. "Longitudinal influence of microglial activation and amyloid on neuronal function in Alzheimer's disease." Brain V. 138, (2015):3685–3698.

Fanning S, et al. "Parkinson's disease: proteinopathy or lipidopathy?" NPJ Parkinsons Dis V. 6 No. 3 (2020):1–9.

Fauser J K, et al. "Induction of apoptosis by the medium-chain length fatty acid lauric acid in colon cancer cells due to induction of oxidative stress." Chemotherapy. V. 59 (2013): 214–24.

Feinman RD, et al. "Dietary carbohydrate restriction as the first approach in diabetes management: Critical review and evidence base." Nutrition V. 31 (2015): 1–13.

Fernández-Gamba A, et al. "Insulin-degrading enzyme: structure-function relationship and its possible roles in health and disease." Curr Pharm Des V. 15 No. 31 (2009):3644–3655.

Ferrero J, et al. "First-in-human, double-blind, placebo-controlled, single-dose escalation study of aducanumab (BIIB037) in mild-to-moderate Alzheimer's disease." Alzheimers Dement (NY) V. 2 No. 3 (2016):169–176.

Fery F, et al. "Ketone body turnover during and after exercise in overnight-fasted and starved humans." Am J Physiol Endocrinol Metab V. 245 (1983): 318–325.

Fife, B. Coconut Cures. Colorado Springs, CO: Picadilly Books, Ltd., 2005.

Fifel K, et al. "Circadian and Sleep Dysfunctions in Neurodegenerative Disorders-An Update." Front Neurosci V. 14 (2021):627330.

Fiorentini D, et al. "Magnesium: biochemistry, nutrition, detection, and social impact of diseases linked to its deficiency." Nutrients V. 13 No. 4 (2021):1136.

Fischer T, et al. "Long-term ketone body therapy of severe multiple acyl-CoA dehydrogenase deficiency: a case report." Nutrition V. 60 (2019):122–8.

Folch J, et al. "The involvement of peripheral and brain insulin resistance in late onset Alzheimer's dementia." Front Aging Neurosci V. 11 (2019):236.

Folch J, et al. "The implication of the brain insulin receptor in late onset Alzheimer's disease dementia." Pharmaceuticals (Basel) V. 11 No. 1 (2018):11.

Fontham ET, et al. "Environmental tobacco smoke and lung cancer in non-smoking women. A multicenter study." JAMA V. 271 No. 22 (1994):1752–9.

Forouhi NG, et al. "Dietary fat and cardiometabolic health: evidence, controversies, and consensus for guidance." BMJ V. 361 (2018):k2139.

Forssner G. "Über die einwirkung der muskelarbeit auf die acetonkörperausscheiding bei kohlenhydratarmer kost." Skand Arch Physiol V. 22 (1909): 393–405.

Fortier M, et al. "A ketogenic drink improves cognition in mild cognitive impairment: Results of a 6-month RCT." Alzheimers Dement V. 17 No. 3 (2021):543–552.

Frazier HN, et al. "Broadening the definition of brain insulin resistance in aging and Alzheimer's disease." Exp Neurol V. 313 (2019):79–87.

Frost GR, et al. "The role of astrocytes in amyloid production and Alzheimer's disease." Open Biol V. 7 No. 12 (2017):170228.

Fu J, et al. "Nonpharmacologic interventions for reducing blood pressure in adults with prehypertension to established hypertension." J Am Heart Assoc V. 9 No. 19 (2020):e016804.

Galvin JE, et al. "The AD8: The Washington University Dementia Screening Test." Published online at https://hign.org/sites/default/files/2020-06/Try_This_Dementia_14.pdf

Garcez M, et al. "Lauric acid prevents production of IL-8 and IL-13 and increase of tryptophan/kynurenine ratio in LPS-stimulated human astrocytes." AAIC (2021): Poster and audio presentation (Hillebrandt, 2021).

Garwood CJ, et al. "Review: Astrocytes in Alzheimer's disease and other age-associated dementias: a supporting player with a central role." Neuropathol Appl Neurobiol V. 43 No. 4 (2017):281–298.

Gasparini L, et al. "Effect of energy shortage and oxidative stress on amyloid precursor protein metabolism in COS cells." Neurosci Lett V. 231 No. 2 (1997):113–7.

Gathright EC, et al. "The impact of transcendental meditation on depressive symptoms and blood pressure in adults with cardiovascular disease: A systematic review and meta-analysis." Complement Ther Med V. 46 (2019):172–179.

Gawdi R, et al. "Physiology, Blood–brain barrier." StatPearls Publishing Treasure Island, Florida (2021).

GBD 2017 Risk Factor Collaborators. "Global, regional, and national comparative risk assessment of 84 behavioural, environmental and occupational, and metabolic risks or clusters of risks for 195 countries and territories, 1990–2017: a systematic analysis for the Global Burden of Disease Study 2017." Lancet V. 392 No. 10159 (2018):1923–1994.

GBD 2019 Risk Factors Collaborators. "Global burden of 87 risk factors in 204 countries and territories, 1990–2019: a systematic analysis for the Global Burden of Disease Study 2019." Lancet V. 396 No. 10258 (2020):1223–1249.

Giau VV, et al. "Gut microbiota and their neuroinflammatory implications in Alzheimer's disease." Nutrients V. 10 No. 1765 (2018): Online.

Gibson GE, et al. "Benfotiamine and cognitive decline in Alzheimer's disease: results of a randomized placebo-controlled phase IIa clinical trial." J Alzheimers Dis V. 78 No. 3 (2020):989–1010.

Gill S, et al. "A Smartphone App Reveals Erratic Diurnal Eating Patterns in Humans that Can Be Modulated for Health Benefits." Cell Metab V. 22 No. 5 (2015):789–798.

Global Burden of Disease Collaborative Network. Institute for Health Metrics and Evaluation (IHME), Global Burden of Disease Study 2017 (GBD

2017) Results. Seattle, United States: 2018. http://ghdx.healthdata.org
/gbd-results-tool

Gray LR, et al. "Regulation of pyruvate metabolism and human disease." Cell
Mol Life Sci. 2014; V. 71 No, 14 (2014):2577-2604.

Grimm MO, et al. "The impact of vitamin E and other fat-soluble vitamins on
Alzheimer's disease." Int J Mol Sci V. 17 No. 11 (2016):1785.

Gugliucci A. "Formation of fructose-mediated advanced glycation end-
products and their roles in metabolic and inflammatory diseases." Adv
Nutr V. 8 No. 1 (2017):54–62.

Guilbaud A, et al. "How can diet affect the accumulation of advanced glycation end-products in the human body?" Foods V. 5 No. 6 (2016):84.

Gutierrez-Mariscal FM, et al. "Coenzyme Q10 supplementation for the reduction of oxidative stress: clinical implications in the treatment of chronic
diseases." Int J Mol Sci V. 21 No. 21 (2020):7870.

Guyenet SJ, et al. "Increase in adipose tissue linoleic acid of US adults in the
last half century." Adv Nutr V. 6 No. 6 (2015):660–4.

Guyenet, S. "By 2606 the US diet will be 100 percent sugar." Whole Health
Source: Nutrition and Health Science www.wholehealthsource.blogspot
.com February 18, 2012.

Hall CB, et al. "Cognitive activities delay onset of memory decline in persons
who develop dementia." Neurology V. 73 (2009):356–61.

Hallberg SJ, et al. "Effectiveness and safety of a novel care model for the management of type 2 diabetes at 1 year: an open-label, non-randomized, controlled study." [published correction appears in Diabetes Ther 2018 Mar
5]. Diabetes Ther V. 9 No. 2 (2018):583–612.

Hamelin L, et al. "Distinct dynamic profiles of microglial activation are
associated with progression of Alzheimer's disease." Brain V. 141 No. 6
(2018):1855–1870.

Hamilton LK, et al. "Neural stem cells and adult brain fatty acid metabolism:
Lessons from the 3xTg model of Alzheimer's disease." Biol Cell V. 110 No.
1 (2018):6–25.

Hamilton LK, et al. "Aberrant Lipid Metabolism in the Forebrain
Niche Suppresses Adult Neural Stem Cell Proliferation in an Animal Model of Alzheimer's Disease." Cell Stem Cell V. 17 No. 4
(2015):397–411.

Hamosh M, et al. "Lipids in milk and the first steps in their digestion." Pediatrics. V. 75 (1985): 146–150

Han YM, et al. "Beta-hydroxybutyrate and its metabolic effects on age-associated pathology." Exp Mol Med V. 52 No. 4 (2020):548–555.

Harvey CJ, et al. "The effect of medium chain triglycerides on time to nutritional ketosis and symptoms of keto-induction in healthy adults: A randomised controlled clinical trial." J Nutr Metab (2018):2630565.

Harwood DG, et al. "The effect of alcohol and tobacco consumption, and apolipoprotein E genotype, on the age of onset in Alzheimer's disease." Int J Geriatr Psychiatry V. 25 No. 5 (2010):511–8.

He F, et al. "Passive Smoking Exposure in Living Environments Reduces Cognitive Function: A Prospective Cohort Study in Older Adults." Int J Environ Res Public Health V. 17 No. 4 (2020):1402.

Heravi AS, et al. "Vitamin D and calcium supplements: helpful, harmful, or neutral for cardiovascular risk?" Methodist Debakey Cardiovasc J V.15 No. 3 (2019):207–213.

Hergesheimer RC, et al. "The debated toxic role of aggregated TDP-43 in amyotrophic lateral sclerosis: a resolution in sight?" Brain V.142 No. 5 (2019):1176–1194.

Hibbeln JR, et al. "Relationships between seafood consumption during pregnancy and childhood and neurocognitive development: Two systematic reviews." Prostaglandins Leukot Essent Fatty Acids V. 151 (2019):14–36.

Hillebrandt HL, et al. "Cognition may improve with medium-chain triglyceride supplementation: A pilot study." AAIC (2021): Poster and audio presentation.

Hillebrandt HL, et al. "Postprandial ketone body levels increase following medium-chain triglyceride oil consumption." AAIC (2021): Poster and audio presentation.

Hirata Y, et al. "Elaidic Acid Potentiates Extracellular ATP-Induced Apoptosis via the P2X7-ROS-ASK1-p38 Axis in Microglial Cell Lines." Biol Pharm Bull V. 43 No. 10 (2020):1562–1569.

Hirata Y, et al. "Trans-Fatty acids promote proinflammatory signaling and cell death by stimulating the apoptosis signal-regulating kinase 1 (ASK1)-p38 pathway." J Biol Chem V. 292 No. 20 (2017):8174–8185.

Hirsch MJ, et al. "Relations between dietary choline or lecithin intake, serum choline levels, and various metabolic indices." Metabolism V. 27 No. 8 (1978):953–60.

Holdsworth DA, et al. "A Ketone Ester Drink Increases Postexercise Muscle Glycogen Synthesis in Humans." Med Sci Sports Exerc V. 49 No. 9 (2017):1789–1795.

Hopp SC, et al. "The role of microglia in processing and spreading of bioactive tau seeds in Alzheimer's disease." J Neuroinflammation V. 15 No. 1 (2018):269.

Hosley-Moore, E. "Doctor says an oil lessened Alzheimer's effects on her husband." St. Petersburg Times October 29, 2008. Newport MT.

Hoyer S, et al. "Cerebral blood flow and brain metabolism findings in neuropsychiatric patients." Nervenarzt V. 37 No. 7 (1966):322–324.

Hoyer S, et al. "Blood flow and oxidative metabolism of the brain in patients with dementia (author's transl)." J Neurol V. 210 No. 4 (1975):227–237.

Hoyer S, et al. "Cerebral excess release of neurotransmitter amino acids subsequent to reduced cerebral glucose metabolism in early-onset dementia of Alzheimer type." J Neural Transm V. 75 No. 3 (1989):227–232

Hoyer S, et al. "Alzheimer disease—no target for statin treatment. A mini review." Neurochem Res V. 32 No. 4–5 (2007):695–706.

Hoyer S. "Abnormalities of glucose metabolism in Alzheimer's disease." Ann NY Acad Sci V. 640 (1991):53–58.

Hoyer S. "Brain metabolism and the incidence of cerebral perfusion disorders in organic psychoses." Deutsche Zeitschrift für Nervenheilkunde V. 197 No. 4 (1970): 285–92.

Hoyer S. "Causes and consequences of disturbances of cerebral glucose metabolism in sporadic Alzheimer disease: therapeutic implications." Adv Exp Med Biol V. 541 (2004):135–152.

Hoyer S. "Glucose metabolism and insulin receptor signal transduction in Alzheimer disease." Eur J Pharmacol V. 490 No. 1–3 (2004):115–25.

Hoyer S. "Senile dementia and Alzheimer's disease. Brain blood flow and metabolism." Prog Neuropsychopharmacol Biol Psychiatry V. 10 No. 3–5 (1986):447–478.

Hoyer S. "The aging brain. Changes in the neuronal insulin/insulin receptor signal transduction cascade trigger late-onset sporadic Alzheimer disease (SAD). A mini-review." J Neural Transm (Vienna) V. 109 No 7–8 (2002):991–1002.

Hsu HW, et al. "Environmental and Dietary Exposure to Copper and Its Cellular Mechanisms Linking to Alzheimer's Disease." Toxicol Sci V. 163 N. 2 (2018):338–345.

Huat TJ, et al. "Metal Toxicity Links to Alzheimer's Disease and Neuroinflammation." J Mol Biol V. 431 No 9 (2019):1843–1868.

Hughes D, et al. "Association of Blood Pressure Lowering with Incident Dementia or Cognitive Impairment: A Systematic Review and Meta-analysis." JAMA V. 323 No. 19 (2020):1934–1944.

Hughes SD, et al. "The ketogenic diet component decanoic acid increases mitochondrial citrate synthase and complex I activity in neuronal cells." J Neurochem V. 129 No. 3 (2014):426–33.

Huttenlocher PR, et al. "Medium-chain triglycerides as a therapy for intractable childhood epilepsy." Neurology V. 21 (1971):1097–1103.

IDF. International Diabetes Federation Diabetes Atlas. (2017): https://www.diabetesatlas.org.

IHME, Institute for Health Metrics and Evaluation: http://www.healthdata.org/

Illam SP, et al. "Polyphenols of virgin coconut oil prevent pro-oxidant mediated cell death." Toxicol Mech Methods V. 27 No. 6 (2017):442–450.

IOM (Institute of Medicine). Dietary Reference Intakes: The Essential Guide to Nutrient Requirements (2006). Washington, DC: The National Academies Press. PDF available at http://nap.edu/11537.

Irwin DJ, et al. "Parkinson's disease dementia: convergence of α-synuclein, tau and amyloid-β pathologies." Nat Rev Neurosci V. 14 No.9 (2013):626–636.

Irwin MR, et al. "Implications of sleep disturbance and inflammation for Alzheimer's disease dementia." Lancet Neurol V. 18 No. 3 (2019):296–306.

Itzhaki RF, et al. "Microbes and Alzheimer's Disease." J Alzheimers Dis V. 51 No. 4 (2016):979–984.

Jabekk PT, et al. "Resistance training in overweight women on a ketogenic diet conserved lean body mass while reducing body fat." Nutr Metab (Lond) V. 7 (2010):17.

Jaiswal N, et al. "High fructose-induced metabolic changes enhance inflammation in human dendritic cells." Clin Exp Immunol V. 197 No. 2 (2019):237–249.

James BD, et al. "Late-life social activity and cognitive decline in old age." J Int Neuropsychol Soc V. 17 No. 6 (2011):998–1005.

Janson J, et al. "Increased risk of type 2 diabetes in Alzheimer disease." Diabetes V. 53 (2004): 474–481.

Jarrett SG, et al. "The ketogenic diet increases mitochondrial glutathione levels." J Neurochem V. 106 No. 3 (2008):1044–51.

Jenkins DJA, et al. "PURE Study Investigators. Glycemic index, glycemic load, and cardiovascular disease and mortality." N Engl J Med V. 384 No. 14 (2021):1312–1322.

Jensen T, et al. "Fructose and sugar: A major mediator of non-alcoholic fatty liver disease." J Hepatol V. 68 No. 5 (2018):1063–1075.

Jensen, T. "The consumption of fats in Denmark 1900–2000. Long term changes in the intake and quality." Anthropology of food(S7) (2012).

Jeong W, et al. "ApoE4-Induced Cholesterol Dysregulation and Its Brain Cell Type-Specific Implications in the Pathogenesis of Alzheimer's Disease." Mol Cells V. 42 No. 11 (2019):739–746.

Jernerén F, et al. "Brain atrophy in cognitively impaired elderly: the importance of long-chain ω-3 fatty acids and B vitamin status in a randomized controlled trial." Am J Clin Nutr V. 102 No. 1 (2015):215–21.

Johnson, Steven. New York Times April 27, 2021. Online at https://www.nytimes.com/2021/04/27/magazine/global-life-span.html

Kabara JJ, et al. "Fatty acids and derivatives as antimicrobial agents." Antimicrob Agents Chemother V. 2 No. 1 (1972):23–28.

Kadir A, et al. "Cardiac ketone metabolism." Biochem Biophys Acta Mol Basis Dis V. 1866 No. 6 (2020):165739.

Kandimalla R, et al. "Therapeutics of Neurotransmitters in Alzheimer's Disease." J Alzheimers Dis V. 57 No. 4 (2017):1049–1069.

Kashiwaya Y, et al. "A ketone ester diet exhibits anxiolytic and cognition-sparring properties and lessens amyloid and tau pathologies in a mouse model of Alzheimer's." Neurobiology of Ageing V. 34 No. 6 (2013): 1530–9.

Kashiwaya Y, et al. "D-b-Hydroxybutyrate protects neurons in models of Alzheimer's and Parkinson's disease," PNAS V. 97 No. 10 (2000): 5440–5444.

Keane KN, et al. "Molecular events linking oxidative stress and inflammation to insulin resistance and β-cell dysfunction." Oxid Med Cell Longev (2015):181643.

Kephart WC, et al. "The 1-week and 8-month effects of a ketogenic diet or ketone salt supplementation on multi-organ markers of oxidative stress and mitochondrial function in rats." Nutrients V. 9 No. 1019 (2017):1–22

Keys A. "Atherosclerosis: a problem in newer public health." J Mt Sinai Hosp V. 20 (1953): 118.

Keys A. "Coronary heart disease in seven countries." Circulation V. 41, Suppl, 1 (1970):1–211.

Khabbush A, et al. "Neuronal decanoic acid oxidation is markedly lower than that of octanoic acid: A mechanistic insight into the medium-chain triglyceride ketogenic diet." Epilepsia V. 58 No. 8 (2017):1423–1429.

Khaw KT, et al. "Combined impact of health behaviours and mortality in men and women: the EPIC-Norfolk prospective population study." PLoS Med V. 5 No. 1 (2008):e12.

Khaw KT, et al. "Randomised trial of coconut oil, olive oil or butter on blood lipids and other cardiovascular risk factors in healthy men and women." BMJ Open V. 8 (2018):e020167.

Kim R, et al. "Association of physical activity and APOE genotype with longitudinal cognitive change in early PD." Neurology (2021):10.

Kimura I, et al. "Short-chain fatty acids and ketones directly regulate sympathetic nervous system via G protein-coupled receptor 41 (GPR41)." Proc Natl Acad Sci U S A V. 108 No. 19 (2011):8030–5.

Kirkland AE, et al. "The role of magnesium in neurological disorders." Nutrients V. 10 No. 6 (2018):730.

Kivimäki M, et al. "Association of alcohol-induced loss of consciousness and overall alcohol consumption with risk for dementia." JAMA Netw Open V. 3 No. 9 (2020):e2016084.

Koepsell H. "Glucose transporters in brain in health and disease." Pflugers Arch V. 472 No. 9 (2020):1299–1343.

Koeslag JH, et al. "Post-exercise ketosis." Physiol Vol 301 (1980): 79–90.

Kondrashova M N, et al. "Synthesis of the sodium salt of beta-hydroxybutyric acid from acetoacetic ester." Biull Eksp Biol Med. V. 51 (1961): 104–105.

Koutnik A. Andrew Koutnik's Blog.
https://www.andrewkoutnik.com/blog/2018/8/22/part-1-what-is-type-1-diabetes

https://www.andrewkoutnik.com/blog/2018/9/8/part-2

https://www.andrewkoutnik.com/blog/2018/9/8/part-3-optimal-blood-glu cose-control

Kow FP, B Adlina, S Sivasangari, et al. "The impact of music guided deep breathing exercise on blood pressure control - A participant blinded randomised controlled study." Med J Malaysia (2018):233–238.

Kramarow EA, et al. "Dementia Mortality in the United States, 2000–2017." National Vital Statistics Reports V. 68 No. 2 (2019):1–28.

Kristoferitsch W, et al. "Secondary dementia due to Lyme neuroborreliosis." Wien Klin Wochenschr v. 130 No. 15–16 (2018):468–478.

Kuo CY, et al. "Association between obstructive sleep apnea, its treatment, and Alzheimer's disease: systematic mini-review." Front Aging Neurosci V. 12 (2021):591737.

L'Episcopo F, et al. "Microglia polarization, gene-environment interactions and wnt/β-catenin signaling: emerging roles of glia-neuron and glia-stem /neuroprogenitor crosstalk for dopaminergic neurorestoration in aged parkinsonian Brain." Front Aging Neurosci V. 10 (2018:12.

La AL, et al. "Long-term trazodone use and cognition: a potential therapeutic role for slow-wave sleep enhancers." J Alzheimers Dis V. 67 No. 3 (2019):911–921.

Lands, William. Fish, Omega-3 and Human Health. 2nd edition (2005), AOCS Press, Urbana, Illinois.

Lappano R, et al. "The lauric acid-activated signaling prompts apoptosis in cancer cells." Cell Death Discovery. V. 18 No. 3 (2017):17063

Law K S, et al. "The effects of virgin coconut oil (VCO) as supplementation on quality of life (QOL) among breast cancer patients." Lipids Health Dis. V. 13 (2014):139.

Legrand P, et al. "The complex and important cellular and metabolic functions of saturated fatty acids." Lipids V. 45 No. 10 (2010):941–946.

Lennerz BS, et al. "Management of type 1 diabetes with a very low-carbohydrate diet." Pediatrics V. 141 No. 6 (2018):e20173349.

Lennerz BS, et al. "Carbohydrate restriction for diabetes: rediscovering centuries-old wisdom." J Clin Invest V. 131 No. 1 (2021):e142246.

Lermyte F, et al. "Emerging approaches to investigate the influence of transition metals in the proteinopathies." Cells. V. 8 No. 10(2019):1231.

Lerner KC. "Clinical Trial Synopsis QB-0011: Madison Memory Study: a randomized, double-blinded, placebo-controlled trial of apoaequorin in community-dwelling, older adults." (2016) Published by Quincy Bioscience at https://quincybioscience.com/research.

Leroi I, et al. "Impact of an intervention to support hearing and vision in dementia: The SENSE-Cog Field Trial." Int J Geriatr Psychiatry V. 35 No. 4 (2020):348–357.

Li C, et al. "Effects of slow breathing rate on heart rate variability and arterial baroreflex sensitivity in essential hypertension." Medicine (Baltimore) V. 97 No. 18 (2018):e0639.

Li Q, et al. "A ketogenic diet and the treatment of autism spectrum disorder." Front Pediatr V. 11 No. 9 (2021):650624.

Lilienfeld S. "Galantamine—a novel cholinergic drug with a unique dual mode of action for the treatment of patients with Alzheimer's disease." CNS Drug Rev V. 8 No. 2 (2002):159–76.

Lim S, et al. "COVID-19 and diabetes mellitus: from pathophysiology to clinical management." Nat Rev Endocrinol V. 17 No. 1 (2021):11–30.

Lin L, et al. "Genetically encoded sensors enable micro- and nano-scopic decoding of transmission in healthy and diseased brains." Mol Psychiatry V. 26 No. 2 (2021):443–455.

Lin TK, et al. "Anti-inflammatory and skin barrier repair effects of topical application of some plant oils." Intern J Molecul Sci V. 19 No. 1 (2018):70.

Lipinski B, et al. "The role of iron-induced fibrin in the pathogenesis of Alzheimer's disease and the protective role of magnesium." Front Hum Neurosci V. 7 (2013):735.

Liskiewicz A, et al. "Sciatic nerve regeneration in rats subjected to ketogenic diet." Nutr Neurosci V. 19 (2016):116–124.

Lollis SS, et al. "Cause-specific mortality among neurosurgeons." J Neurosurg V. 113 No. 3 (2010):474–478.

Lopatko Lindman K, et al. "A genetic signature including apolipoprotein Eε4 potentiates the risk of herpes simplex-associated Alzheimer's disease." Alzheimers Dement V. 5 (2019):697–704.

Lopatko Lindman K, et al. "Herpesvirus infections, antiviral treatment, and the risk of dementia-a registry-based cohort study in Sweden." Alzheimers Dement V. 7 No. 1 (2021):e12119.

Lopez-Rodriguez AB, et al. "Acute systemic inflammation exacerbates neuroinflammation in Alzheimer's disease: IL-1β drives amplified responses in primed astrocytes and neuronal network dysfunction." Alzheimers Dement 2021: Jun 3. Epub ahead of print.

Lorscheider F. "The Dental amalgam mercury controversy – inorganic mercury and the CNS; Genetic linkage of mercury and antibiotic resistances in intestinal bacteria." Toxicology V. 97 No. 1–3 (1995):19–22.

Loucks EB, et al. "Mindfulness-Based Blood Pressure Reduction (MB-BP): Stage 1 single-arm clinical trial." PLoS ONE V. 14 No. 11 (2019): e0223095.

Lowry JA. "Oral chelation therapy for patients with lead poisoning." WHO Committee Report (2010) https://www.who.int/selection_medicines/committees/expert/18/applications/4_2_LeadOralChelators.pdf

Lying-Tunell U, et al. "Cerebral blood flow and metabolic rate of oxygen, glucose, lactate, pyruvate, ketone bodies and amino acids." Acta Neurol Scandinav. V. 63 (1981): 337–50.

Ma Y, et al. "Blood pressure variability and cerebral small vessel disease: A systematic review and meta-analysis of population-based cohorts." Stroke V. 51 No. 1 (2020): 82–89.

Making Mercury History, (2017). Video online at https://www.unep.org/news-and-stories/video/making-mercury-history.

Malapaka RRV, et al. "Identification and mechanism of 10-carbon fatty acid as modulating ligand of peroxisome proliferator-activated receptors." J Biol Chem V. 287 No. 1 (2012):183–195.

Mann GV. "Diet and coronary heart disease." AMA Arch Intern Med V. 104 (1959): 95–103.

Manzar H, et al. "Cellular consequences of coenzyme Q10 deficiency in neurodegeneration of the retina and brain." Int J Mol Sci V. 21 No. 23 (2020):9299.

Marcos-Pardo PJ, et al. "Association among adherence to the Mediterranean diet, cardiorespiratory fitness, cardiovascular, obesity, and anthropometric variables of overweight and obese middle-aged and older adults." Nutrients V. 12 No. 9 (2020):2750.

Martínez Steele E, et al. "Ultra-processed foods and added sugars in the US diet: evidence from a nationally representative cross-sectional study." BMJ Open V. 6 No. 3 (2016):e009892.

Mates E, et al. "A retrospective case series of thiamine deficiency in non-alcoholic hospitalized veterans: an important cause of delirium and falling?" J Clin Med V. 10 No. 7 (2021):1449.

Matschke J, et al. "Neuropathology of patients with COVID-19 in Germany: a post-mortem case series." Lancet Neurol V. 19 No. 11 (2020):919–929.

Mattson MP, et al. "Intermittent metabolic switching, neuroplasticity and brain health." Nat Rev Neurosci V. 19 No. 2 (2018):63–80.

Mattson MP, et al. "Hallmarks of Brain Aging: Adaptive and Pathological Modification by Metabolic States." Cell Metab V. 27 No. 6 (2018):1176–1199.

McCleery J, et al. "Pharmacotherapies for sleep disturbances in dementia." Cochrane Database Syst Rev V. 11 No. 11 (2016):CD009178.

McGrattan AM, et al. "Diet and inflammation in cognitive ageing and Alzheimer's Disease." Curr Nutr Rep V. 8 No. 2 (2019):53–65.

Mehmel M, et al. "Nicotinamide riboside-the current state of research and therapeutic uses." Nutrients V. 12 No. 6 (2020):1616.

Mehta HB, et al. "Association of hypoglycemia with subsequent dementia in older patients with type 2 diabetes mellitus." J Gerontol A Biol Sci Med Sci V. 72 No. 8 (2017):1110–1116.

Meng XF, et al. "Midlife vascular risk factors and the risk of Alzheimer's disease: a systematic review and meta-analysis." J Alzheimers Dis V. 42 No. 4 (2014):1295–310.

Mensink RP, et al. "Effects of dietary trans fatty acids in high-density and low-density lipoprotein cholesterol levels in health subjects." NEJM V. 323 (1990): 439–445.

Mente A, et al. "Urinary sodium excretion, blood pressure, cardiovascular disease, and mortality: a community-level prospective epidemiological cohort study." Lancet V. 392 (2018): 496–506.

Metcalfe-Roach A, et al. "MIND and Mediterranean diets associated with later onset of Parkinson's disease." Mov Disord (2021): Epub ahead of print.

Mielke MM, et al. "Serum ceramides increase the risk of Alzheimer disease: the Women's Health and Aging Study II." Neurology V. 79 (2012): 633–641.

Mijajlović MD, et al. "Post-stroke dementia - a comprehensive review." BMC Med V. 15 No. 1 (2017):11.

Miklossy J. "Alzheimer's disease - a neurospirochetosis. Analysis of the evidence following Koch's and Hill's criteria." J Neuroinflammation. V. 8 (2011):90.

Miller V, et al. "Fruit, vegetable, and legume intake, and cardiovascular disease and deaths in 18 countries (PURE): a prospective cohort study." Lancet V. 390 (2017):2037–49.

Miranda Orr, et al. "Results from a pilot study: the effects of nicotinamide riboside on cognitive impairment." Alzheimers Dement V. 16 Suppl. 9 (2020):e044746. Poster presentation.

Monda V, et al. "Short-Term Physiological Effects of a Very Low-Calorie Ketogenic Diet: Effects on Adiponectin Levels and Inflammatory States." Int J Mol Sci V. 21 No. 9 (2020):3228.

Monteiro C, et al. "The UN Decade of Nutrition, the NOVA food classification and the trouble with ultra-processing." Public Health Nutrition V. 21 No.1 (2018): 5–17.

Mooldijk SS, et al. "Letter to the Editor, Reacting to: 'APOE ε4 carriers have a greater propensity to glycation and sRAGE which is further influenced by RAGE G82S polymorphism.'" J Gerontol A Biol Sci Med Sci V. 75 No. 10 (2020):1906–1907.

Morrill SJ, et al. "Ketogenic diet rescues cognition in ApoE4+ patient with mild Alzheimer's disease: A case study." Diabetes & Metabolic Syndrome: Clinical Research & Reviews V. 13 (2019): 1187e–1191e.

Myette-Côté É, et al. "Prior ingestion of exogenous ketone monoester attenuates the glycaemic response to an oral glucose tolerance test in healthy young individuals." J Physiol V. 596 No. 8 (2018):1385–1395. Erratum in: J Physiol V. 597 No. 22 (2019):5515. Abstract corrected.

Nafar F, et al. "Coconut oil attenuates the effects of amyloid-beta on cortical neurons in vitro." J Alzheim Dis V. 39 (2014): 233–23.

Nafar F, et al. "Coconut oil protects cortical neurons from amyloid beta toxicity by enhancing signaling of cell survival pathways." Neurochem Int V. 105 (2017):64–79.

Nasrabady SE, et al. "White matter changes in Alzheimer's disease: a focus on myelin and oligodendrocytes." Acta Neuropathol Commun V. 6 No. 1 (2018):22.

Nedergaard M. "Garbage truck of the brain." Science V.340 No. 6140 (2013):1529–1530.

Neth BJ, et al. "Modified ketogenic diet is associated with improved cerebro-spinal fluid biomarker profile, cerebral perfusion, and cerebral ketone body uptake in older adults at risk for Alzheimer's disease." Neurobiol Aging V. 86 (2020):54–63.

Netzer CT. The Complete Book of Food Counts. Random House Publishing Group, New York NY, ninth edition, 2012.

Newport MT, et al. "A new way to produce hyperketonemia: use of ketone ester in a case of Alzheimer's disease." Alzheimers Dement V. 11 No. 1 (2015):99–103.

NHIS. "Early release of selected estimates from the 2019 national health interview survey." https://www.cdc.gov/nchs/data/nhis/earlyrelease/EarlyRelease202009-508.pdf

NIA. "Video: How Alzheimer's changes the brain." (2021). https://www.nia.nih.gov/health/video-how-alzheimers-changes-brain?utm_source=AD video&utm_medium=web&utm_campaign=rightrail

Nielsen LB. "Atherogenecity of lipoprotein(a) and oxidized low density lipoprotein: Insight from in vivo studies of arterial wall influx, degradation and efflux." Atherosclerosis V. 143 (1999):229–243.

Nielsen R, et al. "Cardiovascular effects of treatment with the ketone body 3-hydroxybutyrate in chronic heart failure patients." Circulation V. 139 (2019):2129–41.

NIH. "Dietary supplement fact sheets for health professionals." Search for nutrient at https://ods.od.nih.gov/factsheets/list-all/

NIH on Sodium. Https://www.nhlbi.nih.gov/health-topics/all-publications -and-resources/tips-reduce-salt-sodium

Nikisch G, et al. "Three-year follow-up of a patient with early-onset Alzheimer's disease with presenilin-2 N141I mutation - case report and review of the literature." Eur J Med Res V. 13 No. 12 (2008):579–84.

Nonaka Y, et al. "Lauric acid stimulates ketone body production in the KT-5 Astrocyte Cell Line." J Oleo Science V. 65 No. 8 (2016): 693–699.

Norins LC. "Licensed anti-microbial drugs logical for clinical trials against pathogens currently suspected in Alzheimer's disease." Antibiotics (Basel) V. 10 No. 3 (2021):327.

Norins LC. "White paper: It's time to find the Alzheimer's germ." (2018) https://alzgerm.org/whitepaper/

Norwitz NG, et al. "Multi-loop model of Alzheimer disease: an integrated perspective on the Wnt/GSK3β, α-synuclein, and type 3 diabetes hypotheses." Frontiers in Aging Neuroscience V. 11 No. 184 (2019): Published Online.

Norwitz NG, et al. "Precision nutrition for Alzheimer's prevention in ApoE4 Carriers." Nutrients V. 13 No. 4 (2021):1362.

Nuber S, et al. "A stearoyl-CoA desaturase inhibitor prevents multiple Parkinson's disease-phenotypes in α-synuclein mice." Ann Neurol V. 89 No. 1 (2021):74–90.

Nugent S, et al. "Brain and systemic glucose metabolism in the healthy elderly following fish oil supplementation." Prostaglandins Leukot Essent Fatty Acids V. 85 No. 5 (2011):287–91.

Ogino E, et al. "Current and past leisure time physical activity in relation to risk of Alzheimer's disease in older adults." Alzheimers Dement V. 15 No. 12 (2019):1603–11.

Ohtsu A, et al. "Advanced glycation end-products and lipopolysaccharides stimulate interleukin-6 secretion via the RAGE/TLR4-NF-κB-ROS pathways and resveratrol attenuates these inflammatory responses in mouse macrophages." Exp Ther Med V. 14 No. 5 (2017):4363–4370.

Oliveira-de-Lira L, et al. "Supplementation-dependent effects of vegetable oils with varying fatty acid compositions on anthropometric and biochemical parameters in obese women." Nutrients V. 10 No. 7 (2018):932.

Olsen SJ, et al. "Decreased influenza activity during the COVID-19 pandemic—United States, Australia, Chile, and South Africa, 2020." MMWR Morb Mortal Wkly Rep V. 69 No. 1305 (2020):1305–1309.

Ooi SL, et al. "Transcendental meditation for lowering blood pressure: An overview of systematic reviews and meta-analyses." Complement Ther Med V. 34 (2017):26–34.

Ooi TC, et al. "Intermittent fasting enhanced the cognitive function in older adults with mild cognitive impairment by inducing biochemical and metabolic changes: a 3-year progressive study." Nutrients V. 12 No. 9 (2020):2644.

Ouk M, et al. "The use of angiotensin-converting enzyme inhibitors vs. angiotensin receptor blockers and cognitive decline in Alzheimer's disease: the importance of blood-brain barrier penetration and APOE ε4 carrier status." Alzheimers Res Ther V. 13 No. 1 (2021):43.

Oulhaj A, et al. "Omega-3 fatty acid status enhances the prevention of cognitive decline by b vitamins in mild cognitive impairment." J Alzheimers Dis V. 50 No. 2 (2016):547–57.

Our World in Data: "Number of deaths by risk factor, World, 2017." (2017) Online at https://ourworldindata.org/grapher/number-of-deaths-by-risk -factor?country=~OWID_WRL from http://ghdx.healthdata.org/gbd-re sults-tool.

Owen OE, et al. "Brain metabolism during fasting." J Clin Invest V. 46 (1967): 1589–1595.

Ozemek C, et al. "Impact of therapeutic lifestyle changes in resistant hypertension." Prog Cardiovasc Dis V. 63 No. 1 (2020):4–9.

Page KA, et al. "Medium-chain fatty acids improve cognitive function in intensively treated type 1 diabetic patients and support in vitro synaptic transmission during acute hypoglycemia." Diabetes V. 58 No. 5 (May 2009): 1237–1244.

Pan X, et al. "Powerful beneficial effects of benfotiamine on cognitive impairment and beta-amyloid deposition in amyloid precursor protein/ presenilin-1 transgenic mice." Brain V. 133 Pt. 5 (2010 May):1342–51.

Pase MP, et al. "Sugary beverage intake and preclinical Alzheimer's disease in the community." Alzheimers Dement V. 13 No. 9 (2017):955–964.

Passmore R, et al. "The modification of post-exercise ketosis (the Courtice-Douglas effect) by environmental temperature and water balance." Exp Physiol (1958): 352–361.

Pastore A, et al. "Why does the Aβ peptide of Alzheimer share structural similarity with antimicrobial peptides?" Commun Biol V. 19 No. 3 (2020):135.

Patrick RP. "Role of phosphatidylcholine-DHA in preventing APOE4-associated Alzheimer's disease." FASEB J V. 33 No. 2 (2019):1554–1564.

Peedikayil FC, et al. "Effect of coconut oil in plaque related gingivitis - A preliminary report." Niger Med J V. 56 No. 2 (2015):143–7.

Peever J, et al. "The Biology of REM Sleep." Curr Biol V. 27 No. 22 (2017):R1237–R1248.

Peng B, et al. "Role of alcohol drinking in Alzheimer's disease, Parkinson's disease, and amyotrophic lateral sclerosis." Int J Mol Sci V. 21 No. 7 (2020):2316.

Penke B, et al. "Protein folding and misfolding, endoplasmic reticulum stress in neurodegenerative diseases: in trace of novel drug targets." Curr Protein Pept Sci V. 17 No. 2 (2016):169–82.

Perez Ortiz JM, et al. "Mitochondrial dysfunction in Alzheimer's disease: role in pathogenesis and novel therapeutic opportunities." Br J Pharmacol V. 176 No. 18 (2019):3489–3507.

Phillips MCL, et al. "Low-fat versus ketogenic diet in Parkinson's disease: A pilot randomized controlled trial." Mov Disord V. 33 No. 8 (2018):1306–1314.

Phillips MCL, et al. "Randomized crossover trial of a modified ketogenic diet in Alzheimer's disease." Alzheimers Res Ther V. 13 No. 1 (2021):51.

Plaschke K, et al. "Insulin-resistant brain state (IRBS) changes membrane composition of fatty acids in temporal and entorhinal brain cortices of rats: relevance to sporadic Alzheimer's disease?" J Neural Transm (Vienna). 2010 Dec;117(12):1419–22.

Prata J and CH, 2021. From interviews with Carol Prata on February 7, 2018, and August 10, 2021.

Preti L. "Die muskelarbeit und deren ketogene wirkung." Biochem Z V. 32 (1911): 231–234.

Prior I, et al. "Cholesterol, coconuts, and diet on Polynesian atolls: a natural experiment: the Pukapuka and Tokelau Island studies." Amer J Clin Nutr V. 34 (1981):1552–1561.

PubChem. "Thiamine mononitrate." Accessed July 21, 2021, at https://pubchem.ncbi.nlm.nih.gov/compound/10762.

Qiu C, et al. "Prevention of cognitive decline in old age-varying effects of interventions in different populations." Ann Transl Med V. 7 Suppl. 3 (2019):S142.

Rajan KB, et al. "Blood pressure and risk of incident Alzheimer's disease dementia by antihypertensive medications and APOE ε4 allele." Ann Neurol V. 83 No. 5 (2018):935–944.

Rajmohan R, et al. "Amyloid-Beta and Phosphorylated Tau Accumulations Cause Abnormalities at Synapses of Alzheimer's disease Neurons." J Alzheimers Dis V. 57 No. 4 (2017):975–999.

Ramakrishnan R, et al. "Accelerometer measured physical activity and the incidence of cardiovascular disease: evidence from the UK Biobank cohort study." PLoS Med V. 18 No. 1 (2021): e1003487.

Ramani A, et al. "SARS-CoV-2 targets neurons of 3D human brain organoids." EMBO J V. 39 No. 20 (2020):e106230.

Reiman EM, et al. "Functional brain abnormalities in young adults at genetic risk for late-onset Alzheimer's dementia." Proc Natl Acad Sci USA V. 101 No. 1 (2004):284–289.

Reiman EM, et al. "Brain imaging and fluid biomarker analysis in young adults at genetic risk for autosomal dominant Alzheimer's disease in the presenilin 1 E280A kindred: a case-control study." Lancet Neurol V. 11 No. 12 (2012):1048–1056.

Reisberg B. "Functional Assessment Staging (FAST)." Psychopharmacology Bulletin V. 24 (1988): 653–659.

Rennie MJ, et al. "The metabolic effects of strenuous exercise: a comparison between untrained subjects and racing cyclists." ExpPhysiol (1974): 201–212.

Rexach JE, et al. "Tau pathology drives dementia risk-associated gene networks toward chronic inflammatory states and immunosuppression." Cell Rep V. 33 No. 7 (2020):108398.

Riederer P. "Siegfried Hoyer 1933–2014." J Neural Transm (Vienna) V. 121 No. 6 (2014):565–567.

Rioux V, et al. "Saturated fatty acids: simple molecular structures with complex cellular functions." Curr Opinion in Clin Nutri Metab Care V. 10 No. 6 (2007): 752–758.

Rodriguez-Rodriguez P, et al. "Tau hyperphosphorylation induces oligomeric insulin accumulation and insulin resistance in neurons." Brain V. 140 No. 12 (2017):3269–3285. Erratum in: Brain V. 141 No. 5 (2018):e43.

Román GC, et al. "Epigenetic factors in late-onset Alzheimer's disease: MTHFR and CTH gene polymorphisms, metabolic trans-sulfuration and methylation pathways, and B vitamins." Int J Mol Sci V. 20 No. 2 (2019):319.

Rorbach-Dolata A, et al. "Neurometabolic evidence supporting the hypothesis of increased incidence of type 3 diabetes mellitus in the 21st Century." Biomed Res Int (2019):1435276. Published 2019 Jul 21.

Rosenberg A, et al. "Multidomain interventions to prevent cognitive impairment, Alzheimer's disease, and dementia: from FINGER to World-Wide FINGERS." J Prev Alzheimers Dis V. 7 No. 1 (2020):29–36.

Rosenberg A, et al. "Multidomain lifestyle intervention benefits a large elderly population at risk for cognitive decline and dementia regardless of baseline characteristics: the FINGER trial." Alzheimers Dement V. 14 No. 3 (2018):263–270.

Rosenfeldt AB, et al. "High intensity aerobic exercise improves information processing and motor performance in individuals with Parkinson's disease." Exp Brain Res V. 239 No. 3 (2021):777–786.

Roy M, et al. "Fascicle- and glucose-specific deterioration in white matter energy supply in Alzheimer's Disease." J Alzheimers Dis V. 76 No. 3 (2020):863–881.

Ruegsegger GN, et al. "Altered mitochondrial function in insulin-deficient and insulin-resistant states." J Clin Invest V.128 No. 9 (2018):3671–3681.

Rusek M, et al. "Ketogenic diet in Alzheimer's disease." Int J Mol Sci V. 20 No. 16 (2019):3892.

Sacks FM, et al. "Dietary fats and cardiovascular disease: A presidential advisory from the American Heart Association." Circulation V. 136 No. 3 (2017):e1–e23.

Sáez-Orellana F, et al. "Alzheimer's disease, a lipid story: involvement of peroxisome proliferator-activated receptor α." Cells V. 9 No. 5 (2020):1215.

Saito ER, et al. "Alzheimer's disease alters oligodendrocytic glycolytic and ketolytic gene expression." Alzheimers Dement V. 17 No. 9 (2021):1474–1486.

Salas-Salvadó J, et al. "Effect of a lifestyle intervention program with energy-restricted Mediterranean diet and exercise on weight loss and cardiovascular risk factors: one-year results of the PREDIMED-Plus Trial." Diabetes Care V. 42 No. 5 (2019):777–788.

Salkovic-Petrisic M, et al. "What have we learned from the streptozotocin-induced animal model of sporadic Alzheimer's disease, about the therapeutic strategies in Alzheimer's research." J Neural Transm (Vienna) C. 120 No. 1 (2013):233–52.

Salkovic-Petrisic M, et al. "Modeling sporadic Alzheimer's disease: the insulin resistant brain state generates multiple long-term morphobiological abnormalities including hyperphosphorylated tau protein and amyloid-beta." J Alzheimers Dis V. 18 No. 4 (2009):729–50.

Saltz BL, et al. "Recognizing and managing antipsychotic drug treatment side effects in the elderly." J Clin Psychol V. 6, Suppl. 2 (2004): 14–19.

Sambon M, et al. "Neuroprotective effects of thiamine and precursors with higher bioavailability: focus on benfotiamine and dibenzoylthiamine." Int J Mol Sci V.22 No. 11 (2021):5418.

Sanjeev G, et al. "Late-life cognitive activity and dementia." Epidemiology V. 27 No. 5 (2016):732–42.

Sasada T, et al. "Chlorinated water modulates the development of colorectal tumors with chromosomal instability and gut microbiota in Apc-deficient mice." PLoS One V. 10 No. 7 (2015):e0132435.

Sato K, et al. "Insulin, ketone bodies, and mitochondrial energy transduction." FASEB Journal V. 9 (1995): 651–658.

Sato Y, et al. "Soluble APP functions as a vascular niche signal that controls adult neural stem cell number." Development V. 144 No. 15 (2017):2730–2736.

Scarmeas N, et al. "Mediterranean diet and Alzheimer disease mortality." Neurology V. 69 No. 11 (2007):1084–1093.

Schnier C, et al. "Antiherpetic medication and incident dementia: Observational cohort studies in four countries." Eur J Neurol (2021): Epub ahead of print.

Schoeler NE, et al. "K.Vita: a feasibility study of a blend of medium chain triglycerides to manage drug-resistant epilepsy." Brain Communications V. 3 No. 4 (2021):fcab160.

Schöll M, et al. "Glucose metabolism and PIB binding in carriers of a His163Tyr presenilin 1 mutation." Neurobiol Aging V. 32 No. 8 (2011):1388–99.

Schootemeijer S, et al. "Current Perspectives on Aerobic Exercise in People with Parkinson's Disease." Neurotherapeutics V. 17 No. 4 (2020):1418–1433.

Schultz ST, et al. "Breastfeeding, infant formula supplementation, and Autistic Disorder: the results of a parent survey." Int Breastfeed J V. 1 (2006):16.

Senyilmaz-Tiebe D, et al. "Dietary stearic acid regulates mitochondria in vivo in humans." Nat Commun V. 9 No. 1 (2018):3129.

Shahmoradian S. H. et al. "Lewy pathology in Parkinson's disease consists of crowded organelles and lipid membranes." Nat Neurosci V. 22 (2019):1099–1109.

Sienski G, et al. "APOE4 disrupts intracellular lipid homeostasis in human iPSC-derived glia." Sci Transl Med V.13 No 583 (2021):eaaz4564.

Simeone TA, et al. "Regulation of brain PPARgamma2 contributes to ketogenic diet anti-seizure efficacy." Exp Neurol V. 287 Pt. 1 (2017): 54–64.

Simopoulos AP. "An Increase in the Omega-6/Omega-3 Fatty Acid Ratio Increases the Risk for Obesity." Nutrients V. 8 No. 2 (2016):128.

Slutsky I, et al. "Enhancement of learning and memory by elevating brain magnesium." Neuron V. 65 No. 2 (2010):165–77.

Smith AD, et al. "Homocysteine-lowering by B vitamins slows the rate of accelerated brain atrophy in mild cognitive impairment: a randomized controlled trial." PLoS One V. 5 No. 9 (2010):e12244.

Smith WD. "Hippocrates, Greek Physician." Encyclopedia Britannica (2020) Online: https://www.britannica.com/biography/Hippocrates.

Smolders L, et al. "Natural choline from egg yolk phospholipids is more efficiently absorbed compared with choline bitartrate; outcomes of a randomized trial in healthy adults." Nutrients V. 11 No. 11 (2019):2758.

Snowden SG, et al. "Association between fatty acid metabolism in the brain and Alzheimer disease neuropathology and cognitive performance: A nontargeted metabolomic study." PLoS Med V. 14 No. 3 (2017):e1002266.

Snowden SG, et al. "Neurotransmitter Imbalance in the Brain and Alzheimer's Disease Pathology." IOS Press V. 72 No. 1 (2019): 35 – 43.

Snowdon DA, et al. "Serum folate and the severity of atrophy of the neocortex in Alzheimer disease: Findings from the Nun study." Am J Clin Nutr V. 71 (2000):993–998.

Snowdon, DA. Aging with Grace: What the Nun Study Teaches Us About Leading Longer, Healthier, and More Meaningful Lives. Bantam Books, New York, New York (2002).

Soaking Nuts and Seeds (2022) at https://traditionalcookingschool.com/food-preparation/how-and-why-to-soak-and-dehydrate-nuts-and-seeds.

Sochocka M, et al. "The Gut Microbiome Alterations and Inflammation-Driven Pathogenesis of Alzheimer's Disease-a Critical Review." Mol Neurobiol V. 56 V. 3 (2019):1841–1851.

Soscia SJ, et al. "The Alzheimer's disease-associated amyloid beta-protein is an antimicrobial peptide." PLoS One V. 5 No. 3 (2010):e9505.

Soto-Mota A, et al. "Safety and tolerability of sustained exogenous ketosis using ketone monoester drinks for 28 days in healthy adults." Regul Toxicol Pharmacol V. 109 (2019):104506.

Soto-Mota A, et al. "Why a d-β-hydroxybutyrate monoester?" Biochem Soc Trans 2020 V. 48 No. 1 (2020):51-59.

Soto-Mota A, et al. "Exogenous ketosis in patients with type 2 diabetes: Safety, tolerability and effect on glycaemic control." Endocrinol Diabetes Metab V. 4 No. 3 (2021):e00264.

SPRINT MIND Investigators for the SPRINT Research Group, Williamson JD, et al. "Effect of intensive vs standard blood pressure control on probable dementia: a randomized clinical trial." JAMA V. 321 No. 6 (2019):553–561.

SPRINT Research Group, Wright JT Jr, et al. "A randomized trial of intensive versus standard blood-pressure control." N Engl J Med V. 373 No. 22 (2015):2103–16.

Srour B, et al. "Ultra-processed food intake and risk of cardiovascular disease: prospective cohort study (NutriNet-Santé)." BMJ V. 365 (2019):l1451.

Staf RT, et al. "Intellectual engagement and cognitive ability in later life (the "use it or lose it" conjecture): longitudinal, prospective study." BMJ V. 363 (2018):k4925.

Stancu IC, , et al. "Aggregated Tau activates NLRP3-ASC inflammasome exacerbating exogenously seeded and non-exogenously seeded Tau pathology in vivo." Acta Neuropathol V. 137 No. 4 (2019):599–617.

Stirland LE, et al. "Passive smoking as a risk factor for dementia and cognitive impairment: systematic review of observational studies." Int Psychogeriatr V. 30 No. 8 (2018):1177–1187.

Stoykovich S, et al. "APOE4, the door to insulin-resistant dyslipidemia and brain fog? A case study." Alzheimer's and Dementia V. 11 (2019):264–269.

St-Pierre V, et al. "Plasma ketone and medium-chain fatty acid response in humans consuming different medium-chain triglycerides during a metabolic study day." Front Nutr V. 6 (2019):46.

Strollo PJ, et al. "Upper-Airway Stimulation for Obstructive Sleep Apnea." NEJM V. 370 (2014):139–49.

Stubbs B J, et al. "On the metabolism of exogenous ketones in humans." Frontiers in Physiology. V. 8 No. 848 (2017): 1–13.

Stubbs BJ, et al. "A ketone ester drink lowers human ghrelin and appetite." Obesity (Silver Spring) V. 26 No. 2 (2018):269–273.

Stumpf SK, et al. "Ketogenic diet ameliorates axonal defects and promotes myelination in Pelizaeus-Merzbacher disease." Acta Neuropathol V. 138 (2019):147–161.

Sturchio A, et al. "High cerebrospinal amyloid-b 42 is associated with normal cognition in individuals with brain amyloidosis." EClinical Medicine (The Lancet) (2021): Published online ahead of print.

Sultan S, et al. "Low Vitamin D and Its Association with Cognitive Impairment and Dementia." J Aging Res (2020):6097820.

Sun Y, et al. "Metabolism: A Novel Shared Link between Diabetes Mellitus and Alzheimer's Disease." J Diabetes Res (2020):4981814. Published 2020 Jan 29.

Swaminathan S, et al. "Associations of cereal grains intake with cardiovascular disease and mortality across 21 countries in Prospective Urban and Rural Epidemiology study: prospective cohort study." BMJ V. 372 (2021):m4948.

Swerdlow R, et al. "Brain glucose and ketone body metabolism in patients with Alzheimer's disease." Clin Res. V. 37 No. 461A (1989)

Swerdlow RH. "Bioenergetic medicine." British Journal of Pharmacology V. 171 (2014):1854–1869.

Tariq S, et al. "A longitudinal magnetic resonance imaging study of neurodegenerative and small vessel disease, and clinical cognitive trajectories in non-demented patients with transient ischemic attack: the PREVENT study." BMC Geriatr V. 18 No. 1 (2018):163.

Taylor MK, et al. "Dietary neuroketotherapeutics for Alzheimer's disease: An evidence update and the potential role for diet quality." Nutrients V. 11 No. 8 (2019):1910.

Taylor MK, et al. "A high-glycemic diet is associated with cerebral amyloid burden in cognitively normal older adults." Am J Clin Nutr V. 106 No. 6 (2017):1463–1470.

Tham YY, et al. "Lauric acid alleviates insulin resistance by improving mitochondrial biogenesis in THP-1 macrophages." Mol Biol Rep V. 47 No. 12 (2020):9595–9607.

Thau-Zuchman O, et al. "A new ketogenic formulation improves functional outcome and reduces tissue loss following traumatic brain injury in adult mice." Theranostics V. 11 No. 1 (2021):346–360.

Thaweboon S, et al. "Effect of oil pulling on oral microorganisms in biofilm models." Asia J Public Health V. 2 (2011):62–6.

Thevenet J, et al. "Medium-chain fatty acids inhibit mitochondrial metabolism in astrocytes promoting astrocyte-neuron lactate and ketone body shuttle systems." FASEB J. V. 30 No. 5 (2016):1913–26.

Thormar H, et al. "Inactivation of enveloped viruses and killing of cells by fatty acids and monoglycerides." Antimicrob Agents Chemother V. 31 No. 1 (1987):27–31.

Todd KL, et al. "Ventricular and Periventricular Anomalies in the Aging and Cognitively Impaired Brain." Front Aging Neurosci V. 9 (2018):445.

Toledo JB, et al. Alzheimer's Disease Neuroimaging Initiative and the Alzheimer Disease Metabolomics Consortium. "Metabolic network failures in Alzheimer's disease: A biochemical road map." Alzheimers Dement V. 13 NO. 9 (2017):965–984.

Tong M, et al. "Nitrosamine exposure causes insulin resistance diseases: relevance to type 2 diabetes mellitus, non-alcoholic steatohepatitis, and Alzheimer's disease." J Alzheimers Dis V. 17, No. 4 (2009): 827–844.

Travica N, et al. "Vitamin C Status and Cognitive Function: A Systematic Review." Nutrients V. 9 No. 9 (2017):960.

Travica N, et al. "Plasma Vitamin C Concentrations and Cognitive Function: A Cross-Sectional Study." Front Aging Neurosci V. 11 (2019):72.

Tsai MC, et al. "Increased risk of dementia following herpes zoster ophthalmicus." PloS One V. 12 (2017):e0188490

Turner N, et al. "Enhancement of muscle mitochondrial oxidative capacity and alterations in insulin action are lipid species dependent: potent tissue-specific effects of medium-chain fatty acids." Diabetes V. 58 No. 11 (2009):2547–5.

Tzeng NS, et al. "Anti-herpetic medications and reduced risk of dementia in patients with herpes simplex virus infections-a nationwide, population-based cohort study in Taiwan." Neurotherapeutics V. 15 (2018):417–429.

USDA 1992 Pyramid. "A brief history of USDA food guides." Online: https://choosemyplate-prod.azureedge.net/sites/default/files/ABriefHistoryOfUSDAFoodGuides.pdf

USDA FoodData Central. https://fdc.nal.usda.gov/

Valerio F, et al. "The neurological sequelae of pandemics and epidemics." J Neurol 2020:1–27.

Van Cauter E, et al. "Metabolic consequences of sleep and sleep loss." Sleep Med V. 9 Suppl. 1(2008):S23–8.

Van den Brink AC, et al. "The Mediterranean, Dietary Approaches to Stop Hypertension (DASH), and Mediterranean-DASH Intervention for neurodegenerative delay (mind) diets are associated with less cognitive decline and a lower risk of Alzheimer's disease—a review." Adv Nutr V. 10 No. 6 (2019):1040–1065.

Van der Auwera I, et al. "A ketogenic diet reduces amyloid beta 40 and 42 in a mouse model of Alzheimer's disease." Nutr Metab (Lond) V. 2 (2005):28.

Van Hove JLK, et al. "D, L-3-hydroxybutyrate treatment of multiple acyl-CoA dehydrogenase deficiency (MADD.)" Lancet V. 361 (April 2003): 1433–1435.

Vandenberghe C, et al. "A short-term intervention combining aerobic exercise with medium-chain triglycerides (MCT) is more ketogenic than either MCT or aerobic exercise alone: a comparison of normoglycemic and prediabetic older women." Appl Physiol Nutr Metab V. 44 No. 1 (2019):66–73.

Vandenberghe C, et al. "Caffeine intake increases plasma ketones: an acute metabolic study in humans." Can J Physiol Pharmacol V. 95 No. 4 (2017):455–458.

Vandenberghe C, et al. "Tricaprylin alone increases plasma ketone response more than coconut oil or other medium-chain triglycerides: an acute crossover study in healthy adults." Curr Dev Nutr V. 1 No. 4 (2017):e000257.

Vandoorne T, et al. "Intake of a ketone ester drink during recovery from exercise promotes mTORC1 signaling but not glycogen resynthesis in human muscle." Front Physiol. V. 8 (2017):310.

VanItallie TB, et al. "Treatment of Parkinson disease with diet-induced hyperketonemia: a feasibility study." Neurology V. 64 (February 2005): 728–730.

VanItallie TB. "Parkinson's disease: Primacy of age as a risk factor for mitochondrial dysfunction." Metab Clin Exper V. 57 Suppl. 2 (2008):S50–S55.

Varesio C, et al. "Ketogenic dietary therapies in patients with autism spectrum disorder: facts or fads? A scoping review and a proposal for a shared protocol." Nutrients V. 13 No. 6 (2021):2057.

Veech R L, et al. "Ketone bodies mimic the life span extending properties of caloric restriction." IUBMB Life. V. 69 No. 5 (2017): 305–14.

Veech RL, et al. "Ketone bodies, potential therapeutic uses." IUBMB Life V. 51 No. 4 (2001):241–7.

Veech RL, et al. "The 'great' controlling nucleotide coenzymes." IUBMB Life V. 71 No. 5 (2019):565–579.

Velazquez R, et al. "Choline as a prevention for Alzheimer's disease." Aging (Albany NY) V. 12 No. 3 (2020):2026–2027.

Vendel Nielsen L, et al. "Effects of elaidic acid on lipid metabolism in HepG2 cells, investigated by an integrated approach of lipidomics, transcriptomics and proteomics." PLoS One V. 8 No. 9 (2013):e74283.

Venkataraman A, et al. "Alcohol and Alzheimer's Disease—Does Alcohol Dependence Contribute to Beta-Amyloid Deposition, Neuroinflammation and Neurodegeneration in Alzheimer's Disease?" Alcohol V. 52 No. 2 (2017):151–158.

Vidmar Golja M, et al. "Folate insufficiency due to MTHFR deficiency is bypassed by 5-methyltetrahydrofolate." J Clin Med V. 9 No. 9 (2020):2836.

Vijayakumar M, et al. "A randomized study of coconut oil versus sunflower oil on cardiovascular risk factors in patients with stable coronary heart disease." Indian Heart J V. 68 No. 4 (2016):498–506.

Vijayan M, et al. "Stroke, vascular dementia, and Alzheimer's disease: molecular links." J Alzheimers Dis V. 54 No. 2 (2016):427–43.

Volek JS, et al. "Carbohydrate restriction has a more favorable impact on the metabolic syndrome than a low-fat diet." Lipids V. 44 (2009): 297–309.

Volk BM, et al. "Effects of step-wise increases in dietary carbohydrate on circulating saturated fatty acids and palmitoleic acid in adults with metabolic syndrome." PLoS One V.9 No.11 (2014): e113605.

Wallace TC, et al. "Choline: The underconsumed and underappreciated essential nutrient." Nutr Today v. 53 No. 6 (2018):240–253.

Wallin C, et al. "Mercury and Alzheimer's disease: Hg (II) ions display specific binding to the amyloid-β peptide and hinder its fibrillization." Biomolecules V. 10 No. 1 (2019):44.

Wang C, M Zhang, et al. "ApoE-isoform-dependent SARS-CoV-2 neurotropism and cellular response." Cell Stem Cell (2021):S1934–5909(20)30602 -0. Ahead of print.

Wang X, et al. "Associations of cumulative exposure to heavy metal mixtures with obesity and its comorbidities among U.S. adults in NHANES 2003–2014." Environ Int V. 121 Pt. 1 (2018):683–694.

Wang Y, et al. "Maternal dietary intake of choline in mice regulates development of the cerebral cortex in the offspring." FASEB J V. 30 No. 4 (2016):1566–78.

Washington PM, et al. "Polypathology and dementia after brain trauma: Does brain injury trigger distinct neurodegenerative diseases, or should they be classified together as traumatic encephalopathy?" Exp Neurol V. 275 Pt. 3 (2016):381–388.

Watt JA, et al. "Comparative efficacy of interventions for reducing symptoms of depression in people with dementia: systematic review and network meta-analysis." BMJ V. 372 (2021):n532.

Wear D, et al. "Ubisol-Q10, a nanomicellar and water-dispersible formulation of coenzyme-Q10 as a potential treatment for Alzheimer's and Parkinson's disease." Antioxidants (Basel) V. 10 No. 5 (2021):764.

Weinstein G, et al. "Association of metformin, sulfonylurea and insulin use with brain structure and function and risk of dementia and Alzheimer's disease: Pooled analysis from 5 cohorts." PLoS One V. 14 No. 2 (2019):e0212293.

Whelton PK, et al. "2017 ACC/AHA/AAPA/ABC/ACPM/AGS/APhA/ASH/ASPC/NMA/PCNA Guideline for the Prevention, Detection, Evaluation, and Management of High Blood Pressure in Adults A Report of the American College of Cardiology/American Heart Association Task Force on Clinical Practice Guidelines." Hypertension V. 71 (2018):e13–e115.

Whitfield KC, et al. "Thiamine fortification strategies in low- and middle-income settings: a review." Ann N Y Acad Sci (2021). Epub ahead of print.

WHO. "Smallpox." (2014) https://www.who.int/biologicals/vaccines/smallpox/en/

Wiers CE, et al. "Ketogenic diet reduces alcohol withdrawal symptoms in humans and alcohol intake in rodents." Sci Adv V. 7 (2021): eabf6780.

Willett WC, et al. "Intake of trans fatty acids and risk of coronary heart disease among women." Lancet V. 884, No 5 (1993): 581–585.

Willett WC, et al. "Trans fatty acids: are the effects only marginal?" Am J Public Health V. 84 No. 5 (1994):722–724.

Williamson JD, et al. "SPRINT Research Group. Intensive vs standard blood pressure control and cardiovascular disease outcomes in adults aged ≥75 years: a randomized clinical trial." JAMA V. 315 No. 24 (2016):2673–82.

Wilson RS, et al. "Cognitive activity and incident AD in a population-based sample of older persons." Neurology V. 59 No. 12 (2002):1910–4.

Wishart DS. "Metabolomics for investigating physiological and pathophysiological processes." Physiol Rev V. 99 No. 4 (2019):1819–1875.

Wojtunik-Kulesza K, et al. "An attempt to elucidate the role of iron and zinc ions in development of Alzheimer's and Parkinson's diseases." Biomed Pharmacother V. 111 (2019):1277–1289.

Wu Y, et al. "BHBA treatment improves cognitive function by targeting pleiotropic mechanisms in transgenic model of Alzheimer's disease." FASEB 2019:1–18.

Xie L, et al. "Sleep drives metabolite clearance from the adult brain." Science V. 342 No. 6156 (2013):373–7.

Xu W, et al. "Accelerated progression from mild cognitive impairment to dementia in people with diabetes." Diabetes V. 60 (2010):2958–65.

Yamanaka R, et al. "Magnesium is a key player in neuronal maturation and neuropathology." Int J Mol Sci V. 20 No. 14 (2019):3439.

Yang JK, et al.. "Binding of SARS coronavirus to its receptor damages islets and causes acute diabetes." Acta Diabetol V. 47 No. 3 (2010):193–9.

Yang Q, A Vijayakumar, BB Kahn. "Metabolites as regulators of insulin sensitivity and metabolism." Nat Rev Mol Cell Biol V. 19 No. 10 (2018):654–672.

Yashin A, et al. "Antioxidant activity of spices and their impact on human health: a review." Antioxidants (Basel) V. 6 No. 3 (2017):70.

Yassine HN, et al. "Association of docosahexaenoic acid supplementation with Alzheimer disease stage in apolipoprotein E ε4 carriers." JAMA Neurol V. 74 No. 3 (2017):339–347.

Yates LA, et al. "Cognitive leisure activities and future risk of cognitive impairment and dementia: Systematic review and meta-analysis." Int Psychogeriatr V. 9 (2016):1–16.

Yin JX, et al. "Ketones block amyloid entry and improve cognition in an Alzheimer's model." Neurobiol Aging V. 39 (2016):25–37.

Youm YH, et al. "The ketone metabolite β-hydroxybutyrate blocks NLRP3 inflammasome-mediated inflammatory disease." Nat Med V. 21 No. 3 (2015):263–269.

Yu JT, et al. "Evidence-based prevention of Alzheimer's disease: systematic review and meta-analysis of 243 observational prospective studies and 153 randomised controlled trials." J Neurol Neurosurg Psychiatry V. 91 No. 11 (2020):1201–1209.

Yurko-Mauro K, et al. "Beneficial effects of docosahexaenoic acid on cognition in age-related cognitive decline." Alzheimers Dement V. 6 No. 6 (2010):456–64.

Zhang H, et al. "Meat consumption and risk of incident dementia: cohort study of 493,888 UK Biobank participants." Am J Clin Nutr (2021):1–10. Online ahead of print.

Zhang T, et al. "Does aluminum exposure affect cognitive function? a comparative cross-sectional study." PLoS One V. 16 No. 2 (2021):e0246560.

Zhao N, et al. "Apolipoprotein E4 Impairs Neuronal Insulin Signaling by Trapping Insulin Receptor in the Endosomes." Neuron V. 96 No. 1 (2017):115–129.

Zhao WQ, et al. "Insulin resistance and amyloidogenesis as common molecular foundation for type 2 diabetes and Alzheimer's disease." Biochem Biophys Acta V. 1792 No. 5 (2009):482–96.

Zhong G, et al. "Smoking is associated with an increased risk of dementia: a meta-analysis of prospective cohort studies with investigation of potential effect modifiers." PLoS One V. 10 No. 3 (2015):e0118333.

Zilkens RR, et al. "Severe psychiatric disorders in mid-life and risk of dementia in late-life (age 65–84 years): a population-based case-control study." Curr Alzheimer Res V. 11 No. 7 (2014):681–93.

INDEX

Page numbers in italics refer to photographs.

ABOUT THE AUTHOR

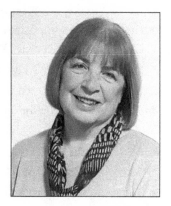

Mary T. Newport, MD

MARY T. NEWPORT, MD, grew up in Cincinnati, Ohio, USA, and was educated at Xavier University and University of Cincinnati College of Medicine, both in Cincinnati, Ohio. She is board certified in pediatrics and neonatology, and completed her training at Children's Hospital Medical Center in Cincinnati and Medical University Hospital in Charleston, SC. She practiced neonatology in Florida for thirty years and was founding medical director of two newborn intensive care units in the Tampa Bay area. More recently, Dr. Newport has practiced at the opposite end of the spectrum, providing care for hospice patients in the Tampa Bay area of Florida for nearly three years, and in-home health risk assessments thereafter. She writes and speaks in the U.S. and around the world on ketones as an alternative fuel for the brain for Alzheimer's and other disorders.

Dr. Newport was caregiver for fifteen years for her husband of forty-three years, Steven Jerry Newport, who suffered from early-onset Alzheimer's disease and died on January 2, 2016. They have two daughters and a grandson. Dr. Newport's previous books include Alzheimer's Disease: What If There Was a Cure? The Story of Ketones (2011; second edition 2013), The Coconut Oil and Low Carb Solution for Alzheimer's, Parkinson's, and Other Diseases (2015), and The Complete Book of Ketones: A Practical Guide to the Ketogenic Diet and Ketone Supplements (2019).

Dr. Newport has been an invited speaker on the subject of ketones as an alternative fuel for the brain for symposia, conferences, and webinars throughout the USA, Australia, Canada, France, Greece, Germany, India, Italy, Japan, Singapore, and Thailand. In the U.S., she has given presentations and webinars for University of South Florida, American College of Nutrition, Institute for Human and Machine Cognition, American Oil Chemists Society, Fellowship in Anti-Aging and Regenerative Medicine, International College of Integrative Medicine, Metabolic Health Summit, Restorative Medicine, and Weston A. Price Foundation, and has given numerous lectures for university students, foundations, and for the public.

For more information, view her website and blog at http://coconutketones.com and follow her on Facebook at https://www.facebook.com/CoconutOilandAlzheimers/?ref=hl.

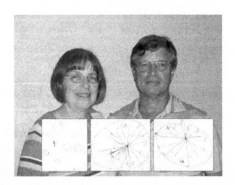

Mary and Steve Newport and Steve's clocks before and after coconut oil. The photo appeared in a news article in the St. Petersburg Times October 29, 2008, and the article and photo went viral. With permission from Eve Hosley-Moore.

ABOUT THE GRAPHIC DESIGNER

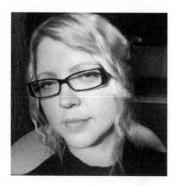

Joanna Newport, Graphic Designer.

JOANNA NEWPORT is the daughter of Steve and Mary Newport and received a Bachelor of Fine Arts in Graphic Design at the International Academy of Design and Technology, Tampa, Florida, in 2008. She is a freelance graphic designer and created more than 100 figures and tables for Clearly Keto for Healthy Brain Aging and Alzheimer's Prevention and for Dr. Mary Newport's previous three books and various presentations. Joanna and her husband, Forrest Rand, helped provide years of in-home care for her father Steven Newport, who suffered from early-onset Alzheimer's disease and Lewy body dementia.

CPSIA information can be obtained
at www.ICGtesting.com
Printed in the USA
JSHW021914271022
32203JS00001B/1